A History
of the
Senses

A History of the Senses

From Antiquity to Cyberspace

Robert Jütte

Translated by James Lynn

polity

First published in 2005 by Polity Press

Published with the assistance of Inter Nationes, Bonn.

The publisher would like to acknowledge the assistance of Ian Cooper in the preparation of this book.

Polity Press
65 Bridge Street
Cambridge CB2 1UR, UK

Polity Press
350 Main Street
Malden, MA 02148, USA

ISBN 0 7456 2957 1
ISBN 0 7456 2958 X (paperback)

A catalogue record for this book is available from the British Library.

Typeset in 10.5 on 12.5 pt Sabon
by Graphicraft Limited, Hong Kong
Printed and bound in Great Britain by
Athenaeum Press Ltd., Gateshead, Tyne & Wear

For further information on Polity, visit our website: www.polity.co.uk

Contents

List of Illustrations   vii

Tuning Up: Conspicuous Manifestations –
(Un-)Timely Reflections   1

Part I   Senses and Historicity

1   Approaching the Suprahistorical   8

Part II   The Traditional Order of the Senses:
From Antiquity to the Early Modern Era

2   Conceptions: The Sensorium   20

3   Classifications: The Hierarchy of the Senses   54

4   Representations: Allegories   72

5   Practices: The Senses and their Ailments   102

Part III   From the World of the Senses to the World of Reason
(Eighteenth and Nineteenth Centuries)

6   Philosophical Sensualism in the Age of Sensibility   126

7   The Senses and Aesthetics   142

Contents

8   The Education of the Senses   157

9   The Transformation of the Senses by Industrialization
and Technology   180

10 Experimental Physiology and the Separation of
the Senses   218

Part IV   The 'Rediscovery' of the Senses in the Twentieth Century

11 Touching – or The New Pleasure in the Body   238

12 Tasting – or What Do Fast Food and Nouvelle
Cuisine Have in Common?   253

13 Scenting – or From Deodorization to Reodorization   265

14 Listening Effects – or The Art and Power of Noises   281

15 Ways of Seeing – or The Human Rights of the Eye   295

16 Psi Phenomena – or The Exploration of Extra-Sensory
Perception   309

Prospects

17 Cyberspace and the Future of the Senses   324

Notes   336
Index   378

List of Illustrations

2.1   The system of the five senses in ancient Indian
      medicine   22
2.2   Symbolic correlations of the sense organs in
      the Chinese tradition   27
2.3   Medieval representation of Aristotle's doctrine
      of the senses (Wellcome Library, London)   37
4.1   Inventory of iconographic symbols of the five senses   74
4.2   The senses on the way to heaven and hell
      (Universitätsbibliothek Erlangen-Nürnberg)   79
4.3   The Triumph of Faith over the Senses (1667)
      (Museo Nacional del Prado, Madrid)   81
4.4   The Return of the Prodigal Son (allegory of the five
      senses) (Herzog Anton Ulrich-Museum, Brunswick)   84
4.5   Gabrielle d'Estrées and her sister in the bath
      (c.1592) (Archiv für Kunst und Geschichte, Berlin)   100
5.1   Listening through an ear-trumpet (Medizinhistorisches
      Institut und Museum der Universität Zürich)   117
8.1   Training the senses in infancy (allegory of the five
      senses) (1893) (Medizinhistorisches Institut und
      Museum der Universität Zürich)   160
8.2   The isolation of vision and hearing according to
      L. F. Froriep (1846) (Institut für Geschichte der
      Medizin der Robert Bosch Stiftung, Stuttgart)   163
9.1   Soldiers' quarters (allegory of the five senses) (c.1850)
      (Medizinhistorisches Institut und Museum der
      Universität Zürich)   202

List of Illustrations

13.1 Fresh air for pedestrians (1904) (Verein für Geschichte und Sozialkunde, Institut für Wirtschafts- und Sozialgeschichte, Universität Wien)   268

13.2 Newspaper advertisement for Odol (SmithKline Beecham GmbH, Bühl)   273

16.1 The scientific investigation of the supersensory (Institut für Grenzgebiete der Psychologie und Psychohygiene e.v., Freiburg)   315

16.2 Clairvoyance experiments with ESP cards at the Rhine Institute (Institute for Parapsychology, Rhine Research Center, Durham, North Carolina)   316

17.1 Stelarc with laser eyes, third hand and amplified body (Grove Press, New York; Photo: Polixeni Papapetrou)   329

Tuning Up: Conspicuous Manifestations – (Un-)Timely Reflections

The Lord God gave me five senses to find my way about down here below:
Five bright lanterns to light my dark path; first one goes on, then another –
Yet they never stay focused on one thing together . . .
Come on you lamps, let's have some light –!
Kurt Tucholsky, *The Five Senses* (1925)

With the growth of interest in the body that is such a striking feature of the everyday culture of the present, the five senses are back in fashion. A decade ago, social critics were lamenting the 'disappearance of the senses' (Dietmar Kamper/Christoph Wulf) and the 'de-sensualization' of the world (Hugo Kükelhaus/Rudolf zur Lippe), but meanwhile the picture has changed. Notwithstanding the turbulence and uncertainty at the beginning of a new millennium, the rediscovery of the senses has become a highly profitable business. Human sensory perception has now conquered the world of advertising. The global character of the phenomenon can be witnessed on the Internet. The end product is a trivialization that literally knows no bounds, a process that does not so much make the senses more acute as numb and deaden them. For who can have any interest in purportedly unique visual, aural, gustatory, tactile and olfactory experiences that dissolve into crude advertising copy the moment they are examined more closely?

Canny exhibition curators, whose job is to keep track of the *Zeitgeist* and respond to the latest popular taste, realized several years ago that 'the senses' was a theme that could entice people of all ages and educational levels into the museums. It all began with an initiative to give blind people access to the fine arts by allowing them to touch the exhibits. In Great Britain alone, there were more than thirty such 'hands-on' exhibitions in the 1980s. The target groups of museums seeking to attract visitors with the prospect of new sensory experiences are no longer just the blind or partially sighted. At an exhibition entitled 'The Sense of the Senses', held in the Federal Exhibition Hall in Bonn in early 1997, the Basel Museum of Design took stock of a widely noted series of exhibitions such as 'Aroma, Aroma' (1995) and 'Touch Me' (1996), in which the theme of human perception was illustrated by the senses.

Meanwhile, in Germany and abroad, other museums have acquired the 'taste' too. In the winter of 1998–9, an exhibition entitled 'Théâtres des Sens' drew tens of thousands of visitors to the Palais de la Découverte in Paris. That same year, the Hunterian Museum in Glasgow put on an exhibition with the somewhat ambiguous title 'Senses in Touch'. It addressed both 'blinded and partially sighted visitors' and people with normal vision. This 'multi-sensory exhibition employing physical objects and computer-generated materials' was intended to help both groups to grasp the significance of the senses. Since then, a travelling exhibition devoted to the five senses has even been advertised on the Internet (www.science-project.org/travelling/senses.htm). The exhibition features installations such as a reaction gauge ('test your response to lights and sounds'), a 'touch test', a 'smell table' and 'feely boxes'. In 2001, a touring exhibition called 'Coming to our Senses' ran for several weeks at an art gallery in Dundee. Here, the visitors could not only view but also smell, hear and touch the works, among which was a giant mobile by Bree Croon, festooned with brightly coloured and elaborately decorated beach balls which could be touched, squeezed and moved about. During the exhibition, experiments with the various senses were conducted at the workshops led by the contributing artists.

Museums that are unable to appeal to, or whet the appetites of, all five senses of their visitors' are offering instead to train senses such as smell and touch, which are supposedly underdeveloped, although they have in fact simply atrophied in post-industrial society. Since the beginning of the 1990s, the grounds of the Museum of Medical History in Ingolstadt have contained a so-called Scent and Touch Garden. According to the museum's brochure, its purpose is not only to meet the needs of handicapped or blind visitors, but also to offer the sighted person a chance to 'develop his sense of smell and touch'.

—— 2 ——

Originally conceived as a way of integrating the handicapped, the place promptly developed into an attraction with far wider appeal. The garden is now an established port of call during official tours of the town. A Garden of the Five Senses has been opened at Valloires in France, where children are supposed to learn an alternative approach to botany by tasting, smelling or touching fruit and flowers. Cleveland Public Library also includes a Sensory Garden which offers visitors a delightful outdoor experience during the growing season. Meanwhile, on the Internet, an American garden centre is advertising under the slogan 'Gardening for the Senses'.

The new buzzword of museum culture cropped up again at an exhibition of food culture at the Hamburg Speicherstadtmuseum in 1999. A review of the exhibition quotes the words of one of the organizers: 'Normally, a museum uses only the sense of sight. Our exhibition is intended to engage all the senses' (*Frankfurter Allgemeine Zeitung*, 30 March 1999). However, the sensory experience of colonial produce that had long lost its exotic character was confined to emissions of the smells of products such as sugar, beer, wine and tobacco through a plastic tube fixed to the ceiling of a former storehouse. As though you couldn't get the same thing in a pub or café!

And speaking of adventure and leisure culture, a Greek manufacturing company is currently advertising its furniture on the Internet under the slogan 'when senses meet wishes' (*epiplo to syn polyzos*). An American furniture store that also sells accessories and giftware promises its customers 'an ambience of rawhide and roses; a blend that will bewitch all your senses'. A German mail-order firm selling natural furniture is promoting 'living with all the senses'. And just to make sure the potential buyer knows why it makes sense to buy natural textiles and furniture made of real wood, he is informed that, 'from one moment to the next, living is a constant succession of millions of impressions of *all* the senses. It's not just a matter of how your furniture and furnishings look, but also of how they feel to the touch.' The company even offers to look after your olfactory requirements, for they will send you a wooden box containing seven samples of scent. 'These scents all have a practical use: in the bedroom, in the linen cupboard . . .', says their leaflet discreetly. It is presumably up to the purchaser to decide where the lavender blossoms will disperse their fragrance. On the other hand, the 'aphrodisiac Eros-Oil' included with them is no doubt intended for one room only.

Given the immense, now almost incalculable, range of products on the health-care market, it is clearly no longer enough to advertise activity holidays, thermal cures and fitness and beauty treatments. The aptly named Six Senses Spa, an international hotel chain with luxury holiday complexes in Bali, the Maldives and Java, promises its guests a unique experience 'formed by the three primary senses of sight, sound and touch'. A Canadian hotel is trying to lure guests with a 'Discover your Senses in Four Days' spa package. Yellowstone National Park has also entered the act with its promotion of the natural beauties of the area as 'a feast for the senses' – not neglecting the sense of smell, which is taken care of by a geyser!

The magic word 'senses' is often used in connection with that other fashionable word 'wellness'. One American spa hotel offers aroma-therapy massages which 'awaken your senses with your choice of a custom blend of essential oils.' Nowadays, hotel brochures can no longer afford merely to list such leisure-time fixtures as jacuzzis, saunas or steam baths. At a four-star hotel in Malaysia, comforts such as these now trade under the shimmering title of Body Senses Wellness Centre.

In the age of multimedia, it is possible to have sensory (and not just sensory-erotic) experiences on the Internet. There is, for instance, a website that describes various games involving the playing of roles, though naturally none of them can actually be played on a PC. Besides practical suggestions on how to activate your fellow players' visual and auditory senses, the site tells you of the difficulty of dealing with the sense of smell during role play, and suggests ways of improvising smells. The author of the home page (http://www.handshake.de/user/willie/adp/adpkaese.html) tells us:

> It is perhaps easiest to achieve the smell of a burned-out village. The group of players, whose characters are about to return home tired out by their successful adventure, should be sent out of the room and the door closed behind them. Once they have gone, place a bit of wood or paper in an ashtray or something similar. On re-entering the room, the group will receive an immediate impression of what has been happening in its native village – which takes you straight to the beginning of a fresh adventure.

One day perhaps, just before the news reports of civil wars in Africa or ethnic cleansing in the Balkans, our subscription channels will give us instructions on how to enhance the realism and vividness of these camera-documented atrocities when viewing them on our living-room TV. Other role-playing games such as 'Shadowrun', which is extremely popular in Britain and America, also appeal to the use of the senses. The gamemaster describes the world the characters see, functioning as their eyes, ears and other senses. A role play entitled 'Luna Rising' is based on humans with the ability to expand their senses across vast interstellar distances – even across time itself!

Finally, let us turn to a more serious approach to the subject. It all began with the large international conference-cum-exhibition entitled 'The Sense of the Senses' – held, as we have seen, in the Federal Exhibition Hall in Bonn in 1997. The participants included well-known psychologists, art historians, sociologists and philosophers, and scholars working in the fields of theatre, music and media, as well as writers and artists with an acknowledged interest in the subject. Oskar Negt spoke about 'Obstinacy and the Dispossession of the Senses'. Thomas Macho and Dietmar Kamper lectured under the intriguing motto 'Either Sense or the Senses'. Among some remarkable, if not particularly sensible, papers was the one given by Hans Moravec, head of a robotics laboratory at the Carnegie Mellon University in Pittsburgh. His contribution bore the symptomatic caption 'The Senses Have No Future'. So there we have it: now it's the senses' turn to have no future. Since then, there have been several successor conferences. In 1998, the University of New South Wales in Australia organized one devoted to 'Cinema and the Senses'. Hollywood sent its best regards, for this was the release year of the film *Senseless*, an American comedy (!) about a man who loses his senses and then regains them. But before pictures learned how to move, the senses had already had to adjust to a new medium in the form of the printed book. So the obvious next step was to organize a conference on 'Audio-Visuality Before and After Gutenberg' (Kunsthistorisches Museum and IKF Vienna, 1998). In the announcement of the conference, which was circulated on the Internet, the relevance of this topic to the present was argued as follows: 'The conference aims to observe physically bounded perception in the process of transition to scriptuality under the conditions of orality/physicality (brain memory–script memory), and to compare this early media revolution with later media revolutions, the transition from a culture of the manuscript to book printing (script memory–print memory), and from book printing to the new media (print memory–electronic memory).' One does not need to be a prophet to predict that the Vienna conference will hardly be the last on the subject of the 'senses'. Persons more qualified than I have reflected on the sensorial side of conferences. The master of the campus novel David Lodge detected it quite early on, and portrayed it in his novel *Small World* (1984). The academic legions of the future will undoubtedly continue to reflect on how to remain in touch with the *Zeitgeist*. In doing so, it seems highly likely that they will at some point encroach on the 'empire of the senses' itself – although certainly without raising moral or political objections, to say nothing of advancing into the kind of areas captured on celluloid by the Japanese film director Nagisa Oshima in his film of the same name (1976).

Nowadays, a visit to the Old Town of Marrakesh is enough to get you transported to the 'Realm of the Senses' – at least according to a travel item in *The Guardian* of 14 October 2000. And the Internet edition of *Straight Times* extols New Zealand as another 'realm of the senses': 'Imagine sinking into a pool of hot spring water, surrounded by native forest and snow-capped mountains, and the only sound you hear is the distant call of the birds.' But for most users of the Internet, the true 'Realm of the Senses' has more to do with eroticism than with landscape. Take, for instance, the following recipe for the intensification of pleasure: 'Just smother your lover in chocolate syrup, and enter the realm of the senses.' Or pertinent ads such as 'Let's explore the realm of the senses together. Call . . .' And if you don't know what 'aural sex' is, let the Internet enlighten you: 'There's a lot to be said for aural sex. Our sense of hearing can trigger immediate and intense stimulation. For example, as lovemaking progresses, we take quicker, deeper breaths. Hearing this from our partners or ourselves can be a real turn-on' (www.excite.com/home/health/healthy_sex).

In the face of such a rich and colourful selection of pleasures and leisure-time options, a historian of culture would have to be blind to ignore a subject that was being offered him on a plate: a historical survey of the senses beginning with antiquity and ending with the present.

— Part I —

Senses and Historicity

— 1 —

Approaching the Suprahistorical

The *forming* of the five senses is a labour of the entire history of the world
down to the present.

Karl Marx, *Economic and Philosophical Manuscripts* (1844)

Anyone who sets out to explore the material world of the past and
present is faced with an almost impenetrable tangle of stubbornly
surviving images, metaphors, themes and representations. Many are
part of a long tradition and have been reused and recycled again and
again. It is only by dint of effort, and with the aid of a critically
trained eye, that the historian can get a purchase on this apparently
suprahistorical subject and begin to distinguish between the historicity of a physical experience (in this case sense perception) and the
form in which it has been preserved or handed down. Furthermore,
it is sometimes by no means easy to determine whether a particular
transformation is due to a change in the form in which the senses are
used, or whether one is dealing with a complete change of discourse
and therefore with the rise of new rhetorical figures.

If he is aiming not simply to compile a more or less structured
archive of sense impressions but also to show how human perception
has changed over time, the historian is well advised to take account
of the expert opinions of specialists in the history of the body. According to Barbara Duden, the medical historian must be especially alert
to the 'reality-creating powers of imagination and perception at a
particular time',[1] and avoid proceeding from the assumption of an
'unhistorical (biological) physical substance' which is only of interest
to history after it has been shaped by culture. This means that we
have to break with the aprioristic assumption of the 'naturalness' of
sense perception, which is a move that historians of medicine often
find difficult to make, for they tend on the one hand to construe their
object as the history of a problem or idea, and on the other hand to

leave questions of 'natural history' to anthropologists or biologists. It is therefore hardly surprising that this discipline, which in many ways remains attached to the methodology of an older and more conventional history of science, continues to regard the senses as largely a matter for the history of physiology. The work of the Münster medical historian Karl E. Rothschuh (1908–1984) is one example of this. Although it dwells at some length on the concept of 'sensibility', his history of physiological concepts is concerned only marginally with the physiology of the senses. Besides new discoveries, Rothschuh attributes the changes of concepts and methods within this fundamental subject of medical science to 'changes of thought'.[2] He also believes that the medical or scientific historian who is interested in the history of physiology 'should not stop at a descriptive morphology of the historical succession of analytical trends and discoveries' but also try to pinpoint both 'the reasons for this historical change and progress' and 'its determining moments', which will enable him to proceed beyond a pure history of ideas.[3]

But long before this older history of medicine adopted the senses as the object of a disciplinary history (and physiology was the obvious candidate here) and began to concede a measure of importance to the influence of social factors, the radical challenge of Karl Marx (1818–1883) was already on the table. In contrast to the somewhat contemplative or philosophical understanding of sensuousness of Ludwig Feuerbach (1804–1872), Marx demanded nothing less than a universal human sensorial appropriation of the objective world:

Man appropriates his comprehensive essence in a comprehensive manner, that is to say, as a whole man. Each of his *human* relations to the world – seeing, hearing, smelling, tasting, feeling, thinking, observing, experiencing, wanting, acting, loving – in short, all the organs of his individual being, like those organs which are directly social in their form, are in their *objective* orientation, or in their *orientation to the object*, the appropriation of the object, the appropriation of human reality.[4]

So there can be no such thing as a natural history of the senses, only a social history of human sense perception:

For not only the five senses but also the so-called mental senses, the practical senses (will, love etc.), in a word, the *human* sense, the human

—— 9 ——

nature of the senses, comes to be by virtue of *its* object, by virtue of *humanised* nature. The *forming* of the five senses is a labour of the entire history of the world down to the present. The *sense* caught up in crude practical need has only a *restricted* sense. For the starving man, it is not the human form of food that exists, but only its abstract existence as food. It could just as well be there in its crudest form, and it would be impossible to say wherein this feeding activity differs from that of animals.[5]

In the context of the history of the sense of taste to which Marx alludes here, this implies that the common human predilection for all things sweet can hardly be regarded as a universal historical phenomenon. As the American cultural historian Sidney W. Mintz has shown, its origins lie not in some biological disposition or genetic mutation, but in colonialism and the mass import of raw sugar to Europe which first made it possible.[6]

The suggestion of Walter Benjamin (1892–1940) that the history of the senses should be considered dialectically, and examined in terms of the relations between biological constants and historical variables, moves in a similar methodological direction.[7] Benjamin chooses the alteration of vision by moving images as an example of how the 'materialist' historiography that is merely sketched in his essay 'On the Concept of History' might appear in practice (i.e., when applied to the senses): 'For the entire spectrum of optical, and now also acoustical perception, the film has brought about a similar deepening of apperception.'[8]

The all-embracing or 'total' history of the socialization of the senses of the kind envisaged by Marx, and to some extent by Benjamin, has still not advanced beyond the initial stages. Such work as might be mentioned in this context consists for the most part of the numerous recent studies of the 'scopic regime', or history of the gaze, which are much indebted to Marshall McLuhan (1911–1980) and above all to Michel Foucault (1926–1984). These mainly historically orientated special studies have sought to identify the social and political developments behind the rise of 'new' ways of seeing that have radically transformed this particular form of sense perception. With the sense of vision as their paradigm, they have shown how mutations of forms of perception are products of a complex, dynamic process that is determined both by the logic of political systems and by cultural and economic factors. A particularly important figure in this context is the American art historian Jonathan Crary,[9] with his controversial claim that the neutral and heterogeneous gaze of the observer was already in place several decades before the actual invention of photography. He relates this development to the long-term effects of new physiological theories, as well as to the invention of new optical instruments (e.g., the stereoscope) in the early nineteenth century.

More than half a century ago, Lucien Febvre (1878–1956), co-founder of the *Annales* school, whose importance for the science of history extends well beyond the borders of France, urged his colleagues to produce a history of human feelings. In the article 'History and Psychology', written for the *Encyclopédie française*, he mentions, among other topics, the change in the sense of time (the experience of the change from day to night and from summer to winter) and changing conceptions of security needs. Febvre also touches on the methodological difficulties that a historian choosing such a diffuse subject matter would inevitably face: 'the danger, namely, of trying to pass directly (and unproblematically) from our own feelings and ideas to feelings and ideas for which similar, or even the same, words have often been used for centuries, and whose apparent and deceptive similarities have given rise to serious misconceptions.'[10] Here we might think of a key concept such as 'nerves',[11] whose importance is not confined to the history of medicine or psychiatry, and whose meaning has altered decisively since the nineteenth century under the influence of social processes (headword 'urbanization') and scientific developments (headword 'psychoanalysis').

In another pioneering essay on the history of mentalities written in 1941, Lucien Febvre touches on some of the basic problems surrounding a history of sensibility (*sensibilité*) or the emotions (*émotions*). His examples are the ambivalence of collective representations and the variable relationship between feeling and reason. What Febvre says here about historical investigations of the emotions also applies in large measure to any future history of the senses: 'They [the emotions] imply interpersonal relations and collective forms of behaviour. They are doubtless based on organic causes that differ from person to person and may often arise from events concerning, or deeply affecting, one person only.' But, as Febvre stresses, the form in which they are expressed is at the same time 'the product of a particular series of experiences of social life, of comparable and

—— 11 ——

simultaneous responses to the pressure of identical situations and similar contacts.'[12]

At roughly the same time the German-Jewish sociologist Norbert Elias (1897–1990) was attempting to determine the sources of the *Process of Civilization* (first published in 1939). Elias traced the establishment of new standards of shame and embarrassment back to a regulation of individual affect, either by means of external compulsion or through the practice of self-discipline, that had been in evidence since the late Middle Ages. In the course of this work Elias, who was forced to emigrate in 1933, found his attention drawn to the conditioning of sensory experience (senses of sight and smell). Compared to the influential if not entirely uncontroversial project of Elias (who later taught in England), Lucien Febvre's conjectures on civilizational progress must be regarded as uncompleted work. He never undertook the longer study that might have underpinned his much-cited claim that, over the course of history, it was possible to discern a gradual repression of feelings by the operations of reason. Although the time-scales of the process may differ, his thesis is reminiscent of the brief reflection on evolutionary history that Sigmund Freud (1856–1939) typically tucked away in one of the notes to his famous essay *Civilization and its Discontents*: 'The diminution of the olfactory stimuli seems itself to have been a consequence of man's raising himself from the ground, of his assumption of an upright gait; this made his genitals, which were previously concealed, visible and in need of protection, and so provoked feelings of shame.'[13]

Febvre's suggestion of an investigation of the 'mental tools' (*outillage mental*), among which he included the use of the senses, doubtless encouraged the emergence of the history of *mentalités*. However, it did not lead to a systematic 'history and anthropology of sense perception', whose method and content were at least presented in outline a few decades later by the French social historian Alain Corbin, though he did not actually produce the study.[14] As its title suggests, Diane Ackerman's *A Natural History of the Senses* is concerned principally with the physiological basis of sense, although the author's breadth of reading is impressive and she includes passing references to numerous points of contact between her subject matter and literature, history and anthropology.[15]

Thus, the history of sense perception exists only in an incomplete state, with much of it consisting of individual historical treatments of the senses of sight,[16] hearing[17] and smell.[18] Touch[19] and taste,[20] on the other hand, have attracted relatively little attention from historians or historically orientated scholars in adjacent disciplines. What is lacking completely, however, is a methodologically ambitious and *comprehensive* account – whether of individual epochs or of the whole period from antiquity to the present – based on an exhaustive study of the sources. Only in histories of philosophy,[21] art[22] and medicine[23] do we occasionally come upon more or less complete surveys (mainly in the form of encyclopaedia articles and anthologies) of the ensemble of the senses (usually five) over a longer or shorter period of time.

The writing of a history of the sensory value systems of past and present cultures and the changing hierarchy of sensory ideas and practices is both an original and a risky undertaking, whose diachronic implementation confronts the historian with huge, though not necessarily insurmountable, problems. There may be certain conceptual difficulties, but not the least of the problems is the absence of a written record. However, an account of the kind proposed here need not be defeated by a lack of source material, as existing mental-historical and historical-anthropological studies have demonstrated clearly enough. The history of the senses, too, can draw on a wealth of evidence, from which the historicity of our senses, their hierarchy, their modes of use, and their frames of reference may be ascertained. These sources consist of normative texts, such as conduct books and health manuals, moral-theological and philosophical treatises and, not least, so-called self-documentations that give us glimpses of cultural practices and the experience of possessing a body. They provide selective information on the role and development of individual senses and their variable hierarchy (including the importance attached to them). The detailed personal records of the Cologne city councillor Hermann Weinsberg (1518–1597) are one example of this kind of individual testimony. At the close of each decade of his life, Weinsberg performed a meticulous description of his ageing body and current state of health, during which he devoted particular attention to his senses. The following observation appears under the heading of 'hearing' in the year that he turned sixty: 'My hearing is beginning to fail me somewhat. I feel something buzzing and ringing in my head. I wonder if there is some matter there that is causing this. Yes, as the body grows old with the years, the five senses of man grow old too.'[24] We must, of course, beware of assuming that Weinsberg's impressive

—— 13 ——

description of his own bodily sensitivities was simply typical of the sixteenth century, when, under the influence of the Renaissance, people were reputedly discovering their identities for the very first time. Yet notwithstanding their singularity, sources of this type supply important clues both to historians of everyday life and to chroniclers of the mental attitudes of the past, whose methods have been compared by Carlo Ginzburg, one of the pioneers of 'microhistory', to the difficult, but in the end successful, detective work of a Sherlock Holmes.

It goes without saying that the information supplied by biographical and other sources is, for the most part, only fragmentary, and may also be scarcer in one epoch than in another, but this should not alarm the historian who ventures onto the terrain of the history of mentalities.[25] Despite the obvious difficulty of assembling a persuasively comprehensive corpus of source material for a period extending all the way from antiquity to the present, I have opted for a largely diachronic account of culturally influenced systems of emotion and perception and the sensory functions and practices connected with them. The elements and forms that remain the same, and those that change, will be demonstrated by means of thematic longitudinal sections and cross-sections of particular epochs. The latter are temporally variable and do not always adhere to conventional periodizations (antiquity, Middle Ages, early modern age, modernity).

The next part of this study, which covers the period from antiquity to the early modern age, shows first that the 'economy of the senses' is a mirror image of the society in question, meaning that in any given hierarchy or classification of the senses it is possible to discern mental outlines and reproductions of the social hierarchy and value system to which it is attached. The firmly entrenched schema of the society of feudal estates, which was not fundamentally challenged until the French Revolution, when it was replaced by bourgeois society, therefore corresponds to a precisely defined realm of the senses, which acquired what was to become its classical form, namely the number five, in Greek antiquity. Here, therefore, we are looking at a phenomenon of 'longue durée', or long duration, which justifies the large period of time covered by this section. In the succinct formulation of the French medievalist Jacques LeGoff, 'the history of mentalities is the story of the slowness of history.'[26] Nevertheless, we must not overlook the fact that there are different forms of duration and that they tend to merge with each other to form a historical patchwork. The explanation of these interlockings is one of the most difficult tasks of the history of mentalities in general and the senses in particular. The shorter excursions are therefore intended to clarify both the breaks and the continuities and the so-called simultaneity of the asynchronous.

In addition to the concepts and representations with which particular groups and cultures construct their very divergent realities and sensory worlds, I have, wherever feasible on the basis of the available sources, taken careful account of the notion of 'appropriation' introduced into modern historiography by the French social historian Roger Chartier.[27] In these pages, therefore, practices and uses are just as much a part of sensory history as discourses of order and classification. The permanent danger (e.g., of accident) to the sensory functions and their restoration (by therapeutic intervention) is an obvious focus of enquiry here, not least because of the plentiful supply of source materials, but also because the topic has received relatively little attention from medical history.

Towards the end of the eighteenth century, the heterogeneous character of the senses acquired the status of a general principle with the advent of so-called sensualism. In general terms, this meant that the individuation of the senses shifted from the sense organs as a whole to the sense impressions of the nervous system, the so-called stimuli. In the time of Goethe (1749–1832) irritability and sensitivity were phenomena that were not solely the interest of a few doctors and scientists. The educated bourgeoisie participated in this discourse, alongside philosophers, artists and literati. In his *Ästhetica in nuce*, for example, Johann Georg Hamann (1730–1788) pleaded the importance of purging the natural use of the senses of the unnatural use of abstractions. Aestheticization entailed the 'civilizing' or 'disciplining' of the senses. This process had already begun long before the so-called Interim Age (*c*.1750–1850) that has acquired such importance in the history of concepts.

We shall also turn our attention to what Alain Corbin has called 'collective hyperaesthesia', which is a phenomenon that has been the subject of a good deal of recent research. It refers to that oversensitivity of the nerves of the feelings and senses that we encounter in the literature and art of the nineteenth century. Although some of the senses were temporarily revalued during this period, the reign of the eye and the sense of vision began at a much earlier date with the invention and distribution of the camera obscura, and continues unbroken to this day. A further item of consideration is the extent to which this process, together with the dulling of certain senses (smell and touch, for instance) that has been a constant subject of observation and complaint since the nineteenth century, was also a consequence of urbanization and industrialization. The late eighteenth and early nineteenth century is, after all, the period when the physiological exploration of the sense organs by natural and medical scientists becomes increasingly important. It is during these years that the foundations of our modern, experimentally tested knowledge of the structure and function of the human sensory apparatus are laid. These scientific discoveries are associated principally with the name of one man, Johannes Müller (1801–1858), who published two pioneering works on the physiology of the senses in 1826, and was awarded the chair of anatomy and physiology in Berlin just a few years later.

At the turn of the millennium, the human senses, which have hitherto been explained scientifically as physical sensations or systems of perception, or interpreted psychologically and revalued by philosophy, are undergoing a strange renaissance. While traditional concepts of the body continue to circulate in people's minds, they are now having to compete with the knowledge disseminated by modern biology and medicine via the media (e.g., exhibitions on the senses aimed at the promotion of health and well-being). If advertisements for the most diverse products (from cars to toothpaste) are being addressed directly to the five senses, either individually or in their totality, and museums have taken to providing 'sensuous experiences', now is undoubtedly the moment to reascertain the role of the senses in the modern world and to enquire into the changes and continuities. This 'rediscovery' of the senses, which is in some ways a mere few decades old, certainly has a lot to do with commercialization, but it is also a response to the growing needs of a post-industrial leisure society, in which the senses are befuddled by artificial worlds and overstrained by incessant stimulation.

We shall therefore pay special attention to the 'use value' of a particular sense along with its social and cultural manifestations. Why, for instance, are more and more supermarkets sprinkling their customers with music and enticing them inside with clouds of perfume? The historian, whose task is to observe long-term changes within the human 'economy of the senses', must try not only to isolate the causes of this now inescapable shopping-mall 'bombardment' of the senses but also to describe and analyse its consequences (conditioning and satiation are just two of the key words here).

Finally, we shall hazard a look at a phenomenon that was hardly specific to the twentieth century but became a subject of scientific investigation during it. I am referring to premonitions, visions, dream predictions, second sight, apparitions, ghosts. The new (borderline) science of parapsychology is now trying to discover explanations for experiences that human beings have had since primeval times. Here we shall be focusing more on the problem of 'extra-sensory perception' (telepathy, clairvoyance, prophecy) than on the physically inexplicable human manipulation of matter (psychokinesis). We shall also discuss the methods, goals and results of the research in this field that is currently under way in Germany and the United States.

The incorporeal world of the age of computers and the Internet has radically altered sense perception. Without reversing the traditional role of the historian as a 'backwards-facing prophet' (Friedrich Schlegel), we shall conclude with a brief consideration of the virtual sensory reality of the daily offerings of the much-sung 'information highway'. It is now no longer just the information scientists and technology-obsessed artists who tumble about in cyberspace. More and more museum experts and historians are busily generating virtual worlds. The University of Stuttgart is conducting an interdisciplinary research project that involves a multimedia presentation of a work of art in its intellectual-historical context. The central subject is the famous Herrenberg altar by Jerg Ratgeb (*c.*1480/85–1526), now in the collection of the Stuttgart Staatsgalerie. This unusual project is a collaboration of architects, information scientists and technology-struck, multimedia-friendly historians of art and regional history, and its aim is to produce a new overview of Jerg Ratgeb's works in a virtual, artistic space composed of four projections (front, right, left and above).

In cyberspace, sense impressions are displaced outwards from the body and thus displaced from the traditional sense organs, giving a new and highly topical significance to Karl Marx's sentence 'since arms and legs function in their own specific way, the eye and the ear – organs which take man away from his individuality and make him the mirror and echo of the universe – must have a still greater right to activity, and consequently must be *intensified* arm-and-leg activity.'[28]

Part II

The Traditional Order of the Senses: From Antiquity to the Early Modern Era

— 2 —

Conceptions: The Sensorium

They may be subjected to three forms of scrutiny: physical, logical and
moral. The physical explanation concerns the internal composition of the
senses, their nature and God's intention in creating them.

Zedler's Universal Lexicon (1743)

The idea that perception or sensation may be localized in certain physical organs has a long tradition. It pervades many cultures, although
not all of them set the number of these organs at the sacred or magical
figure of five. As we shall see, however, the division of the sensorium
into five (and not six, seven or eight) has undoubtedly proved to be
the most influential and most frequently applied method of assigning
cognitive functions to individual parts or organs of the body.

The process of this accumulation of knowledge, at the end of which
stands a more or less completely articulated system of sensory physiology, is marked by the influence of both medical thought and the
philosophy of nature. Its beginnings are notoriously difficult to trace.
This applies both to the dominant conceptions of the body in the
regions of the Christian West, which are rooted in Graeco-Roman
antiquity, and the comparable conceptions of other cultural regions
that continue to this day to shape the therapeutic practices of medical
systems developed there in the course of centuries, or indeed millennia
(*ayurveda*, traditional Chinese medicine).

Indian natural philosophy

Let us turn first to ancient Indian medicine or natural philosophy
as it appears in the *Vedas*.[1] The *Vedas* are the most ancient Indian
religious texts and consist for the most part of hymns, liturgical chants,
sacrificial formulas and magic spells. According to Indian tradition,

the *Veda* consists of several parts: the *Ṛgveda* (Veda of Verses), the *Sāmaveda* (Veda of Chants), the *Yajurveda* (Veda of the Sacrificial Formulas) and the *Atharvaveda* (Veda of the Spells). The oldest parts of the *Vedas* were composed around 1500 BC. Each *Veda* is accompanied by a body of prose writing of later date. The medical learning of the *Vedas* is to be found mainly in the *Saṁhitās* (Collections), which form the oldest stratum of the corpus of Vedic texts, and in the *Upaniṣads* (Esoteric Doctrines), which are generally thought to date back to between 500 and 1000 BC.

In the *Ṛgveda*, the oldest of the Vedic texts, there is as yet no collective name for the senses. The word *indriya* does not acquire this meaning until later, and refers initially to the god Indra in his quality of light. The *Atharvaveda* (VI, 9, 5–6) contains a hymn to the fire god which enumerates a series of mental abilities in a way that suggests a precise differentiation of individual senses: 'The light sits firmly (in my heart) especially to enable me to see . . . The holes of my ears fly outwards (in many directions), my gazes go outwards, this light passes outwards.'[2] Although the *Ṛgveda* already has a verb for 'touch' or 'feel', there is again no expression for the corresponding sensation, *sam-sparśa* (feeling), until the *Atharvaveda*. The same applies to the perception of taste. The oldest Vedic texts are still unfamiliar with the later collective name *rasa*. Only the word for 'smell' (*ghanda*) is already present in these most ancient strata of the *Ṛgveda*.

These still decidedly vague ideas about the body acquired precision and definition only with the passage of time and after empirical and rational elements had begun to enter Indian medicine. The culmination of this long process is the teachings of the *Ayurveda* (The Wisdom of Long Life), whose principal texts are named after the three legendary Indian physicians Caraka, Suśruta and Vāgbhaṭa. These medical texts, which are also called *saṁhitās* (collections), date back to between AD 350 and AD 600, and they enable us to reconstruct the ancient Indian conceptions of the physiology of the senses towards the end of the Vedic period with a fair degree of accuracy.

In the *Ayurveda*, which forms an appendix to the *Atharvaveda*, the idea of a tight dovetailing of macrocosm and microcosm also plays a key role. The connections between the body, the senses, the mind and the self, or the soul, are cosmological in nature (see figure 2.1). Creation, and with it humanity, begins with the undeveloped (*avyakta*) primeval matter (*prakṛti*), which is composed of the three *gunas*

—— 21 ——

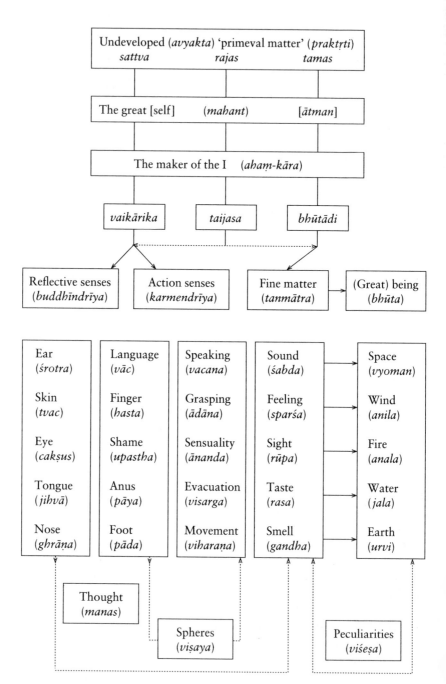

Figure 2.1 The system of the five senses in ancient Indian medicine (*Source*: Reinhold F. G. Müller, *Grundsätze altindischer Medizin* (Copenhagen, 1951), p. 83)

(qualities, shaping powers): *sattva* (spiritual being), *rajas* (blindness) and *tamas* (darkness). This primeval matter gives rise first to *mahant* (the great self), and then to *aham-kāra* (the maker of the I). Through a process of transformation (*vaikārika*), *sattva* acts upon both the five senses of knowledge or *buddhīndrīya* (hearing, touch, sight, taste, smell) and the five senses of action or *karmendrīya* (speaking, holding, begetting, evacuating, walking). The quality of *rajas*, which is associated mainly with demons, snakes and ghosts, produces a heated (*taijasa*) effect and influences both the sensory apparatus and the finer components of the individual senses (*tanmātra*), as well as the five elements (*mahābhūta*) usually associated with them. The translation of *bhūta* as 'element' is a little problematic, since the word actually means 'what has become'. The sense of this can be derived from its corresponding old Indian synonym *dhātu* (root substance), which is a collective term for space, wind, fire, water and earth. The application of these conceptions of the divine macrocosm to the microcosm of the human body produces the following account of the Creation: the Self gives birth to space, from space comes wind, from wind comes fire, from fire comes water, from water comes earth, from earth come plants, from plants come food and from food comes man, with the god of light Brahman, who is Lord of the Fire of Heaven (*brahman*), figuring as the initiator of the entire process of transformation. For their part, the five primeval substances engender seven core components (*śara*) of the human body: sperm, marrow, bone, fat, flesh, blood and skin.

Besides the five senses mentioned, there is an additional *ati-indriya* (super-sense). This highest or, if you like, sixth sense is *manas* (spirit), which is occasionally called *sattva* or *cetas* (literally: 'the emission of beams'). In order for *manas* to activate the senses, the *ātman* or self must be adjusted to its particular goal (*artha*). Thus, *śruta* (that which has been heard or beamed outwards) must meet the object corresponding to its purpose, for which the usual word is *śabda* (sound, noise, word). The bodily organ involved is called *karṇa*, which literally means 'hole through which the stream of hearing passes'. It seems fair to assume, therefore, that the sense organs as such attracted relatively little attention in ancient Indian medicine and natural philosophy. They are envisaged simply as the meeting points (*adhiṣṭhāna*) of the qualities or objects assigned to them (skin – sensation; nostrils – smells; tongue – tastes; eyes – shapes; ear – sounds).

—— 23 ——

Both the early Vedic texts and the ayurvedic texts of a later period deal most extensively with the sense of taste. But it is important to bear in mind that the concept in question (*rasa*) did not originally serve as a collective term for various kinds of taste, but was simply a general word for a liquid or a (body-)fluid. The earliest textual strata of the *Ṛgveda* are at first dominated exclusively by the taste of sweetness. A progressive differentiation can then be observed as we move forward in time. For every 150 instances of 'sweet' in the texts comprising the *Atharvaveda* there is a place describing a salty or a pungent taste. In the oldest medical texts, which are written in Sanskrit, there was a considerable division of opinion concerning the number of different kinds of taste. The number six eventually prevailed and was canonized, so to speak, by the celebrated ancient Indian physician Punarvasu Atreya in the ayurvedic corpus of the *carakasaṃhitā*: sweet (*madhura*), sour (*amla*), salty (*lavaṇa*), pungent (*kaṭu*), bitter (*tikta*) and tangy or tart (*kaṣāya*). In another medical compendium, the *suśruta-saṃhitā*, these tastes are associated with the five *mahābhūta* or primal substances (space, wind, fire, water, earth) as well as the three pathological sources of error or *doṣa* (air, bile, phlegm). Sour, salty and pungent have a positive effect on bile; sweet, bitter and dry, on the other hand, are negative. Phlegm may be positively affected by the qualities sweetness, sourness or saltiness, but the effects of the other kinds of taste are negative. This idea is connected not least with the theory of the effects of the three *doṣa* on digestion, or the human metabolism. Thus, it was thought that phlegm (*kapha*) played a part in eating, that gall (*pitta*) had an active role in the process of metabolizing food, and that the wind (*vāyu*) was involved in the conversion of food into excrement.[3] It is therefore not surprising that the theory of the different types of taste (*rasa*) traditionally occupies an important place in ayurvedic medicine, since it forms the basis of dietetics and the selection of medicines in cases of sickness. Thus, one of the Vedic texts dealing with the characteristics, taste and effects of garlic notes that, 'In respect of taste and digestion, it is described as pungent, but on the other hand it is also noted as sweet for digestion; it smells mild but is difficult to digest, but due to its strength it is hot; it is also known to be sexually stimulating.'[4] As a place in the *suśruta-saṃhitā* indicates, the ancient Indians were fully aware that taste sensations can vary according to whether they are received at the tip, middle or back of the tongue.

The extent to which rational reflection and empirical knowledge have become more important in the *Ayurveda* than in the prehistoric period of the Vedas is not only attested by its teachings on taste. Traces of this type of thought are found everywhere in the medical texts named after the three great legendary Indian physicians.

Chinese natural philosophy

In ancient China, too, the human organism was perceived as a miniature copy of the universe. According to Chinese thought, man is an organic part of nature and is closely interrelated with the cosmos. This cosmic-magical conception is reflected in the *I Ching* (Book of Changes), for example, which dates back to the first millennium BC. There, the sky is compared to the human head and the earth to the stomach.

The *yin–yang* principle and the doctrine of the five elements or phases of transformation are undoubtedly among the oldest and most important building blocks of Chinese natural philosophy. The end of the Chou dynasty (1122–255 BC) saw the development of a dualistic system of thought that connected together numerous natural phenomena and abstract ideas, and envisaged the human organism as the site of a permanent struggle between conflicting elements, just like the natural world that surrounded it. The two polarized forces, in which universal energy reveals itself, are denoted by the symbols *yin* and *yang*, which originally meant the shadow side (*yin*) and the sunny side (*yang*) of a hill. *Yin* is conceptually associated with cold, cloudy, rain, femininity, inside, darkness; *yang* with sunshine, heat, spring, summer and masculinity. In view of these chains of association, it is hardly surprising that *yin* is considered to symbolize negativity and *yang* positivity.[5] These two forces must be maintained in a state of equilibrium; otherwise the cosmic order and with it the human organism will be disrupted. So a displacement in either direction betokens disharmony and illness. In the fifth section of *The Yellow Emperor's Classic of the Interior*, for example, we read:

The Yellow Emperor spoke: '(The two categories) *yin* and *yang* are the underlying principle of heaven and earth; they are the web that holds all ten thousand things secure; they are the father and mother to all transformations and alterations; they are the source and beginning of all creating and killing; they are the palace of the sun, moon and stars. . . . When treating sickness, one must penetrate to their source.'[6]

Tsou Yen (*c.*300 BC) is associated with the second natural-philosophical reflection, namely the doctrine of the five phases of transformation. Tsou Yen abandoned the ordering of the hosts of natural phenomena exclusively according to the dualistic principle, and invented five series of correspondences, whose starting points were the five 'elements' (metal, wood, water, fire and earth). However, the latter cannot be elided with the sometimes similarly designated basic elements familiar to cultures such as ancient Greece, namely earth, air, fire and water, plus a *quintessentia* or fifth essence representing a kind of substratum of the others. As Joseph Needham points out, Chinese thought envisaged the five elements as 'five powerful forces in ever-flowing cyclical motion, not passive and inert primary substances'.[7] They are held in a complex relationship of mutual conquest or creation. Water, for instance, conquers fire; fire in turn creates ash (= earth). For medicine this means that the elements can both support and oppose, as becomes apparent in the following excerpt from the twenty-second section of *The Yellow Emperor's Classic of the Interior*:

> The Yellow Emperor asked the following question: 'If, during medical treatment, one desires to establish correspondences between the body of man, on the one hand, and the regular progression of the four seasons and the five phases, on the other hand, how is it possible to act in accordance [with these principles] and what would be regarded as contrary conduct?'. . . . Ch'i Po replied: 'The five phases are metal, wood, water, fire and soil. They alternate in succession between a position of pre-eminence and one of insignificance. [This transformation] provides us with an understanding of life and death, an insight into creation and decay, as well as helping us to determine the influences in the five depots, the times during which [an illness] is minor or serious, and the ultimate prognosis for life and death.'[8]

The doctrine of the five elements or the five phases of transformation is the basis of the idea that there are many numerical correspondences between nature and the human body (see figure 2.2). These classifications are not easy to date. Some, such as the astronomical

Figure 2.2 Symbolic correlations of the sense organs in the Chinese tradition

Elements *hsing*	Direction *fang*	Sense organ *kuan*	Tastes *wei*	Smells *chou*	Yin–yang	Internal organ *tsang*	Part of body *thi*
Wood	East	Eye	Sour	Goatish	Yin in yang or lesser yang	Spleen	Muscles
Fire	South	Tongue	Bitter	Burning	Yang or greater yang	Lung	Pulse (blood)
Earth	Centre	Mouth	Sweet	Fragrant	Equal balance	Heart	Flesh
Metal	West	Nose	Acrid	Rank	Yang in yin or lesser yin	Kidneys	Skin and hair
Water	North	Ear	Salt	Rotten	Yin or greater yang	Liver	Bones (marrow)

Source: Joseph Needham, *The Shorter Science and Civilisation in China*, ed. Colin A. Ronan (Cambridge, 1978), table 9 (selection)

correlations, may date back to the ninth century BC. The psycho-physical correspondences, which also include the sense organs, were presumably elaborated during the time of Tsou Yen (*c.*300 BC). However, some of these correlations were queried at a fairly early stage, one of the doubters being Wang Chung in the first century AD: 'The horse is connected with *wu* (fire), the rat with *tzu* (water). If water really conquers fire [it would be much more convincing if] rats normally attacked horses and drove them away.'[9] Yet, despite such criticism, these symbolic correspondences have determined Chinese scientific thinking and medical practice for centuries.

It is noticeable not only that the Chinese perception of the world is determined by such key concepts as order or structure, but also that the correspondences between the individual parts of the macrocosm and microcosm are arranged largely according to a numerical scheme based on the number five. Needham sees this as an instance of a connection between number mysticism and associative thinking that is typical not only of Chinese natural philosophy. Space, for instance, is not perceived as something abstract, but as a spatial continuum divided into five zones (north, south, east, west and centre). This is connected in turn with the five elements and the five senses. The correspondences between the various parts of the universe, which has to be imagined as a gigantic organism, may be likened to the phenomenon of resonance. The aptness of this musical or phonetic metaphor is endorsed by a work entitled *Chun Chiu Fan Lu* [String of Pearls from the Annals of Spring and Autumn] written by Tung Chung in the second century BC: 'All things reject whatever is different [to themselves] and follow what is akin. Thus it is that if [two] *chi* [matter-energy] are similar they will coalesce; if notes correspond they resonate. Sounds which correspond totally enter into resonance. . . . They sound by themselves. There is nothing miraculous, but the Five Notes being in relation; they are what they are according to the Numbers [whereby the world is constructed].'[10]

In the macrocosm, as in the microcosm, therefore, everything has its fixed place and acts on other things, and this influence must be envisaged as a giving and taking, a reciprocal interplay of natural forces. Since this complex system of correspondences embraces the points of the compass, heavenly bodies, colours, smells, the time of day and the seasons, as well as food and tonal pitch, it is hardly surprising that Chinese doctors began at an early stage to develop a dietetics and therapeutics that took account of these natural laws. Furthermore, they were convinced of its capacity to assist diagnosis. This gave rise to the idea that, by examining such things as the pulse, the smell of the breath, the colour and temperature of the skin, and the condition of the bodily orifices and the sense organs, they would be able to diagnose any irregularity in the influences of *yin* and *yang*, and pinpoint the affected digestive organs and alimentary tracts. In this context the fifth section of *The Yellow Emperor's Classic of the Interior* notes that: 'possessing acrid and sweet [volatile] influences and [material] flavors and producing dissipation, belongs to *yang*. That which is sour and bitter and produces discharge or drainage belongs to *yin*.'[11]

The correspondence system of the twelve 'organs' is also important in the sensory-physiological ideas of traditional Chinese medicine. A distinction is commonly drawn between so-called depots (*tsang*) and palaces (*fu*). The first group includes kidneys, liver, heart, spleen, lungs and the heart-enclosing network; the second category consists of stomach, small intestine, large intestine, triple burner and bladder. The way in which the human senses and their appurtenant bodily orifices, together with the 'depots' and 'palaces', were included in the associational series of the *yin–yang* dualism and the five phases of transformation is shown by a section entitled the *Huang-ti nei-ching su-wen* in the classic of Chinese medicine from which we have already quoted liberally:

> Ch'i Po replied: 'The stomach is the sea in which liquid and solid foods collect; it is the great source that sustains the six palaces. The five [material] flavors enter through the mouth and are stored in the stomach. . . . this means that all [volatile] influences and [material] flavors destined for the five depots and six palaces originate in the stomach, and – following their transformation there – can be felt at the "influence-opening". The five [volatile] influences enter through the nose and are stored in the heart and lungs. When the heart and lungs are affected, the nose cannot function properly.'[12]

Both pulse-diagnosis and a refined form of olfactory diagnosis of the relative seriousness of an illness continue to this day to play an important role in traditional Chinese medicine.[13]

The maintenance of healthy senses occupies a central place in a chapter of the famous textbook *Ku-chin i-t'ung ta-ch'üan* (Comprehensive

System of Medicine of All Times), which was compiled in the six-teenth century AD by Hsü Ch'un-fu. The following instructive comment appears there under the heading 'All Injuries Caused by Evil Originate in the Senses': 'When the correct influences have been weakened, evil [influences seize control of] the senses ... If one's senses are in the proper condition, one is protected from all evil.'[14] Appropriately, therefore, the section describing the therapies for maladies of this kind includes a prescription for 'damage to the senses by wind'.

A problem that tended to preoccupy Chinese philosophers more than physicians was the question of whether sensory perception and intellectual knowledge were in conflict or agreement with each other. According to the Mohist school of Chinese philosophy, named after its founder Mo Ti (479–381 BC), the object of sensory perception is the world as it is comprehended by the various organs or 'five paths'. Conceptual or interpretive knowledge (*chih*) can only be achieved through reflection. Thus, according to the *Mo Tzu* (Book of the Master): 'when one says fire is hot, this is not [only] on account of the heat of the fire; it is [because] I make the assimilation [or correlation] [of the visual sensation of] light [and the tactile sensation of heat].'[15] The conflict between sensory perception and knowledge acquired through the use of reason is accentuated by the so-called dialecticians round Kung-sun Lung, who founded his own school of philosophy in the period when China was dominated by Confucianism. One of their theorems or paradoxes was: 'The eyes do not see.'[16] It expressed their conviction that only reason 'sees', and that this implied something quite different from what 'seeing' was traditionally taken to mean. During the Han period (*c.*206–220), Hsun Tzu, who as a Confucian subscribed to a dualistic philosophy, taught that the senses were determined by, and classified according to, their domains of perception, and could not exchange their functions. In his view, intellectual knowledge presupposed that the natural senses had already categorized their impressions, for only then could reason endow sensory perceptions with meaning. Reason here is perceived as the 'natural ruler'[17] of the five senses.

As the English historian of science Joseph Needham has stressed, the Western and the Chinese macrocosm–microcosm concepts, within which the senses occupy their allotted place alongside other elements and natural phenomena, have their common origin in a cosmic-magical construction of the world.[18] But there are also fundamental differences between the two traditions, above all in their understanding of the universe. The central issue is the much-debated and always burning question of what really keeps the world together. While the classical and later Christian tradition held that the gods, or God the Father as creator, had a guiding hand in the matter, the Chinese thought that the combination of the various parts was generated by a kind of will, albeit a will which was not subordinated to a schematism or mechanism and could occasionally also manifest itself spontaneously.

Graeco-Roman natural philosophy

Like India and China, classical Greece shows no evidence of having initially possessed a collective name for the senses. They are simply enumerated separately. The senses which are usually mentioned explicitly in this context are seeing and hearing and their appurtenant organs, as for instance in the works of the pre-Socratic philosophers Heraclitus (end of sixth century BC) and Parmenides (around 500 BC).[19] The same applies to early Greek literature. In Homer (eighth century BC) and Hesiod (eighth/seventh century BC), the word *idein*, which is the usual term for visual perception, is sometimes also used to mean the recognition and identification of objects.[20] Xenophanes (*c*.570–470 BC) uses mainly the Greek verb *nouein* to denote the senses of seeing and hearing. In one of his fragments he writes of God: 'whole he sees, whole he thinks, and whole he hears.'[21] He evidently means that, unlike mortals, the gods do not require special organs of seeing and hearing in order to have knowledge of things. The following line is taken from Epicharmos (*c*.550–460 BC), whose comedies and epigrams were very popular with the Greeks: 'Reason alone sees, reason alone hears, all else is deaf and blind.'

The pre-Socratics also included Pythagoras (*c*.570–500 BC), the celebrated philosopher and mathematician from Samos, who founded a school which greatly influenced the development of Greek medicine. It is in his work that we find the first stirrings of a physiology of the senses. Pythagoras thought of hearing, for instance, as an outwardly directed event, in the course of which a warm and fine stream of air flowed from the soul. He depicted the process of seeing as a kind of invisible fire that emanated from the eyes and touched the objects of perception and grasped their colours and shapes. Both events, seeing as well as hearing, are thus connected with a particular element. 'The eye perceives the light that comes from fire, the ear perceives the sounds of the air.'[22]

Pythagoras strongly influenced Alcmaeon of Croton (*fl. c.*500 BC), a physician and philosopher who wrote a work entitled *On Nature* that is reputedly the first book in the Greek language to deal almost exclusively with the science of medicine. Alcmaeon clearly possessed a knowledge of anatomy based on animal dissection. His ideas on the functioning of the senses were preserved for posterity by Theophrastus (*c.*372–287 BC), a pupil of Aristotle and the author of an important work on the senses (*De sensibus*):

> Of those who ascribe perception to something other than similarity, Alcmaeon states, to begin with, the difference between men and animals. For man, he says, differs from other creatures 'inasmuch as he alone has the power to understand. Other creatures perceive by sense but do not understand', since to think and to perceive by sense are different processes and not, as Empedocles held, identical. He next speaks of the senses severally. Hearing is by means of the ears, he says, because within them is an empty space, and this empty space resounds. A kind of noise is produced by the cavity and the internal air re-echoes this sound. Smelling is by means of the nostrils in connection with the act of respiration when one draws up the breath to the brain. By the tongue we discern tastes. For since it is warm and soft, the tongue dissolves [substances] with its heat; and because of its loose and yielding texture it readily receives and transmits the [savours]. Eyes see through the water round about. And the eye obviously has fire within, for when one is struck [this fire] flashes out. Vision is due to the gleaming – that is to say, the transparent – character of that which [in the eye] reflects the object; and sight is the more perfect, the greater the purity of this substance. All the senses are connected in some way with the brain; consequently they are incapable of action if [the brain] is disturbed or shifts its position, for [this organ] stops up the passages through which the senses act.[23]

It is worth observing that Empedocles uses the Greek word *pagamai* (flat of the hand or gripper) to denote the senses in general. The idea behind this is that the senses grasp their objects like hands. When he comes to describe the activity of the senses, on the other hand, Empedocles uses the Greek word *athrein*, which originally meant 'to stare at something', and is used in this context to indicate the firmness with which the senses grasp their objects. It is also noticeable that both of the expressions used by Empedocles to describe sensory perception in general refer to the senses of sight and touch. Besides hearing and seeing, he also mentions taste and smell.

According to Theophrastus, Empedocles was one of the Greek natural philosophers who broke with long-established opinion and based their explanations of sensory perception on the principle of 'sameness' rather than 'contrariness'. This states, for example, that the eye contains the elements of water and fire, which according to Empedocles means that we perceive brightness by means of fire and darkness by means of water. This first verifiable example in the Greek tradition of the kind of connection between elements and sense organs that we have already encountered in the ancient Indian and Chinese tradition is later developed further by Empedocles' successors, most notably by Aristotle.

The senses were first fully enumerated by Democritus (*c.*460–370 BC), who was a contemporary of Socrates and the founder of the atomist school of Greek thought. In *Fragment* 11 he states:

> There are two forms of knowledge, one genuine, one obscure. To the obscure belong all the following: sight, hearing, smell, taste, touch. The other is genuine and is quite distinct from this . . . When the obscure form can no longer see, hear, smell, or taste the smaller things or perceive them by touching them, and the investigation has to become more subtle, they are replaced by the genuine form which possesses a more refined organ of knowledge.[24]

Here, and for the first time, a distinction is drawn between sense perception and another, superior form of knowledge. Democritus does not consider the inferior form of knowledge to be fundamentally negative, but he certainly regards it as imperfect. This critical attitude towards the senses as a source of knowledge is confirmed in another section, which has come down to us through the celebrated Greek physician Galen (AD 129–*c.*200): 'After Democritus has expressed his mistrust of sense perception in the sentence: "Although ordinary language tells us that there is colour, sweetness, bitterness, there is in truth only atoms and emptiness", he lets the senses speak out against reason: "Wretched mind, do you, who get your evidence from us, yet try to overthrow us. Our overthrow will be your downfall"'

(*Fragment* 125).[25] Democritus' theory of sense perception, to which Theophrastus later refers in detail (*De sensu*, 49–82), may be summarized as maintaining that nothing exists in the 'real' world except atoms and the empty space between them. When the atoms penetrate the organs of perception, they produce the images which we usually take to be true images of the 'real' world in which we live. In the words of the Hellenist Kurt von Fritz, 'it follows from this that while it is possible to have reliable and definite knowledge of the general structure of the external world, as well as general knowledge of the structure of the objects that give rise to certain sense perceptions, the inferences we are accustomed to make in respect of the presence and structure of certain objects at a given moment will always be uncertain.'[26] Democritus is therefore an agnostic who, while not denying all sensory knowledge, nevertheless insists that the soul or reason (*nous*) has to clarify and, if necessary, correct impressions conveyed by the senses, in order to gain knowledge of the finer or atomic structure of the external world.

While the Greek word *organon* (tool) appears just once (in *Gorgias*) as a term for the seat of sense perception in the work of the pre-Socratics, Plato (427–347 BC) explicitly describes the senses as organs of the soul in the *Theaetetus*[27] and, in so doing, establishes the concept permanently in the vocabulary of Western sensory physiology. The place in question deals with the alleged equivalence of knowledge and perception – a view supported by Socrates' fictional interlocutor Theaetetus. Via the familiar maieutic question-and-answer game, the latter finally comes to recognize that we perceive things not with the senses but with our eyes and ears. Or, as Socrates puts it succinctly: 'Yes, my son. It would be a very strange thing I must say, if there were a number of perceptions sitting inside us as if we were Wooden Horses, and there were not some single form, soul or whatever one ought to call it, to which all these converge – something *with* which, *through* those things, as if they were instruments, we perceive all that is perceptible' (*Theaetetus*, 184d). With this, Plato draws a sharper distinction than any of his predecessors between sense perception and the act of thought. In contrast to Aristotle, he attributes the faculty of synthesis, or the capacity to process diverse sense impressions, to human reason or the soul, and not to some higher sense (*sensus communis*). His argument is simply that, 'while the soul considers some things through the bodily powers, there are other things which it considers alone and through itself' (*Theaetetus*,

185e). Thus, the Greek word *organon*, which Plato uses here and elsewhere in the text, refers in the first instance to the physical capacity to perceive rather than to the physiological-biological sense organ in the narrower sense. In giving Socrates the following words, Plato at the same time stresses the uniqueness of each type of perception: 'And are you also willing to admit that what you perceive through one power, you can't perceive through another? For instance, what you perceive through hearing, you couldn't perceive through sight, and similarly, what you perceive through sight you couldn't perceive through hearing?' (*Theaetetus*, 185a).

In the *Timaeus*, Plato deals systematically with the senses, in the order of taste, smell, hearing and vision. Unlike the other senses, the sense of touch is not attached to a specific physical organ. Sensations of pleasure and pain and other qualities perceptible to the senses, such as soft and hard, warm and cold, heavy and light or rough and smooth, feature as 'disturbances that affect the whole body in a common way' (*Timaeus*, 65c). The various sensations of taste (strong, bitter, pungent, biting, salty, sour, sweet) are attributed to stimulations of the tongue. In the case of smell, however, Plato allows just the one distinction between pleasant and unpleasant, 'because a smell is always a "half-breed". None of the elemental shapes, as it happens, has the proportions required for having any odour' (*Timaeus*, 66d). In his view, it is only when certain substances become damp, begin to decompose, or melt and vaporize that smells arise which are then experienced as fragrant or foul. Plato explains aural perception as follows: 'In general, let us take it that sound is the percussion of air by way of the ears upon the brain and the blood and transmitted to the soul, and that hearing is the motion caused by the percussion that begins in the head and ends in the place where the liver is situated' (*Timaeus*, 67b). The sensory stimulus specific to the ear is sound conveyed by air. The sensation produced in the ear is registered in the brain where it leads to the actual perception.

Plato deals in greatest detail with the sense of sight, which he even describes in one place as 'divine'. In the *Timaeus*, the event of seeing is attributed to three different kinds of fire: daylight, the beam of the eye and the fire emitted by things in the outside world. In his view, the act of seeing is based on an interaction between a subject and an object. The movements proceeding from the eye and the object meet at what he calls the middle: 'On such occasions the internal fire joins forces with the external fire, to form on the smooth surface a single fire which is reshaped in a multitude of ways. So once the fire from the face comes to coalesce with the fire from the spirit on the smooth and bright surface, you have the inevitable appearance of all images of this sort' (*Timaeus*, 46a, b).

Since, according to the teaching of Empedocles, like can act only on like (here the fire within the eye and the fire in the objects of the external world), Plato's statement would appear to imply that in darkness the 'beam of sight' would be extinguished and there would be no sense perception. As Plato notes elsewhere, seeing also involves a simultaneous sensitivity to colour. He envisages this process as one in which the human individual perceives neither the object nor its colour as they are in themselves, but merely as something coloured which is then judged and interpreted by the mind.

Plato's theory of sense perception must be considered in the context of the central concept of his philosophy, namely the 'idea' (*eidos*), which derives from the Greek word for 'to see'. By 'ideas', Plato meant the original forms of all the objects we are able to perceive in the external world with the aid of our senses: the 'phenomenal world' of creatures (human beings, animals, plants) and objects, but also abstract concepts (virtue, good and evil). These 'ideas' exist in an eternal, unchanging world. In the phenomenal world, however, they are present only as poor copies and imitations (witness the celebrated image of the cave!). To reach the 'ideas', we need to use the dialectical method. The latter eventually bears the 'eye of the soul', which is 'really buried in a sort of barbaric bog', upwards and on to the 'ideas' (*Republic*, VII, 533d).

Aristotle (384–322 BC) not only extended the epistemologies of the pre-Socratics and expanded the hitherto merely inchoate physiology of the senses, but also advanced them to a state of completion that retained its authority well after the Christian Middle Ages, and also influenced Arabic and Jewish natural philosophy.[28] Unlike Plato, Aristotle ascribes psychical functions to the senses: 'The sense and its organs are the same in fact, but their essence is not the same. What perceives is, of course, a spatial magnitude, but we must not admit that either the having the power to perceive or the sense itself is a magnitude. What they are is a certain ration or power *in* a magnitude' (*De anima* [On the Soul], 424a, 25ff.). Thus perception presupposes the presence of certain physical and mental functions.

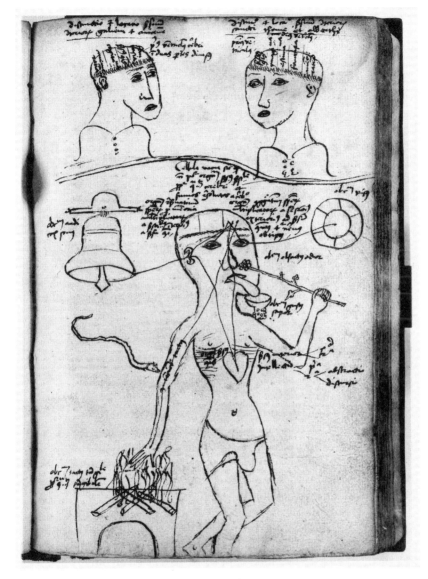

Figure 2.3 Medieval representation of Aristotle's doctrine of the senses; from *Epitomea seu reparationes totius philosophae naturalis Aristotelis*, Cologne, 1496

According to Aristotle, the object of perception, or 'the perceived' (*aistheton*), is of primary importance for sensory knowledge. The ability necessary for perception (*aisthesis*) is located in the various sense organs (*aistheteria*). The Aristotelian doctrine of the senses signals a fresh beginning in Greek natural philosophy in that it emphatically separates sensory knowledge from other events taking place in the soul, and does not derive perception from any direct contact between an object and a sense organ, but posits the presence of a 'medium' as mediator. In *De anima*, for example, which is probably his most important work on the physiology of the senses, Aristotle argues that 'in each case the sense-organ is capable of receiving the sense object without its matter. That is is why even when the sensible objects are gone the senses and imaginings continue to exist in the sense organs' (425b, 24ff.). In another place, Aristotle illustrates this with a concrete example: 'The account holds also of sounds and smells; if the object of either of these senses is in immediate contact with the organ no sensation is produced. In both cases the object sets in movement only what lies between, and this in turn sets the organ in movement' (*De anima*, 419a, 25ff.).

As Aristotle points out, perception differs according to the nature of the soul (human, animal, vegetable). Thus, many animals are said to lack the senses of sight, sound and smell. Even man, the highest being, has only five senses, namely sight, hearing, smell, taste and touch. As we shall see below, this fixed the number of the senses at five for a long time to come. Aristotle is also the first philosopher to construe the sense of touch as a discrete sense, which takes him beyond Plato, who allowed only four senses. The logical conclusion in the third book of *De anima* that there could be no further senses (e.g., a sense for the perception of movement) was only very occasionally called into question by later writers.

In the Aristotelian view, each function is determined by its object. Applied to the senses, this means that each sense organ is assigned to a specific object of perception: 'I call by the name of special object of this or that sense that which cannot be perceived by any other sense than that one and in respect of which no error is possible; in this sense colour is the special object of sight, sound of hearing, flavour of taste' (*De anima*, 418a, 11f.). Similar considerations apply to the animal realm. Aristotle claims, for example, that fish can smell, although their medium is water rather than air, as in the case of human beings. In addition to the individual senses and the various objects of perception to which they refer, Aristotle assumes the existence of a so-called common sense (*sensus communis*): 'But in the case of the common sensibles there is already in use a general sensibility which enables us to perceive them directly; there is therefore no special sense required for their perception' (*De anima*, 425a, 18ff.). The perceptual categories he considers common to all the senses (*sensibilia communia*) are movement, rest, number, shape and, not least, size. Although these conceptual forms are of decisive importance in the process of perception, they do not in his view have the same defini-tional quality as the *sensibilia propria* of the five senses. In contrast to the characteristics of perception that may be grasped 'in them-selves' (*per se*), Aristotle also recognizes predicative responses to per-ceptible objects. In the case of a white object, for example, it is these that enable us not just to grasp its colour by means of our faculty of sight, but also to assign a particular mental attitude to our seeing, such as identifying it as a person dressed in white and known by a certain name.

Aristotle's *De anima* deals with the senses one by one in the order of sight, hearing, smell, taste and touch, placing special emphasis in each case on the object of the perception.

According to Aristotle, the sense of sight, which he treats first, is directed towards what we can perceive with our eyes, with colour being for him 'the special object of sight' (*De anima*, 418a, 9). He assumes, furthermore, that the inner part of the eye is watery and that the eye consists of fire and water. He understands the process of seeing as a qualitative change caused by a movement that proceeds from the visible object and is transmitted via a transparent medium. In his opinion, this transmission is possible only if this medium, which consists of air and water, is luminescent. Neither Aristotle, nor the Greek natural philosophers who preceded and succeeded him, con-nected seeing with the refraction of light. The first to do this was the Arab scholar Ibn Al-Haytham (tenth–eleventh century AD). Instead, Aristotle adopted a theory of seeing based on the effect of an object on a subject (the theory of immission) that only gradually gained acceptance.[29] This was because it had long been thought that the process of seeing was actively controlled by the eyes, which emitted a sort of 'sight-beam' said to consist of fire (Empedocles), light (Plato), atoms (Democritus) or breath (Galen). This idea was still in circulation at the beginning of the modern era and numbered Leonardo da Vinci (1452–1519) among its adherents. However, a contemporary of that universal genius, the Swiss natural scientist Conrad Gessner (1516–1565), considered extramission theory to be already outdated and bluntly declared that 'visio non fit extra mittendo' ('seeing has nothing to do with the emission of rays').[30]

Now to hearing. What the ear perceives, says Aristotle, is sound, 'but the sound we hear is always the sounding of something else, not of the organ itself' (*De anima*, 420a, 17). Again, he posits the existence of a special medium for the perception of sound, which in this case is air: 'All sounds, whether articulate or inarticulate, are produced by the meeting of bodies with other bodies or of air with bodies, not because the air assumes certain properties, as some people think' (*De audibilibus* [On the Audible], 800a, 1ff.). Sound is accordingly perceived by an ethereal sort of organ that Aristotle believed to be located in the tympanum. We should recall here that, since before the early modern era only the eardrum and middle ear had been identified, the inner ear was still unexplored.[31] Around 1600, even a surgeon and anatomist as celebrated as Hieronymus Fabricius de Aquapendente (1533?–1619) had to concede that the anatomy of the ear was far more difficult to describe than that of the eye.[32] So Aristotle remained an authority on the subject for a long time.

The object of the sense of smell is an odour, although Aristotle admits that it is not quite as easy to devise categories for this sense as for a more differentiated perception such as taste. He believes that it is always possible to distinguish between sweet, sharp, bitter, pungent and oily smells. Smelling is again rendered possible by a medium (air or water). Aristotle thought that the air breathed in through the nose and the *pneuma* flowing from the heart into the vessels of the brain were mixed together in the *poroi* (channel-like passages between the nose and the brain). He expounds his ideas on the seat of the organ of smell in *De sensu* (438b, 25f.). Here, the olfactory faculty is sited in the region of the brain. This opinion was later endorsed by Galen, who managed not only to locate the sense of smell anatomically, but also to explain why the detection of smells should take place in that particular place: 'What remains is the organ of smell, which is not in the nasal passages, as the majority believe, but in the tips of the anterior ventricles of the brain, to which the nasal passages ascend; for at this point its ventricles are most vaporous.'[33]

These ideas must be seen in the context of the nowadays rather odd-sounding notion that cerebral fluid can flow into the nose and throat. The Greeks referred to this phlegm discharged by the brain as catarrh. Blessed with the authority of the great Galen, the idea of the nose as the 'cloaca of the brain' (*la cloaca del cerebro*) – in Francesco Sansovino's (1521–1586) graphic phrasing – persisted into the modern era. With its complex, though logically coherent, development of Aristotelian ideas, Galen's theory of smell did much to ensure that the physiological event of sensation as we know it today – stimulation of the nerve, transmission through the corresponding neural conductors and perception in the brain – was not appreciated for centuries.[34] It was not until around 1500, when the dissection of corpses became more common, that the *fila olfactoria* were identified as olfactory nerves. In 1655, the Wittenberg professor of medicine Conrad Victor Schneider (1614–1680) finally succeeded in proving scientifically that the smell receptors were located in the nasal mucous membrane. However, the first accurate dissection of the olfactory nerve branchings from the mucous membrane to the brain was performed towards the end of the eighteenth century by the Italian anatomist Antonio Scarpa (1752–1832).

The object of taste is touchable according to Aristotle. If our tongue is either too wet or too dry, we have no sense of taste. He divides the forms of taste into sweet, bitter, fatty, salty, pungent and burning hot. As late as the seventeenth century, many doctors and natural scientists were still convinced of the basic correctness of Aristotle's theory of taste perception. 'In completing this work, I have followed in the footsteps of Aristotle, the prince of philosophers, who describes taste as a particular form of the sense of touch', states the author of a medical thesis on the physiology of taste (*De gustu*), completed in 1689 under the supervision of Johann Moritz Hoffmann (1653–1727).[35] This doctoral dissertation, written and defended by Bernhard Matthias Franck (1667–1701), was indeed based on an essentially Aristotelian scheme of taste perception. Along with things having no taste, his work differentiates between pungent, sweet, sour, salty, bitter, strong and fatty tastes. As far as its theory of perception is concerned, however, this early modern medical dissertation owes more to René Descartes (1596–1650) than to Aristotle.

The significance of the papillae in the perception of taste also remained unknown until well into the modern era. It was only in 1669 that these parts of the tongue were identified as organs of taste by the Italian anatomist Marcello Malpighi (1628–1694). The existence of taste nerves other than the *nervus lingualis* known since Galen was first confirmed by François Magendie (1783–1855) at the beginning of the nineteenth century.

According to Aristotle, the organ of the sense of touch is not the skin, but the heart. The corresponding medium (the flesh) is thus in the body itself, and not outside it. Aristotle describes the object of the sense of touch as the palpable. The distinction between the palpable and the visible or the resonant lies in the fact that, while the latter are perceived through the agency of the medium, here 'it is as if a man were struck through his shield, where the shock is not first given through the shield and passed onto the man, but the concussion of both is simultaneous' (*De anima*, 423b, 15ff.). For this reason, Aristotle also considers the sense of touch to be much more closely related than the other senses to the four elements, since the properties of the elements (dry, wet, cold, warm) are all palpable.

The Aristotelian doctrine of the fully unified and independent nature of the sense of touch was scarcely ever questioned in subsequent periods. Other components of his physiology of the senses were also accepted. The *De anima* of Albertus Magnus (*c*.1197–1280) follows him in similarly classifying qualities such as hard and soft and rough and smooth as derivatives of the qualities primarily registered by the sense of touch (warm, cold, wet and dry). As we know today, these tactile qualities are, in fact, detected by sensors in the skin that pass on the corresponding stimuli to the brain via the peripheral nerves and the spinal cord. But until the nineteenth century, by which time experimental physiology had made substantial progress, it was impossible to form any definite, let alone correct, idea of the way these stimuli were relayed, even though Albertus Magnus had already drawn attention to the central role of the nerves in the sense of touch.[36]

The sense of touch held on to the special position in the hierarchy of the senses granted to it by Aristotle until well into the Middle Ages, and even into the modern era. Much of this was due to the medieval philosopher and theologian St Thomas Aquinas (1224/5–1274). In his own *De anima*, Aquinas endorsed Aristotle's view that without the sense of touch there could be no other senses. In his pithy formulation, touch is 'the first sense, the root and ground, as it were, of the other senses'.[37]

Compared to Aristotle, the later schools of Greek philosophy have nothing essentially new to report on the subject of the senses. The Sceptics merely doubt whether the senses were truly capable of comprehending real physical qualities. Like the Stoics, the Pneumatics derive the action of the senses from so-called pneuma (air, breath, wind). Each of the five senses has its own special pneuma, which is related among other things to the elements. The pneuma of hearing, for instance, is dry like the earth; the pneuma of smell, on the other hand, is located in the nose and is damp and vaporous.[38] According to the Stoics, the senses do not work afferently, or conducted inwards, but efferently, or directed outwards. The subject of perception is the central controlling organ. Streams of pneuma flow from this to the individual senses and establish connections. This idea acquired anatomical definition when the Alexandrian physician Herophilus (*c.*335–*c.*288 BC) discovered the nerves and assigned them the communicative function of forwarding the pneuma. He located the central organ of sensory perception described by the Stoics in the ventricles of the brain. Chrysippus (*c.*280–*c.*207 BC), on the other hand, who had reformulated the doctrines of the Stoa, refused to adopt this new idea and continued to regard the heart as the seat of the faculty of perception.

Galen, who practised as a physician in Rome at the beginning of the second century AD and became the most important representative of classical medicine after Hippocrates, finally broke with the Aristotelian construction of the heart as the seat of the central organ of perception (*hegemonikon*). He held that sensory perception took place in the brain, or, more precisely, in the cerebral ventricles.[39] Galen recognized seven cerebral nerves in all, and this topography survived until the seventeenth century. Galen describes the optical nerve and other nerves extending from the brain as follows:

> Whoever desires to enumerate simply the processes arising from the brain will say that the first pair of nerves springing from the brain goes to the two nasal cavities, and its course travels along the middle region of the skull. The second pair is that of the optic nerves, and in their course its two components travel one on each side of the first pair. . . . For as we explained previously in our description of the eye, the eye is moved by means of the pair of 'hard' nerves (*oculomotorii*), but perceives the things that it sees by means of the pair of soft nerves (*optici*).[40]

The discovery and description of the optic nerve did not, however, solve the problem of visual perception. Galen developed two separate explanatory models, one pneumatic, the other geometric. The former assumes that the pneuma of the eye receives the first optical impression, and that this stimulus is then conveyed to the brain by the nerve fibres situated between the lens and the retina. According to the model based on Euclid (325–285 BC), on the other hand, light passes through the eye in a straight line to the brain. It was not known until the early modern era that the reception of visual impressions by the retina functions in the manner of a camera obscura. Before then, the centre of seeing was thought to be the eye's lens. Johannes Kepler (1571–1631) was the first to put forward the idea that 'vision occurs through a picture of the visible thing [being formed] on the white, concave surface of the retina.'[41] René Descartes' *Dioptrics*, which appeared alongside his famous *Discourse on Method* in Leiden in 1637, did much to bring Kepler's theory of the retinal image – which has since proved correct – to the attention of the world at large, and it eventually gained general acceptance.

But to return to Galen. This celebrated Greek physician, who bequeathed to posterity an enormous corpus of medical writing, followed Aristotle in holding that, for each of the various forms of sensory perception, there was a corresponding organ. Heat and coldness, for example, were perceived by means of the sense of touch, and colour by the sense of sight. As far as the olfactory sense was concerned, Galen held that one could only smell substances that emitted a kind of vapour, for only the finer constituents of smellable things reached the ventricles of the brain. Since vapour was known to be combined with warmth, anything that could be smelt must possess the quality of warmth. As the medical historian Georg Harig notes, Galen attributes the affinity between taste and smell to perceptual similarities: 'Just as the substances kindred to lingual juices taste sweet or pleasant, so the substances related to the pneuma of the cerebral ventricles produce a pleasant smell. Unlike other sensory perceptions, however, these sensations are often not distinguished terminologically, although they do in fact show just as much variation.'[42]

In late antiquity, the philosopher Plotinus (*c*.203–270), who founded Neoplatonism, stands out among adepts of the senses.[43] Plotinus emphasized the unity of the senses and rejected the periphery–centre model of perception favoured by the pupils of Aristotle and the Stoics. In his view, perception required neither a medium between object and sense organ, nor any other kind of relay within the human or animal organism. The connections were in fact established through 'sympathy', which was a kind of remote contact. So there was no more need to explain visual perception by resorting to a light-beam theory à la Plato. It is also curious to observe Plotinus flirting with materialism with his claim that we grasp the world directly with our senses, and not by means of representations.

In late antiquity, the differences between the various schools of natural philosophy begin to disappear. At the exact interface between ancient pagan and late classical Christian or medieval theories of perception, we encounter Nemesius, who was a practising bishop in Emesa during the fourth century, and who between AD 390 and 400 composed a philosophical-anthropological treatise on the nature of man (*peri physeos anthropu*). Among other things, the book contains a statement of his opinion that the human being was composed of a rational soul and a body. On physiological matters, Nemesius was essentially a follower of Galen. Concerning the senses, he writes: 'there are five sense organs [*aistheteria*], but just one perception [*aisthetesis*], namely that of the psyche, which uses the sense organs to identify the feelings arising from them.'[44] More significant, however, was his distribution of the inner senses (*imaginativum* = perception, *excogitativum* = reason, *memorativum* = memory) across the three chambers of the brain: 'The organs of sense perception are the front ventricles of the brain, the spiritus animalis they contain, the nerves that emerge from the chambers moistened by the spiritus animalis and the tools of the senses in their structure.'[45] The doctrine of the location of the three psychic faculties in the ventricles of the brain remained authoritative for centuries, and was not discarded finally until the publication of Thomas Soemmering's study *Über das Organ der Seele* (On the Organ of the Soul) in 1796. Nemesius of Emesa's anatomical classification, together with his syncretic interpretation of the various classical theories of perception, ensured that he was not without influence on medieval scholasticism, especially as both Albertus Magnus and Thomas Aquinas frequently quoted his treatise on the nature of man.

Besides Nemesius, the Church Father Augustine of Hippo (354–430) is a particularly important figure in early Christian theories of perception. His theory of sensory perception contains both Stoic and Neoplatonic elements.[46] Augustine portrays the activity of the senses as a kind of experience (*notitia*) which approaches the reason from the outside via the senses. Like Aristotle and others before him, Augustine distinguishes five external senses, with which man experiences the world. The *De trinitate*, which contains the key elements of his theory of perception, does not treat each of the senses separately because Augustine believes they are all structured in a similar way. His example is the sense of sight (bk XI, ch. 2). According to this, all visual perception rests on three assumptions: the presence of a visible object, the cognitive act of seeing and, finally, the 'alertness of the mind'.[47] The last-named condition refers to an intentional and active concentration on the object registered by the eye. Here, as elsewhere in his epistemology, we encounter a tripartite division borrowed from the Holy Trinity. It is clear from his commentary on the Book of Genesis that Augustine subscribed to the Platonic extramission or transmission theory of vision: 'The act of seeing is a beam projected from our eyes.'[48] When dealing with the rational activity of the soul, however, Augustine adheres largely to Aristotle's idea of the *sensus communis*. However, he does go on to posit the existence of an additional inner sense (*sensus interior*) which has no equivalent in this form, either in Aristotle or in any of the other Greek writers. Each sensation is reported back to this superior sense by the ordinary five senses. In contrast to reason, however, the function of the *sensus interior* is merely integrational and transmissive. For, in Augustine's view, it is the mind (*mens*) that acquires knowledge of physical objects by using the senses: 'The soul connected to the body experiences sensations by means of a bodily aid, and the name of this bodily aid is, precisely, the sense organ' (*De trinitate*, IX, 2, 2).[49] Perception through the five external senses is thus a sensation that arises when an object touches or stimulates a sense organ and the soul refers this sensory impression to itself.

Medieval natural philosophy

Medieval theories of the senses draw mainly on two classical sources: Aristotle's remarks on the mental faculties and Galen's physiological theory of perception.

Arab scholars played a decisive role in the mediation of this body of knowledge. Foremost among them was Avicenna, otherwise known as Ibn Sînâ (980–1037). His major work, *Canon of Medicine*, was of paramount importance for the development of Western medicine. Avicenna's teachings on pharmacology, pathology and hygiene were based to a large extent on Galen, but he went his own way in other areas, including the physiology of the senses. Even such important Christian scholars as Albertus Magnus and Thomas Aquinas embraced the medical authority of this Muslim physician, astronomer and statesman, and quoted constantly from his works.

Avicenna's doctrine of the inner senses incorporated the divergent Aristotelian and Galenian traditions and, dialectically speaking, raised the theory of perception to a new level. In the introductory remarks on perception in his treatise on the soul (*Risala fi n-nafs*), he writes: 'Perception is either external – the five senses – or internal – the common sense, the imagination, the faculty of judgement, and memory.'[50] In another place, he offers examples of the tri- or quinquepartite division of the inner senses.[51] The first inner sense, which is called *fantasia* in the Latin translation, has the task of comprehending the forms of perceivable objects. Memory serves to preserve the thoughts or concepts grasped by the senses. The imagination restores, in a kind of movement, what has been obliterated from memory. Judgement, on the other hand, has the task of 'assessing the correctness or incorrectness of the inferences of the imagination before they are committed to memory.'[52]

Avicenna deals only briefly with the five external senses. In addition to the objects proper to its character as a particular sensory faculty, each of the five senses grasps five other qualities or modalities: shape, number, size, movement and repose. The same applies to the sense of smell, although Avicenna admits that in the case of human beings, whose sense of smell is not very highly developed, this acute power of discernment is barely or only partially present. The process of smelling is explained as follows: we breathe in the air which has absorbed the smell of an odorous body. This affected air is received by the nose and comes into contact with the frontal part of the brain, where it is identified by the olfactory faculty. In the case of the visual process, Avicenna follows Aristotle's doctrine and rejects the Platonic sight-beam theory.

One of the most important and influential commentaries on Aristotle comes from Ibn Rušd (1126–1198), who is better known under his

Latin name of Averroes. This work was examined critically by Albertus Magnus in his disputation *De unitate intellectus contra Averroem* (1256), and by Aquinas in his polemic *De unitate intellectus contra Averroistas* (1270). The subject of this dispute was largely the thesis that although every human being possessed an individual soul, the latter was more comparable to the soul of an animal, and therefore lacking in rational abilities. According to Averroes, therefore, it is not the individual human soul that is immortal, only the general human intellect. As might be expected, this idea was vehemently opposed by all who believed in the immortality of the individual soul.

However, we are more concerned here with Averroes's further development of the Aristotelian and Galenian doctrine of the pneuma in his great commentary on *De anima*. For it is in this work that the classical concept of *spiritus*, which is distinguished from Augustine's by its focus on the material characteristics of the human soul, first enters the Latin West, where it would exert a lasting influence on theoretical discussions of perception. The peculiarity of Averroes's doctrine of the *esse spirituale*, which combines Aristotelian and Neoplatonic elements, lies in its assumption that the faculty of sense perception is activated by the *spiritus*: a mind that is material in substance and endowed with exceptional acuteness. Averroes bases his elucidation on the senses of sight and smell: 'Just as colour has a twofold being, consisting of a being in a coloured body (which is its physical being) and a being in the transparent *medium*, so smell also has a twofold being, consisting of a being in an odorous body and a being in the *medium*; and the former is called physical being and the latter mental being, the former is natural [being] and the latter external' (*De anima*, II, 97).[53] This implies that objects perceptible to the external senses are distinguished by three different forms: a purely material being (*esse corporale*) in the perceptible object, a purely spiritual being (*esse spirituale*), in so far as these objects are comprehended by the mind, and then a sort of mixed condition of material and mental being in the *medium* – also called the *diaphanum* – that mediates between object and sense organ.

Although ostensibly Aristotelian, Averroes's doctrine of the *sensibilia*, or the contents of human perception, is decidedly original on several counts. First, the five external senses are defined, as in Aristotle, by their particular objective spheres. Colour, for instance, is the actual object perceived by the eye and only by the eye. In this

---

48

context, Averroes introduces the concept of *intentio*. It refers to the individual meaning that may be clearly described by the various perceptual categories into which the object falls. Although we may be able to grasp these discrete *intentiones* with our five senses, says Averroes, the knowledge of the actual essence of an object of perception requires concepts and the capacity to form definitions, which is again the task of the intellect.

With the reception of Aristotelian natural philosophy in the thirteenth century, other aspects of perception begin to enter the limelight of learned enquiry, and there is a vastly increased interest in the physiology of the senses.

One of the great achievements of Albertus Magnus was his use of the teachings of Avicenna and Averroes to bring about a reconciliation between the Aristotelian doctrine of the soul and Galenian physiology. This celebrated theologian's use of the senses of touch and eyesight to exemplify the idea of an immaterial representation of perceptible objects is distinctly Aristotelian. However, Albertus Magnus qualifies Aristotle's conception of the role of the medium in perception with the observation that a movement of the medium (his example is a breath of air) produces different effects on hearing, vision and smell. On the issue of whether perception is an active or a passive process, he sides against Plato, who regarded all sensory perception as active.

On the other hand, his four-stage model of the perceptual process is relatively new, even though it is based essentially on Aristotelian thought and on Avicenna's distinction between inner and outer senses. It asserts that at the first stage of sense perception 'form is abstracted and separated from matter.' At the second stage, form is 'detached from matter and its presence, but not from the contingent properties adhering to it (*appendices*), nor from the conditions of matter.' Examples of the latter are a certain bodily posture, the colour of a face or the shape of a head. 'At this stage of comprehension', says Albertus Magnus, 'we think of someone absent as curly-headed, white, long- or short-fingered, old or young, none of which has much to do with the fact that he is a human being' (*De anima*, II, 4, 3).[54] The third step involves the comprehension not only of perceptible objects but also of those mental 'intentions' that leave no impression on the sensory perceptions, but could not be part of our consciousness without the senses. Albertus Magnus assigns to this class such human qualities as comradeliness or friendship. 'At the fourth and last stage we grasp the "whatness" (*quidditas*) of things, free from any adherent material qualities.'[55] This is the most important function of reason.

Like Aristotle, Albertus Magnus uses a circular argument in his attempt to prove that there are no senses other than the external senses and the common sense:

> From what we shall now demonstrate, it may safely be assumed that there are no senses other than the five senses of sight, hearing, taste, touch and smell. For in using our five senses to perceive everything perceptible to us via the medium connected to us, and everything perceptible by means of the remote medium, we lack no further sensory modalities, for we possess senses solely in order to acquire knowledge of things that are perceptible.[56]

Albertus Magnus concludes with a brief treatment of each of the senses, beginning with sight and ending with the sense of touch, for which he shares Aristotle's high regard. His ideas on sight are worthy of note, for they are clearly influenced by Avicenna and the eminent Arab scholar and natural philosopher Alhazen (*c.*965–1039), who advanced a new theory of visual perception. 'Every act of seeing', writes Albertus Magnus in the treatise entitled *De sensu et sensato* (XIV, 14), 'takes place in the shape of a pyramid, whose base is formed by the perceived object and whose apex is the centre of the lens.'[57] Albertus Magnus's special interest in the eye and the visual process is demonstrated by a wealth of exact observation and natural-philosophical speculation. We find him, for instance, describing the phenomenon of being blinded by light and the difficulty of adapting to daylight after a long period of confinement in darkness. Like Aristotle before him, he also busied himself with the riddle of visual after-images. His work also contains fascinating random observations on the senses, but since none of them seriously challenges the Graeco-Arab doctrines with which we are now familiar there is no need to examine them separately here.

In respect of its treatment of the five outer senses, the perceptual theory of St Thomas Aquinas mentioned above follows largely in the footsteps of Aristotle. Aquinas starts out from the reflection that the higher forms of life are endowed with all five senses. Borrowing from the classical tradition, he describes the external senses as a passive potential and defines and distinguishes them according to their respective formal objects of perception (the smellable, the visible, etc.). In his opinion, perception is based on a common root (*radix*), which gives rise in each case to an individual power of sensation (*vis sentiendi*) in the sense organs on the periphery of the body. He is here referring to the *sensus communis*, which, unlike Avicenna, he counts among the four inner senses. The latter also include the faculties of imagination (*phantasia* or *imaginatio*), memory (*memoria* and *reminiscentia*) and the powers of discrimination specific to perception (*vis cogitativa*).

Aquinas's ranking of the senses is based on the doctrine of *immutatio spiritualis* or mental modification, an incorporeal yet material transcription of sensory stimuli. Thus, a beam of light striking the eye does not produce a physical change. In the case of hearing, smell and taste, on the other hand, a hybrid form of mental and physical change is already present, while in the case of touch a material transcription takes place.[58] In his *Sentencia libri de sensu et sensato*, Aquinas summarizes his theory of the stages in the sentence: 'The greater the capacity of a sensory faculty, the less change there will be in the organ seized by the object.'[59] Since, according to this theory, the visual faculty acquires visual knowledge solely by means of intellectual modification, the sense of sight automatically qualifies for the highest position. In this respect, Thomas Aquinas hardly differs from other Christian writers of the Middle Ages, who, under the influence of Neoplatonic currents of thought, were particularly attentive to the sense of sight. According to Jörg Tellkamp, however, the achievement of the great Aquinas lay precisely in the fact that, 'by following the threads of Aristotle's *De anima*', he developed 'a richly layered theory that accorded the sense of touch a role that was at least equal to that of sight.'[60]

Besides St Thomas Aquinas and Albertus Magnus, the two great Christian scholars of the thirteenth century, there were other scholastics who dealt more or less extensively with theories of perception in general, and the role of the senses in particular. They number Robert Grosseteste (before 1170–1252), Johannes Duns Scotus (1266–1308) and the English Franciscan Roger Bacon (*c.*1214–1292), who was particularly interested in the theory of sight. To follow the various ramifications of these discussions would take us a little too far, however, particularly as the differences are slight, and such minor deviations or reservations as there are centre mainly on the doctrine of the common or inner sense(s).[61]

Natural philosophy in the early modern era

The traditional division of the senses into those that were more mental (seeing and hearing) and those that were more physical (taste, smell and touch) retained its validity until well into the modern era. Yet there were stirrings of protest at quite an early date against the scholastic idea that the soul could be split into different cognitive faculties. Tommaso Campanella (1568–1639), who was known chiefly for a utopian text entitled *The State of the Sun* (1623), countered this idea by stressing the integrity of the mind and by treating the soul of reason and the soul of feeling as equals. This meant that, in contrast to the classical and medieval tradition, the external senses were no longer defined and individuated primarily by their objects but by their organs.[62] Campanella also distanced himself from the hitherto dominant school of thought by describing the five senses not as tools comparable to quill pens, but as 'channels'.[63] He also vehemently opposed the notion of a separate 'inner sense'. According to him, the discriminating function of the outer senses extends also to the common objects of the senses. While his contemporary the Italian physician Girolamo Cardano (1501–1576) embarked on a fresh deductive proof that the senses were five in number, Campanella, like Michel de Montaigne (1533–1592), did not exclude the possibility that one or two human senses might still be unaccounted for. Another contemporary, the Protestant theologian Philipp Melanchthon (1497–1560), remained loyal to the Aristotelian construction, with or without a watertight logical proof, and refused to entertain the slightest doubt that the number of the senses was five.[64]

With its principal representative René Descartes leading the way, the dualistic philosophy of the late seventeenth and early eighteenth centuries finally broke for good with the Aristotelian idea of an intelligent sensorium. Henceforth, the inner senses were allowed only a purely physical or even mechanical function.[65] The 'human machine' dreamed up by Descartes disposes over external sensations, whose stimuli originate in the objects of the external world, as well as inner impressions that originate in the body itself. Descartes' *sensus interni* no longer refers to the common sense but to natural drives such as hunger or thirst. These must be distinguished from the so-called states of mind (*passions de l'âme*), among which he includes feelings such as joy or sadness.

Johannes Kepler (1571–1630) not only ushered in a new era in the history of optics, but also provided the physiology of the senses as a whole with an entirely new theoretical basis. The concept of the sense organ was one example of change. With the sense of sight as its model, Kepler's *Weltharmonik* (Harmony of the World) demonstrated that 'it is through the eyes that the harmonic motions of the planets are perceived. The mind's inborn judgement of quantities indicates how the eye must be, and the eye is therefore the way it is because that is how the mind is, and not the other way round.'[66] With this idea, it became possible for the first time to judge the capacities of the senses according to a precise norm. Applied to the theory of visual perception, it meant that here, for the first time, was a possibility of literally measuring and assessing eyesight, not least in view of the optical aids that were either already available (e.g., spectacles) or would become so in the early modern epoch (e.g., the camera obscura or the telescope). With the aid of these instruments, new, empirically grounded discoveries were made in the physiology of the senses. The microscope, for instance, suddenly revealed properties of bodies (particularly colour structures) that appeared quite different when viewed with just the naked eye. As the historian of philosophy Eckart Scheerer notes: 'Mechanically enhanced vision provided empirical evidence of the existence of secondary qualities that were defined "in relation to our senses", in contrast to the "primary" or "original" properties that matter was said to possess independently of the senses.'[67]

By the beginning of the modern era at the latest, therefore, traditional natural philosophy was having to respond to the technological possibilities of an entirely new form of sensory experience. In doing so, it was confronted by a problem that had received little attention in the past, namely the possibility that the individual senses were heterogeneous in character. One concrete instance of this was the question of whether a person blind from birth, whose sight had been restored by an operation, would be able to distinguish visually between physical forms and objects previously known to him only through the sense of touch. This is an issue to which we will return in more detail in a later context.

—— 3 ——

Classifications: The Hierarchy of the Senses

The number of the senses

The number of the senses is set firmly at five both in the Western tradition and in early Indian and Chinese culture, where this figure had symbolic meanings. In the latter context, we might think of the ancient Indian doctrine of the five fires, or the Chinese idea of the five points of the compass. There are also five points to the pentagram, which consisted of five lines drawn in one stroke of the pen to produce the shape of a star. In antiquity, it was considered to be a representation of the form of the first letter of the Greek alphabet in five different positions (*pentalpha*), while later it came to symbolize the harmony of the cosmos. In the slightly modified form of the pentacle, it was, and still is, said to possess magical or apotropaic powers. In Islam, there are the Five Pillars of Islam (profession of the faith, the five daily prayers, almsgiving, fasting, pilgrimage to Mecca). The Holy Scriptures of Judaism, the Torah, consist of the first five books of the Old Testament (Pentateuch), and there are altogether five containers for the phylacteries worn by pious Jews. Christianity has propagated the parable of the five wise and five foolish virgins (Matt. 25) and venerated the five wounds of Christ as symbolic of the salvation of the world.

The 'fiveness' of the senses is thus very congenial to theological allegoresis, that is, the symbolic interpretation of the sacred scriptures of the most diverse religions, and it is therefore not surprising that the number became canonical. In the writings of the early medieval Church Father Hrabanus Maurus (*c.*780–856), we read that 'there are many places in Holy Scripture where the number five stands for the five physical (external) senses' (*De universo*, VI, 1).[1]

Yet symbolic potency is not enough on its own to explain why the number five has remained binding since antiquity. Its regular use as a kind of formula (e.g., in medieval law: 'and that you will swear by your five senses that . . .')[2] needed to be supplemented by an explanation grounded in fact and logic. This was provided by no less a figure than Aristotle, whose authority was hardly contested until well into the modern era. He it was who provided conclusive proofs based on the natural philosophy of his own time. As Theophrastus makes a point of noting in his *De sensu*, Plato had actually refrained from expressing an opinion as to whether there might be other senses in addition to the usual five, or sometimes four. Not so Aristotle. In the *De anima* (424b, 22ff.), from which we have already quoted at length, he states categorically: 'That there is no sixth sense in addition to the five enumerated – sight, hearing, smell, taste, touch – may be established by the following considerations.'

The later Church Fathers had no doubt that Aristotle had decided the question once and for all. Albertus Magnus followed a similar line of reasoning by basing his own analysis on the point of view of the sense media and their functions. In his commentary on *De anima*, he concludes, with Aristotle, that: 'For all these reasons, I maintain that anyone in possession of organs sufficiently capable of perceiving everything that is perceptible by means of one connected and one remote medium suffers no deficiency of senses. A living being with five senses has at its disposal organs that are fully capable of receiving everything perceptible by means of both a connected and a remote medium' (*De anima*, II, 4).[3] Even in the mid-nineteenth century, at a time when experimental physiology was making new discoveries and the canonical number five was beginning to lose its hold, the now forgotten author of a popular scientific work felt called upon to carry on proving, by time-honoured logical means, that 'it is impossible for there to be any more senses than those already given, because these exhaust all conceivable modifications, and any additional new sense would necessarily be superfluous.'[4]

The Jewish scholar Saadia ben Josef (892–942), who taught in Babylon, was doubtless correct when he maintained in his *Kitab al-amanat wa al-i 'tiqadat* (Book of Beliefs and Opinions) that there had been constant attempts to increase the number of the senses.[5] The figure varies between eight and four, and the senses concerned are mainly variants of the sense of touch, which, because of its variable functions and anatomical-topographical distribution over the whole body, is often counted in the plural. Saadia ben Josef himself wondered if the perception of heaviness and lightness should be counted as a separate sense. The possibility that there was perhaps, after all, a special sixth sense was still being ruled out by scholars in the early modern era, on the grounds that it conflicted with unambiguous statements on the matter in the works of Aristotle, Averroes and Albertus Magnus. In the Jewish tradition of the late Middle Ages, the physician and philosopher Simon Duran (1361–1444), who was a rabbi in Algeria, wrote a work entitled *Magen avot* (Shield of the Fathers) that contains yet another summary of the reasoning behind the dominant view that there could be no more senses than five.[6] The book denies the existence of a sixth perception in any shape or form, and refuses to entertain the idea of any medium for the perception of sensory stimuli other than those already to hand. Abraham ben Meir Ibn Esra (1089–1164), one of the most distinguished of the Spanish-Hebrew poets, grammarians and commentators, even made a joke of the issue when he declared of a fellow writer that his bad poems could clearly only be understood by some sense as yet unknown.

It is interesting that the term 'sixth sense' was not used to mean 'extra-sensory perception' before the end of the eighteenth century. Early examples of this usage can be found in the work of Friedrich Maximilian Klinger (1752–1831), who says of a man that 'he knows how to steal the sixth sense from nature's secret store room', and Christoph Martin Wieland's novel *Agathodämon* (1799), in which someone asks: 'What kind of sixth or seventh sense do we possess with which to prove the reality of the objects with which the world of spirits has been populated?'[7] Other eighteenth-century candidates for the sixth sense include the 'sense of beauty' (Herder) and the sex-drive (Georg Forster).

The equation of the sixth sense with sexual feelings may strike us as a little unusual today, but it may be encountered occasionally in baroque lyric poetry. Daniel Casper von Lohenstein (1635–1683), for instance, writes: 'Ear and tongue channel pleasures intense / my feelings are married to some sixth sense.'[8] Immanuel Kant's question 'whether we must actually assume the existence of a sixth sense proper to sexuality' confirms that the assumption of a 'sex-th' sense was not just a literary topos, but also a subject of serious learned discussion until the early nineteenth century.[9] Brillat-Savarin, whose famous book on the physiology of taste was published anonymously in 1826, takes it for granted that the sixth – and to him most vital – sense was the sense of sex.[10]

Apart from the above, most other occasional deviations from the number five are to be found not in natural-philosophical or medical writings, where Aristotle long remained the final word, but in literature. Here, poetic licence knew no bounds and the numbers were just as likely to fall short of as exceed the canonical figure. In Christoph Martin Wieland's famous novel *Die Abderiten* (The Abderites) we read: 'But my four senses tell me that I am not guilty.' The baroque novelist Grimmelshausen has his eponymous hero Springinsfeld 'return to his seven senses'. *Simplicissimus*, his best-known work, contains the following comic exaggeration: 'In this prostration and confusion of my proper reason and seventeen senses, the only solution was for me to stay . . . permanently invisible.'[11] The number seven occurs frequently, since writers would often generously add on a couple more inner senses. Wieland, for instance, added self-consciousness and common sense. The strong influence of the Aristotelian tradition on classical German literature is nonetheless evident in another passage in Wieland's *Abderiten*:

> 'Now you are trying to deny us our five senses!' 'Heaven forbid!', replied Democritus. 'If you are modest enough to claim no more than five senses, it would be extremely unjust to disturb your peaceful enjoyment of them. Mind you, if you use them all together, five senses are perfectly competent judges in cases where it's a matter of deciding whether something is black, smooth or rough, soft or hard, pleasant or repulsive, bitter or sweet.' (I, 8)

Wieland's satire, in which the Gothamites of antiquity figure as embodiments of eternal 'folly and stupidity', typically incorporates Aristotle's now familiar ruling that the senses are five.

On the other hand, poets and novelists in Germany and elsewhere were manifestly unaware of the discourse surrounding the question of the possibility of other kinds of physical sensation that had been triggered by the intense interest in phenomena such as magnetism, electricity or chemical reaction. Questions such as the existence of an additional sense of heat or temperature, or even of a sense resembling a bat's, were strictly the preserve of the biologists, physicists and physiologists, who were beginning to discover the fascinating realm of the senses towards the end of the eighteenth and the beginning of the nineteenth century.

The classification of the senses

In the course of the centuries, there have been repeated attempts not only to enumerate the senses but also to classify them according to specific criteria. The most obvious rubrics were location in the body, distribution in nature, type of stimulation, the anatomical-physiological peculiarity of the organ in question, and usefulness. The extraordinary diversity of these classificatory schemata emerges in a treatise on the senses written at the beginning of the sixteenth century by the French mathematician and theologian Charles Bouvelles (*c*.1470–*c*.1553). Although this work contains few original ideas, it is a generally excellent digest of the opinions of classical and medieval authors.

The division of the senses into five external and five internal senses is relatively old. As we have seen, it appears for the first time in Avicenna. Bouvelle's study represents a further refinement of Aristotelian doctrine, in which the five physical senses are supplemented by a still largely unspecified rational and perceptual mental activity. This type of thinking reflects the dualistic conception of the immateriality of the intellect and the materiality of the body that we encounter time and again in the Greek, Arab and Hebrew traditions and the writings of the early Church Fathers.

As already noted, the common starting point of the various medieval constructions is the Aristotelian doctrine based on the three rational faculties of perception, although Aristotle does not refer to these explicitly as inner senses. They are the common sense (*koine aisthesis*), the imagination (*phantasia*) and the memory. Specifications of the inner senses differ from author to author, for in contrast to the external senses it is difficult to find a common point of reference among the variable formal objects of the inner senses. Charles Bouvelles, who as a Renaissance scholar was drawing on classical and medieval sources, tried to find a way out of this dilemma by assigning five objects of perception to the five cognitive powers first described by Avicenna and St Thomas Aquinas. It then followed that the five physical senses were the outward signs of these inward powers. Bouvelles further assumed that the sensory power possesses the same number of external organs as there are forms of cognition, namely five. In this way, the numerical symmetry between inner and outer senses acquires a grounding in logic.

However, it is probably correct to assume that the interpretation of the parable of the five foolish and five wise virgins (Matt. 25: 1–13), which makes the nature and function of reason and the senses crystal clear to all, had a far wider impact than complex philosophical constructions of this kind. This allegorical comparison, which is based on the number five (or ten), can in fact be traced back to the early Church Fathers (Origen, Augustine).[12] The division of the senses into five inner senses and five outer senses is also supported by the scriptural exegesis of the Jewish tradition. According to the philosopher and rabbi Moses Albilda, who was active in Thessalonika at the beginning of the sixteenth century and wrote a well-known Bible commentary (*Olat Tamid*, printed in Venice, 1601), the ten curtains of the tabernacle (Exod. 26), which were strung together in two rows of five, symbolized the groups of the five inner and outer senses.[13]

Another classification distinguishes between general senses and particular senses. According to Bouvelles, the former category comprised senses that were not only peculiar to a whole living species (humans or animals), but also distributed over the entire body. As Aristotle had already shown in his *Historia animalum* (IV, 82), this group could contain only one sense, namely touch, which was not assigned to any particular organ. Although the sense of taste was also species-specific and not subject to individual variation, it was nevertheless tied to a particular place in the body (the tongue). Here, of course, Bouvelles was ignoring the fact that elsewhere Aristotle does actually number taste among the general senses.[14] The reason for this, as Avicenna explains in his commentary on Aristotle, is that these two senses are useful and indispensable to life, whereas the others do not satisfy this criterion.[15] In Bouvelles' view, the other senses are not developed to their full potential by all members of a species, only by its perfect individuals.

Bouvelles' distinction between mediate and immediate also originally derives from Aristotle.[16] It is based on the idea that, in the case of the sensations of touch and taste, the objects are brought directly into contact with their corresponding organs, whereas the other three senses enter into contact with their objects only via a medium (air and water). This distinction had already been made by Albertus Magnus, who in his influential commentary *De anima* came to the by no means original conclusion:

> For if all senses perceive by means of an external medium – some senses, of course, touch their perceived objects directly, whereas others that are remote from their objects do not touch them, in which case they are transmitted to them by the media that are at first changed by them – then we may say that we perceive everything through media that are different from and external to us. (II, 3)[17]

According to Bouvelles, we must distinguish thirdly between senses with single organs and senses with dual organs. Touch and taste fall into the former category, while smell (nostrils), sight (eyes) and hearing (ears) all possess two bodily orifices. This distinction dates back to Galen. Nemesius, on the other hand, who was writing in late antiquity, thought of taste as a dual sense, for the tongue might also be split, as in the case of snakes. The argument from honour has a role in this classification. The 'more vital' senses are doubly represented. The Jewish philosopher-physician Joseph Albo (*c*.1380–*c*.1444), who was known for his Talmudic, medical and scientific learning, viewed the doubling of some of the senses as a dispensation of divine providence that was not essentially necessary but nonetheless beneficial.[18] According to him, God had endowed the higher creatures with two eyes, ears and nostrils in order to minimize the risk of the complete loss of these vitally important sense organs. Another argument, deriving probably from the Spanish-Jewish tradition, referred to the aesthetic effects that God had intended with this doubling effect.

Bouvelles' fourth distinction, which is again of older origin, concerns the usefulness of the senses, as opposed to their mere agreeableness.[19] Here, touch and taste are rated as absolutely indispensable senses, since they are essential to the consumption of food. Smell, on the other hand, falls into the category of pleasantness. Under this classification, seeing and hearing are allocated to a group of their own, since Bouvelles believes that their contribution to the *honestas* (honour) of man is greatest. Seeing and hearing were there to serve the higher purpose of educating mankind and providing it with spiritual nourishment. In the Jewish tradition it is typically these nobler senses with their more elevated purpose that are said to be 'doubled' on the Sabbath.[20] According to Moses Almosnino (*c.*1500–*c.*1580), it is no accident that the Bible mentions only sight and hearing (Eccles. 1: 8: 'the eye is not satisfied with seeing, nor the ear filled with hearing'), for they belong to the nobler human senses. No less a figure than the celebrated Jewish physician and philosopher Maimonides (1135–1204) had earlier stressed that the meaning of the Holy Scriptures could only be grasped by the higher senses that served the honour of God. With this, a distinction is broached which we shall consider in the context of the hierarchization of the senses, that is, their ranking according to lower and higher.

The hierarchy of the senses

The hierarchy of the senses is both a cultural construction (and therefore based on ideological premises) and a product of the phylogenetic development of the human species (upright physical posture, species-specific increase in the performance of the brain) and the technological changes that have taken place in the course of the process of civilization (displacement of an oral culture by one that is written, the invention of printing, etc.).[21]

The 'classical' hierarchy of the senses originates with Aristotle and is arranged as follows: *visus* (sight), *auditus* (hearing), *odoratus* (smell), *gustus* (taste), *tactus* (touch). However, as we shall see, this hierarchy has never been entirely undisputed. The battle for 'precedence' among the senses even became a popular motif in the literature of the Renaissance and the baroque. The theme is also taken up in the opera and art of the period (e.g., *Il pomo d'oro* by Marc-Antonio Cesti, 1623–1669, based on the libretto by Francesco Sbarra).

The best-known example of the genre is undoubtedly the comedy *Lingua, or The Combat of the Tongue and the Five Senses for Superiority*, attributed to Thomas Tomkis, which was published in 1607 and frequently reprinted and translated. The action concerns the struggle between the senses for priority. The individual senses are personified and distinguished by their striking apparel. Other allegorical figures appear, including Sleep (*somnus*), Appetite (*apetitus*) and Common Sense (*communis sensus*). At the end of the competition, after each of the senses has sung their own praises and achievements and justified their right of precedence, it is the last-named who pronounces a verdict that leaves everything as it was: '*Visus*, Tactus, and the rest, our former sentence concerning you, wee confirme as irrevocable, and establish the Crowne to you *Visus*, and the Roabe [robe] to you *Tactus*.'[22] Nothing changes, therefore. The sense of sight remains in first place and touch must be contented with the position of runner-up.

There is no Solomonic judgement of this kind in the poem written at the beginning of the eighteenth century by Jacques Le Pansif. The first stanza announces the theme:

> The senses got into a fight
> you couldn't say the cause was slight
> They wanted to get it firmly agreed
> which of them Venus didn't need.[23]

The senses then take their turn in the traditional sequence, with sight going in first and feeling last. There is a decidedly erotic aspect to this competition; for the issue is which of them stands in greater favour with Lady Venus. The poet leaves us in no real doubt that the laurels go to the sense of touch, which is usually ranked last, since he does not consider it necessary to comment on it. Touch has the last and, therefore, decisive word:

> Feeling laughed out loud
> and asked: what use is a bride
> to lie with day after day,
> if we don't feel the urge for this kind of play.

The favour of a woman is also the prize in an allegorical elegy by the German baroque poet Jakob Balde, SJ (1605–1668). As might be expected from an author belonging to the Society of Jesus, the woman in question here is not Venus, but Urania, the muse of astronomy and the embodiment of the soul's awareness of its heavenly destiny. Nonetheless, the subject is again love, albeit platonic rather than sexual, and each of the senses tries to win Urania's favour by writing her three love letters, to which she answers in the negative. The individual senses are seconded in the poem by the painter Cinna (I, 3), a musician (II, 3) and the famous master cook Rumpold (IV, 3). They too all reach for their pens to plead the cause of their clients. The sense of sight is, predictably, the first to present his credentials, and he addresses Urania as follows: 'An especially precious sense, without which you could not read, sends you this greeting . . . We senses are quintuplets, and you too have always appeared to value me most of all. For why else would you lavish so much stolen flattery and tenderness on just one of us? On me, to whom you cry "My light!" '[24] But knowing that sensory perception of any kind can jeopardize the salvation of the soul, Urania refuses to let either *Visus* or any of the other senses charm her into preferring him. So there can be only one winner of this competition: *Urania victrix*, the title heroine of Balde's 'historical-metaphysical poem on the world' (Kühlmann and Seidel).

The five senses are commonly ranked in descending order of merit, beginning with the highest, which is almost always sight, and ending with the lowest, which is usually sensation. The illuminated illustrations to the manuscript of an allegorical poem entitled *Anti-Claudianus* by Alanus ab Insulis (*c*.1128–1202) are a particularly apt expression of this arrangement. Here, *Ratio* (reason) has harnessed five horses (the senses) to the chariot of *Prudentia* (intelligence). The first sense to strike the eye of the viewer is the allegorized sense of sight, which is represented as a horse with blinkered eyes.[25] This way of depicting the senses is hardly unprecedented and is, of course, influenced by a passage in Plato's *Phaedrus* which describes the difficulties confronting the charioteer (*nous*, or reason) as he struggles to steer an unequal pair of horses along the proper path to the higher spheres. A Sanskrit text of the fourth century BC also depicts the horses of the senses being restrained by a charioteer representing reason.[26]

Rankings of the senses in reverse, or ascending order, are much more rare, however. One of the few examples may be found in the work of the Jewish scholar Joseph Albo mentioned above, who defends this arrangement on physiological and genetic grounds.[27] Taking an evolutionary approach, he begins with the lower senses, with touch in the lead, and ends with vision, the 'noblest' of the senses. One occasionally comes upon quite arbitrary rankings that are better understood as simple listings rather than hierarchies. An example is the following enumeration taken from the tenth-century Jewish dogmatics (*Kitab al-Amanat*) of Saadia ben Josef, which clearly follows no particular organizing principle: *nitamin* (things tasted), *nirim* (things seen), *nischmaim* (things heard), *murachim* (things smelt), *memuschaschim* (things felt).[28]

In what follows, we shall present the five senses in their classical sequence, beginning with vision and concluding with touch. In doing so, we shall be on the lookout for occasional promotions and/or demotions of particular senses.

The privileged position of the *sense of sight* is in no way a by-product of the invention of printing and the advent of the modern era. On the contrary, the optical sense has been at the top of the ladder since antiquity. However, the rationalization of this state of affairs has varied enormously. For Aristotle, sight stands highest because of its cognitive value, and the same applies to Plato. One need only think of the famous image of the cave in *The Republic*, which adumbrates the passage from an oral to a visual culture that had already largely been completed by Plato's time. In Ovid's *Metamorphoses*, written around the time of the birth of Christ, this privileging of sight is typically interpreted as a product of human evolution:

> There was as yet no animal which was more akin to the gods than these [the animals], none more capable of intelligence, none that could be master of all the rest. It was at this point that man was born . . . Whereas other animals hang their heads and look at the ground, he [the Creator] made man stand erect, bidding him look up to heaven, and lift his head to the stars. So the earth, which had been rough and formless, was moulded into the shape of a man, a creature till then unknown.[29]

The pre-eminence of vision is thus explained by the central role of this sense in the process of civilization. For Augustine, the visual sense deserves first place because it is the most universal of the senses and the others can all be named after it. As the Church Father argues in more detail in the *Confessions* (X, 35), it is possible to say that one sees something when one is actually hearing it. The sense of sight is also the most objective of the senses, for what we see can be seen in the same way by another person.[30] Isidor of Seville (*c.*570–636), the greatest encyclopaedist of the early Middle Ages, holds the eye superior because man sees further than he hears, and hears further than he smells.[31] Alcuin (*c.*735–804), the Carolingian historian and adviser of Charlemagne, actually derives the precedence of eye from its etymology. Bernard of Clairvaux (1091–1153), the preacher of crusade, considers sight privileged because the eyes are placed higher in the body than the other senses and can identify objects over long distances, which is essentially a restatement of Isidor. The abbess Hildegard of Bingen (1098–1179) offers a similar rationalization: 'This seeing with the eyes is so pleasant, so wonderful, because with it man is able to distinguish between the good and the inferior through knowledge and discernment.'[32]

The privileged position of sight was reflected in the educational norms of the Middle Ages. According to a popular didactic poem by Thomasin von Zerclaere (after 1185–1259?) entitled *Der welsche Gast* (The Strange Guest), one should 'try if one can / to choose the kind of man / who looks better than he sounds.'[33] The church, too, exploited the special status of the eyes. Jerome (*c.*348–420) had earlier declared that: 'It is stated in Holy Scripture that the people shall learn by their eyes as well as their ears.'[34] And in the thirteenth century, John of Genoa accounted for the frequent use of the language of images (e.g., in the richly illustrated Bibles for the poor) by arguing that people were more likely to experience the morally uplifting effects of religion (*devotio*) if they could see things, rather than simply listen to them.[35]

Somewhat similar arguments for the priority of sight can be found in the Hebrew literature of the Middle Ages, which was based, as we have seen, on classical and Arabic sources. To quote all the relevant instances would take up far too much of our space, so we will confine ourselves to a line from Maimonides, physician to the court of the Sultan Saladin, and probably the most famous Jewish thinker of the Middle Ages: 'The most complicated and also the most perfect of the senses is the sense of sight.'[36] Jewish scholars also drew attention to the speed and efficiency of vision, often using examples of the kind already encountered in Aristotle and Theophrastus.

No one seriously challenged the superiority and precedence of the visual sense in the early modern era; indeed the invention of printing decisively assisted the breakthrough of visual culture. Leonardo da Vinci, the universal genius of the Renaissance, was not about to rock the boat and was one of the host of scholars who gave pride of place to vision: 'The sense of sight is the Lord and commander of the others.'[37] In a popular work entitled *Grewel der Verwüstung Menschlichen Geschlechts* (Terrors and Scourges of Humanity, 1610), written a few years before the outbreak of the Thirty Years' War, the Tyrolean author and physician Hippolytus Guarinonius (1571–1654) summarized the argument for the eyes in a form more or less familiar since antiquity: 'The human eyes grasp so much more than any of the other five senses, namely all visible things in different places and directions, such as above, below, behind, to the side, in the middle, and on the outside, even to the boundaries of the earth.'[38]

There is no lack of evidence – stretching all the way back to antiquity – of philosophical, and especially theological, backing for the sense of hearing, which tends to belie its reputation as the 'eternal runner-up', even though statistics may at first seem to tell a different story. In the Old Testament, there are four references to seeing for every two instances of hearing. This discrepancy is even more pronounced in the New Testament, where the ratio is 6:2. The striking differences between the two parts of the Bible are generally attributed to the fact that Christianity was much more exposed to the influences of Hellenism, although the Jewish philosopher Philo of Alexandria (*c*.20 BC–*c*.AD 50), who followed the Greek authorities in describing vision as the best, quickest, truest and keenest of the senses, was certainly one exception to this rule.[39]

The *sense of hearing* is more in demand in matters involving not so much the recognition of truth as the guarantee of salvation and obedience to God's commandments. 'Schma Israel' (Listen, Israel) are the first words of the most important prayer of Judaism, which is at the same time a fundamental profession of faith. This use of hearing in the sense of listening to God and achieving salvation is also encountered, albeit less frequently, in the Gospels, which are the announcement of good tidings from God. The Gospel of St John states, for instance, that 'the dead shall hear the voice of the Son of

God; and they that hear shall live' (John 5: 25). Medieval Judaism continues the tradition of ascribing a leading role to hearing in faith and religious practice. The kabbalist and biblical exegete Bachja ben Ascher (*d.* 1340) condenses the advantages of hearing into four points that are underpinned by numerous examples from Holy Scripture: 1) it favours the poor in spirit who can be taught only by oral instruction; 2) anyone at all can learn by it; 3) only the sense of hearing enables us to recognize things exactly and to clear up any doubts left behind by visual experience; and 4) when oral instruction (consider, for instance, the Hebrew concept of *torah be-al-peh* = oral laws) is supported with stories and examples, listening can acquire a high degree of concreteness.[40]

Although the eyes were the final court of appeal as far as independent perception was concerned, some medieval Arab and Christian scholars were prepared to concede the functional primacy of hearing for religious instruction and the knowledge of divinely revealed truth. Here, seeing and hearing are assigned to different areas of competence and measured according to different scales of value. The medieval German mystic Meister Eckhart (*c.*1260–1327) succinctly reduces this bipartite division of the hierarchy to a formula: 'Hearing brings things to me, but seeing extracts things from me, including the labour of seeing itself. In the eternal life to come, therefore, the bliss we shall enjoy from the power of hearing will exceed that of the power of sight.'[41]

The intermediate position of the *sense of smell* has likewise hardly been questioned since antiquity. As we have seen, Aristotle had placed it between the long-range senses of seeing and hearing and the two short-range senses of taste and touch. In his treatise on the soul, Albertus Magnus followed Avicenna in assuming that the object of perception was present in two forms (material and immaterial), and believed this to be corroborated by the ambivalent position of the sense of smell. He too was unwilling to contemplate a higher ranking, since traditional theory held that the faculty of smell was of minor importance to the inner senses. Albertus Magnus sees confirmation of this in the fact that people almost never dream of smells. Avicenna, who ranked the senses according to their usefulness, with the senses of touch and taste in first position, also places smell in the middle of his somewhat utilitarian hierarchy. Konrad von Megenberg (1309–1374) came up with an interesting variant of this in-between position: 'The sense of smell occupies the middle position between the three, with sight above it, and hearing to one side of it.'[42] Here, smell inhabits a point equidistant from the so-called higher senses. The hierarchical scheme employed by René Descartes, on the other hand, is almost classical. He also puts smell in an intermediate position on the grounds that, although less crude than touch and taste, it lacked the perceptual refinement of hearing, to say nothing of vision. The absolute primacy of smell is rarely postulated, however, and is usually encountered in literary rather than natural philosophical texts. One example is by the Jewish-Spanish poet Abraham Ibn Esra, who, in a commentary on Isaiah 11: 3, emphasized the infallibility of smell compared to other senses.[43] It is also stressed repeatedly (and not only in the Jewish tradition) that smell carries the seal of the Lord (see Gen. 2: 7), which may explain the great importance attached to scent in Christian worship[44] – in the cults surrounding saints, for example, or the ritual use of incense, myrrh and scented chrism. In Judaism there are the spice boxes containing fragrant herbs, which are savoured at the close of the Sabbath as a sign of the difference between the secular weekday and the sacred day of rest. But while noting the widespread regard for the sense of smell in the religions of the world, we should not overlook the fact that, in Christianity at least, there were others, notably the missionary early Church Fathers, who considered it to be a source of temptation, and were prepared to accept it – if at all – only in a purely spiritual form, purged of the dross of profanity.

The inferior status of the *sense of taste*, which has persisted since the time of Aristotle, is based primarily on the consideration that not all animals possess a sense of smell. Taste is often, as in Avicenna, elided with touch to form a single sense. The upshot of this was that the negative qualities of touch, allegedly the very lowest of the senses, were transferred to taste, as for instance in the work of the Jewish scholar Salomo Halevi (end of the sixteenth century), who typically associated it with the pudenda.[45] Contrasting with this are the attempts by theologians such as Aquinas to grant taste a place directly below the faculties of sight and hearing on the sensory scale in the light of the doctrine of the *immutatio spiritualis*, an immaterial form of perception based upon spiritual transformation.

In the Christian West, there was another revaluation of the sense of taste by Isidor of Seville (560–636), in the shape of his equation of *sapor* (taste), the specific formal object of this form of sensory perception, with *sapere* (knowledge) and *sapientia* (wisdom).[46] This paved the way for the distinction between aesthetico-mystical and physiological taste that was to influence subsequent discussion of the role of taste in the Middle Ages and above all in the early modern epoch. Guillaume d'Auvergne (1180–1249), for example, takes *gustus* to mean both the rational knowledge of the object and the sensuous enjoyment of the subject. In this theory, beauty is characterized by its capacity to awaken pleasurable sensations of taste in the observer.[47] In medieval scholasticism, therefore, the concept of taste circulates in both a rational and a sensuous version. But it is not until the sixteenth- and seventeenth-century tracts and commentaries on rhetoric and poetics that a theoretical basis is finally established for aesthetic discrimination, which is then followed by the gradual establishment of taste as an aesthetic category. It goes without saying that the physiology of taste was among the beneficiaries of this semantic shift, in as far as it brought about a revaluation of the sense of taste.

The *sense of touch* is the extremist among the senses, for it has frequently been ranked both at the bottom and at the top of the scale of esteem. This apparent contradiction goes back to its variable status in Aristotle, for, while ranking it fifth in order of merit (after sight, hearing, smell and taste), the treatise on the soul also describes it as a sense that reaches its highest form of development in man (*De anima*, 421a, 22). The Arab scholar Avicenna, whom we have already had occasion to mention in this study, provides one explanation of Aristotle's conflicting statements. As he understood it, what Aristotle meant was that with respect to honour the primacy of the sense of sight applied, but that from the point of view of natural aptitude the sense of touch merited priority. This resolution of the contradiction met with the approval of many medieval scholars. Aquinas developed a complex theory based on Aristotle's doctrine of the soul, in which touch and sight are granted more or less equal rights. In common with Avicenna he thought that, in addition to the traditional hierarchy dominated by vision, there was a second hierarchical order in which the sense of touch played the major perceptual role. With his exhaustive and conclusive argument for the alternative primacy of sensation, Aquinas shows himself to be a decidedly original thinker.

Aquinas opens his case for the superior status, and systematic primacy, of the sense of touch by noting that sensitive life forms define themselves by means of their sense of touch: 'touch [is] the first sense, the root and ground, as it were, of the other senses, the one which entitles a living thing to be called sensitive.'[48] The haptic comprehension of the world is also of central importance for the survival of the individual and the species, since it is the means by which we distinguish between the edible and the inedible – an argument already advanced by Avicenna. With the exception of taste, the other senses merely serve to make life agreeable (*propter bene esse*). Another important argument for the priority of touch, according to Aquinas, is that it is the root (*radix fontalis*) of all sentient activity. It follows from this that the other senses are all derived from it: 'In the first place touch is the basis of sensitivity as a whole; for obviously the organ of touch pervades the whole body, so that the organ of each of the other senses is also an organ of touch, and the sense of touch by itself constitutes a being as sensitive.'[49] Thus, the operations of the other senses are seen as subordinate to *tactus*. Aquinas's third argument for the precedence of touch rests upon its optimal performance in the process of gathering knowledge: 'Therefore the finer one's sense of touch, the better, strictly speaking, is one's sensitive nature as a whole, and consequently the higher one's intellectual capacity. For a fine sensitivity is a disposition to a fine intelligence.'[50] Following Aristotle's idea of the flesh as the medium of touch, Aquinas argues that sensorial beings with 'hard flesh' would not perceive things as well as those with soft flesh (e.g., man) and would therefore be less receptive to perception of any kind.

This remarkable reappraisal of touch may be encountered in the works of other Christian, Muslim and Jewish scholars of the Middle Ages, although their approach was sometimes slightly different and their distinctions less subtle. After the thirteenth century, the Jewish tradition underwent a change that may also be seen later in the allegorical representations of the Renaissance and baroque: the sense of touch falls increasingly into disrepute. The culprit, once more, is Aristotle, or, more precisely, his *Nicomachean Ethics* (III, 8b), where the sense of taste is associated with 'the pleasures of love' and accused of 'disorderliness'. No less a figure than Maimonides, who refers to this passage in his *Guide for the Perplexed* (II, 36), decided to approve it.[51] It was, however, his later translators and commentators who forged a connection between this approving quotation of Aristotle and various places in the Bible (e.g., Deut. 4: 28), thereby helping to ensure that the mental association of touch with sinful behaviour (voluptuousness and unrestrained sex drive) became widespread. Thus, both Abraham ben Schemtov Bibago, who was a doctor at the court of King Juan II of Aragon towards the end of the fifteenth century, and the celebrated Talmudist Moses Isserles (*c*.1525–1572) refer explicitly to the sense of touch as shame (*cherpah*). The Jewish-Spanish writer and philosopher Joseph Schemtov ibn Schemtov (*c*.1468–1490) cites Aristotle as his source without concerning himself with the ambiguities of the passage in the *Nicomachean Ethics*.

Clearly, the association of touch with the sexual urge in the language and visual imagery of the Middle Ages and, above all, the modern era has other origins and roots besides these. In this context, we might consider the poem by Jacques Le Pansif quoted above, as well as the still living Christian tradition, according to which it was Eve who first touched the apple when she seduced Adam.[52] In this way, *tactus* became a symbol of eroticism as such, to which poets and painters of not only the early modern age returned time and again.

4

Representations: Allegories

Our life is a symbol of the life of nature.

Melchior von Diepenbrock, *Pastoral Letter* (1846)

The French social and cultural historian Roger Chartier defines 'representations' as 'images of social life' deriving from strategies of authority and political practice. Chartier uses the concept of representation in a more restricted and historically precise sense than Ernst Cassirer in *The Philosophy of Symbolic Forms* (1923–9), the reason being that he is concerned in the first instance with 'the fundamental historical question of variability and plurality in the comprehension (or incomprehension) of the representations of the social and natural world offered in texts and images.'[1] He is thus less interested in the phenomenon of a figurative mode of thought based on a universal function of the mind. His historical-critical approach can therefore be applied fruitfully to a history of the senses.

In what follows, we shall be concerned above all to trace the invention and entry into tradition of such representations, and to establish their significance in the construction of the social world. In so doing, we will do well to bear in mind the advice of the philosopher Johann Gottlieb Fichte to the student of symbols: 'furthermore, it is clear that these symbolic descriptions of the supersensual must, in all cases, take account of the stage of development of the cognitive capacities of the peoples concerned; so that the origin and development of the symbolic description will vary from language to language.'[2]

Imagery of the senses in general

It is not just since the Renaissance that the equation of certain human characteristics, or social functions and structures, with parts of the body, and particularly the senses, has been both a popular theme within a multitude of discourses, and an expression of the literary and artistic appropriation of the most varied philosophies of the world. Whether symbolic or literal, images of the senses may be encountered all the way back to ancient times (see figure 4.1). The interpretations of Holy Scripture by Jewish and Christian scholars are particularly rich in systematic classifications of the five senses that are essentially figurative. The common, allegorical basis of these images is the number five. It involves both the numerical correspondences between micro- and macrocosm and the systemic connections between the inner and outer human world, including the complex relations between the senses themselves. As Ludwig Schrader has indicated, we need also to distinguish further between vertical and horizontal structural correspondences.[3]

The allegorical interpretation of the Old Testament by Jewish scholars was not intended merely to embellish poetic passages, or to extend and illustrate the prescriptions of religion. These exegetes were striving to come closer to divine truth and to reveal themes related to salvation. The work of Philo of Alexandria is a veritable treasure trove in this respect.[4] He interprets the fiveness of the senses allegorically. One example of his allegorical method is his interpretation of a biblical passage (Gen. 19: 23–5) dealing with the destruction of the five cities (*pentapolis*) of the Jordan Valley. As we know, only the town of Zoar was spared the wrath of God. The war between the five kings (Gen. 14) and the four other kings (whom Philo sees as embodiments of desire, greed, fear and distress) is likewise interpreted allegorically. The two kings who fall into the slimepits and perish there represent the senses of taste and touch, as these are the senses that extend deep into the body. According to Genesis, the three other kings manage to escape. This brings Philo to the assumption that they can only stand for the three remaining senses, commonly described as the long-range senses because of the type of perception they perform. In addition, he resolves the contradiction between two passages in the Bible (Exod. 1: 5 and Deut. 10: 21) by means of a bold speculation on the subject of salvation. In the first account, the patriarch Jacob takes seventy souls or people with him to Egypt, whereas in the second the number is seventy-five. In Philo's view, the difference can only be the five senses. Jacob had first to reject the senses before he could become the founder of Israel.

Figure 4.1 Inventory of iconographic symbols of the five senses

Sense	Animals	Objects	Bible	Mythology	Persons
Sight	Eagle	Telescope, magnifying glass, spectacles, mirror, compass, sextant, astrolabe, sun, moon, stars, globe, torch, painting, portraits, easel, jewellery	Adam and Eve are introduced to paradise	Narcissus	Doctor inspecting urine
	Lynx			Io	Blind man
	Cat			Argus	Geographer
	Owl		Adoration of the Magi	Orassio (nymph)	Astronomer
			Healing of the blind man		Old man (with spectacles)
Hearing	Stag	Lute, harp, cello, violin, horn, trumpet, flute, bagpipes, drum, tambourine, triangle, bells, pianoforte, organ, clock, birdcage, rifle, pistol, music, human ear	God reprimands Adam and Eve	Orpheus and Eurydice	Man (of mature years)
	Wild boar		Sermon of John the Baptist	Ache (nymph)	Musicians
	Mole		The Annunciation		
Smell	Dog	Flower pot (vase, bouquet, flower basket), cornucopia, phial, flowers (particularly roses, carnations, tulips and lilies)	God breathing life into Adam	Juno	Boy
	Vulture		The anointing of Jesus by Mary Magdalene	Osfressia (nymph)	
	Insect		The Magi present frankincense and myrrh	Flora	
Taste	Ape	Sea food (lobster, oysters, etc.), fish, exotic fruit (incl. pomegranates), bread, cheese, game, confectionery, wine, grapes	Eve offers the apple to Adam	Persephone	Dinner party
	Chameleon		Feeding of the 5000	Hebe	Man tasting wine
			Marriage feast at Cana	Geussia (nymph)	Youth
Touch	Bat	Surgical instruments, plasters, coal- and open fire, coins, purse, armour, hammer and anvil, dagger, loom, fishing net, door knocker, deck of cards and chess pieces	Angel expelling Adam and Eve from paradise	Pygmalion	Doctor/Barber
	Pecking parrot/bird			Aphrodite	Lucretia
	Spider		Elijah curses his mockers	Amor and Psyche	Angler
	Tortoise		Peter's draught of fish	Venus-Urania	Lovers
	Scorpion		Christ taken from the cross	Aphea (nymph)	Old man (groping)
	Lizard			Amor	

Philo also finds allegories in the five coats presented by Joseph to his brother Benjamin (Gen. 45: 22) and in the contribution of a fifth of all the produce of Egypt. In the five pillars that stand before the tabernacle (Exod. 26: 37), connecting the exterior with the interior, he spies an allusion to the function of the senses, which are the entrances to the realm of the spirit, that is, to the soul of man.

Philo of Alexandria is by no means the only biblical commentator to pursue manifest connections of this kind. This particular form of symbolic scriptural interpretation based on the fivefold nature of the senses has existed since the beginnings of Jewish biblical exegesis in the period of the Talmud and Midrash (second to seventh centuries AD).[5] The tradition includes Isaac Arama, who died in Thessalonika in 1556, and his interpretation of a familiar Old Testament story (Gen. 27: 18–29) as an interrogation performed by the blind Isaac with his remaining four senses. This important sixteenth-century Talmudic scholar sees an allusion to the five exterior senses even in the simple enumeration of ethical principles contained in Isaiah (33: 15). The rapturous description of spring in the Song of Songs (2: 11) is for him yet another allegory of the human soul.

A contemporary of Arama, Salomo Halevi, another Jewish commentator, interprets a passage in Jeremiah (3: 14–17), in which the contrites are promised return to Zion, as a representation of penitence. The same scholar interprets the ten mighty men mentioned in Ecclesiastes (7: 19) as an implicit reference to the five external and internal senses. For Moses Albilda, the seven-branched candelabra mentioned frequently in the Torah symbolizes the five senses which, together with the common sense, take the intellect into their midst and receive its spiritual enlightenment. Abraham Bibago (*d.* 1489) perceives the longing of the children of Israel for Egyptian food (Num. 11: 4–9), and the five items they mention individually, as a figuration of humanity's pursuit of divinely revealed truth and religious knowledge. On the other hand, the attempt of Moses Isserles (*c.*1525–1572) to associate the despatch of letters ordering the murder of Jews (Esther 3: 13) with the five senses seems a little far-fetched. He bases his allegory on the senses' known proneness to evil. The same writer also interprets the five offerings of food in Leviticus 2 as a reference to the senses, not only because of the numerical correspondences but also in the light of the relations obtaining between them.

As these examples show (five kings, five messengers, five daughters, etc.), the allegorical interpretation of biblical figures appearing in groups of five was particularly widespread in the Jewish tradition. The Jewish historian David Kaufmann demonstrated the pervasiveness of this type of symbolic thought in the Judaism of late antiquity and the Middle Ages:

> The historical substance had evaporated into symbol. The old king of Elam, Kedorlaomar, petrified into the mask of the highest powers of the soul; the nation's sovereign queen was turned into fantasy. Even Jacob and his sons were victims of this allegoristic iconoclasm: Together with her six sons and daughter Dina, the matriarch Lea turns into the shade of the animal soul, leading a brood consisting of the five senses, the common sense and a gate-crashing elf child.[6]

Allegorical 'number games' of this kind were also popular in Christian biblical exegesis. The best known is the parable of the five wise and five foolish virgins mentioned above (Matt. 25). The first reading of this kind dates back to Origen (AD 185–254).[7] The subject is then taken up again in the *Letters* (Epistolae) of Paulinus of Nola (353/4–431). This early Church Father follows Origen in maintaining that the five wise and the five foolish virgins represent, respectively, the purity and depravity of the senses.[8] To judge from the extraordinary number of crucifixion scenes in medieval visual art, the allegorical association of the five wounds of Christ with the five senses was hardly less popular as a theme. The German mystic Heinrich von Seuse (*c*.1295–1366) lists the various forms of sensory torment suffered by Christ on the cross in his *Büchlein der Weisheit* (Little Book of Wisdom), and closes with a prayer to God: 'I therefore implore you to shield my eyes from the sight of abandonment, and protect my ears against lascivious remarks. Lord, remove things tasty to my lips, make me indifferent to the scent of the things of the world and take away the softness of my body.'[9] Nor, in this context, should we overlook the redemptive scheme (five rows of angels – five senses – five wounds of Christ) contained in Hildegard of Bingen's *Scivias*. The popularity of this allegory doubtless owed much to the detailed descriptions of the torments visited upon Christ's senses as he bore the cross to Calvary that we find in works such as the widely circulated *Legenda aurea* of Jacob of Voragine (*c*.1230–1298).

Other examples[10] of such or similar moral-theological reinterpretations of New Testament passages may be found in the works of the Church Fathers, notably in Augustine. His interpretation of the five yoke of oxen in Luke 14: 19 as *curiositas quinque sensus*, or the curiosity satisfied by the five senses, is based on their particular ordering in the text. Meister Eckhart attempts an interpretation of the same passage and also comes up with a reference to the five senses. If it wishes to be invited to God's banquet, the soul must part with their company. Otfrid von Weissenburg (*c*.800–870) explains the division of his harmonization of the Gospels into five parts by arguing that the word of God necessarily purifies the five senses. Peter Damian (1007–1072) takes the five kings of Midian (Num. 31: 8) to refer to the five senses, on the grounds that all human vices originate in the external senses. Slightly more familiar is his comparison of the five senses to the five vulnerable and poorly guarded gates of a city, based on passages in Luke (21: 34) and Isaiah (33: 15–16). Hugo of Saint-Victor (1096–1141) uses a similar metaphor when demonstrating the lurking threat to the salvation of the soul. In the five columned halls comprising the gateway to the Pool of Bethesda (John 5: 3), which accommodated many of the sick, blind, lame and crippled, he sees an image of the five senses, for it was known that sense perception damaged the body and the soul.

Window imagery is even more frequent in medieval Christian biblical exegesis, albeit with reference not to the New Testament but to a passage in the Book of Jeremiah (9: 20). This image also appears in the literature of antiquity, most notably in Cicero's interpretation of the sense organs as windows of the soul (*Tusculan Disputations*, I, 20, 46). It is later adopted by Augustine, Paulinus of Nola and Bernard of Clairvaux and reinterpreted in the light of the doctrine of salvation. It is also taken up by the late medieval poet Tilo von Kulm in a poem entitled *Von siben Ingesigeln* (On the Seven Seals): 'This is the ability of our senses, external and internal, which are the windows of reason through which first of all many and various images are borne by the wind.'[11] The five windows are here equated with the five senses. To avoid being seduced by the things of the world, these loopholes of evil must be opened with caution and kept securely closed when not in use.

The allegorization of the five senses by Hippolytus of Rome (*c*.170–*c*.235/6) refers exclusively to the Old Testament: Genesis = eye,

Exodus = ear, Leviticus = smell, Numbers = taste and Deuteronomy = touch. Guillaume de Thierry (*c*.1080–1149), on the other hand, compares the eyes to the angels, the ears to the patriarchs, the nose to the prophets and the sense of taste to Christ. According to Hrabanus Maurus, the sum of five shekels of silver mentioned in the Old Testament (Lev. 27) signifies the opportunity granted to man fully to realize his potential and to increase his efforts, by analogy with the five senses. Thus, a person who hears better than others will also be more perceptive. This important Church Father also construes the width of the New Temple (Ezek. 40: 25), namely twenty-five cubits, as a symbolic reference to the ability of the senses to multiply themselves. This is again an allusion to the need for man to redouble his efforts and summon all his powers if he wishes to remain on the narrow path of salvation. The same idea is expressed by an anonymous late medieval English poet. In a short verse based on the mysticism of numbers, the author condenses examples familiar from the Old and New Testament into a kind of readily intelligible set of religious instructions for use in achieving the salvation: 'Kepe well X and Flee fro[m] VII / Rule well V and come hevyn [heaven].'[12] In other words: obey the Ten Commandments, steer clear of the Seven Deadly Sins and keep the five senses under a tight rein.

On the other hand, the role of the five senses in the religious art of the Middle Ages is conspicuously marginal. Exceptions simply prove the rule. Here we will mention just the well-known illustration in an illuminated Erlangen manuscript (Codex 8, fol. 130v) produced during the second half of the twelfth century at a monastery in Heilbronn (see figure 4.2).[13] The picture shows a ladder that forks in the middle. One of the branchings continues upwards to heaven, where God sits on his throne and St Peter guards the gates. The other descends into hell, where the Devil and his accomplices are lying in wait. The rungs leading up to the point where the two paths separate are inscribed with the names of the five senses, in the traditional order of touch, smell, taste, hearing and vision. After the fork, the path continues steeply upwards on rungs bearing the names of the four virtues: justice, courage, prudence and moderation. Appropriately, the road to hell is paved here not with the proverbial good intentions, but with the names of the four corresponding vices.

The senses also seldom appear as an ensemble in the secular art of the Middle Ages.[14] The few such works that exist are mainly known

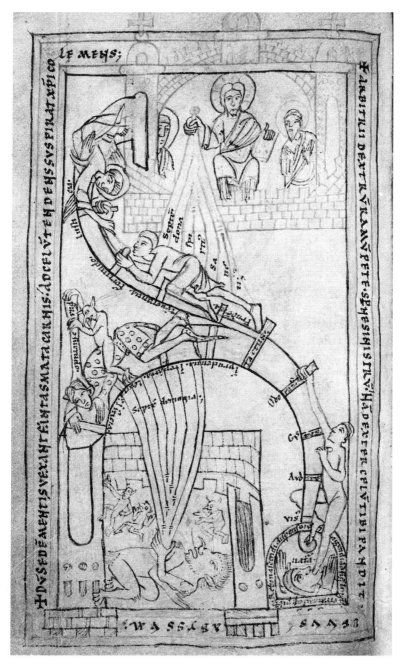

Figure 4.2 The senses on the way to heaven and hell; medieval manuscript from a monastery at Heilbronn

only to experts (the famous *Lady with the Unicorn* in the Musée de Cluny in Paris is a whole cycle of pictures!) and include the Fuller Brooch in the British Museum, which dates from around AD 850 and depicts a set of female figures personifying the five senses, with sight occupying the central position. In contrast to the programmatic religious images of the times, the remaining late medieval secular depictions are concerned less with the links between the senses and sin than with the experience of the senses as something positive, particularly in the form of love. One manifest expression of this profane approach to the 'gateways' of human perception is the coloured illustrations of the so-called *bestiaires d'amour*, late medieval collections of erotically suggestive animal descriptions that were hugely popular in fourteenth- and fifteenth-century France and Germany.

In sharp contrast to these, all religious allegories, whether based on Old or New Testament sources, reflect the prevailing Judeo-Christian theological consensus in their depictions of the senses as treacherous. Their capacity to grasp divine truth is shown as either limited or inadequate. Thus, these texts and images express something approaching downright hostility to the senses, although this attitude is not necessarily typical of the Middle Ages.

The moral-theological justification for the condemnation of the senses was therefore found in biblical passages that could plausibly be associated with the senses. Given the wealth of examples, this survey of the poetical-allegorical treatment of the popular medieval and pre-medieval theme of the depravity of the senses can make no claim to exhaustiveness. But it should now be sufficiently clear that there were religious interests behind the condemnation of the senses, which were orchestrated in the form of a struggle for the souls of the faithful. This is only partially contradicted by the fact that popular medieval religiosity resorted frequently to 'the pleasures of the eye', and placed all the other senses at the service of a more or less mystical experience of God. For along with the apparently dominant motif of the senses as a moral threat, we are reminded again and again that the sense organs were servants of God's sense of beauty and that, in using them, we are serving a divinely ordained purpose.

The end of the Middle Ages and the resulting split within Christianity did not put an end to an ambivalent attitude to the senses that runs like a red thread through the history of the church since Augustine. Important remnants of the traditional ascesis were absorbed into both Catholicism and Protestantism; ascetic and anti-physical trends reappear again and again to denounce the sinfulness of the senses and to propagate the triumph of faith.

The high point of the literary and pictorial representation of this theme was the age of the Counter-Reformation. Two outstanding examples of the continuing development of the traditional motif are typically supplied by Spain, where in the mid-seventeenth century the poet Pedro Calderón (1600–1681) wrote a play entitled *El nuevo palacio del Retiro* and Juan Antonio Escalante (1633–1669) painted what is probably his best-known work (now in the Prado Museum), whose message can be summarized as the triumph of faith (see figure 4.3).[15] In Calderón's play, the personified senses struggle for possession of a bouquet (symbolic of divine knowledge) which *la Fe* (Faith) holds firmly in her hands. Each of them must submit to a test by the sacred host. In Escalante's painting of 1667, Faith (*fides*) is

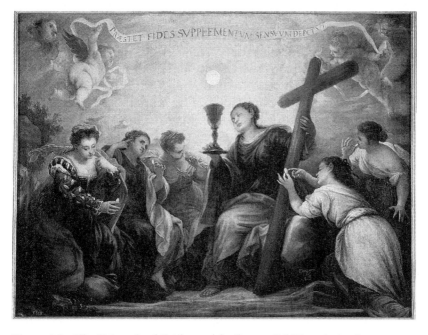

Figure 4.3   The Triumph of Faith over the Senses (1667); painting by Juan Antonio Escalante (1633–1669)

again represented as a woman, who is supporting the cross with her left arm and raising a chalice surmounted by a host with her right hand. The five senses, also female, are grouped around her, and they identify themselves by pointing to the particular senses they represent. For the benefit of the viewer who does not immediately grasp the allegorical allusions, the angels hovering above the scene hold out a banner bearing the Latin sentence 'Praestet fides supplementum sensuum defectui', which freely translated means 'May faith compensate for the shortcomings of the senses.' The picture is an iconographic example of the Counter-Reformation's sometimes violent critique of the material world. Another such specimen is the engraving by Philipp Galle of a work by Erasmus Quellinus (*d.* 1678) in which the viewer can make out a similar kind of epigram ('Faith is the path to salvation, whereas the senses must be left behind'). The image thus bears the now familiar message that salvation comes from faith and piety alone, and that the senses play no part in it.[16] However, there were others, such as one of the fellow Jesuits of Ignatius Loyola (1491–1556), who considered that the senses and religion could indeed work together in a manner pleasing to God. In his instructions to the missionaries of the Jesuit order, written in 1549, he points the path to salvation: 'From time to time we should also devote ourselves to pious works of a more sensorial nature, such as visiting the sick and imprisoned and providing help to the poor; such acts are a sweet savour unto God [2 Cor. 2: 15].'[17]

This kind of allegorical-religious thematization of the relations between the senses and faith is, of course, by no means confined to the Counter-Reformation. The undisputed popularity of the subject in the Calvinist Netherlands of the late sixteenth century suggests that, in this respect at least, there may be some truth in Max Weber's controversial theory of secular asceticism.

In the early modern era, allegories featuring the five senses in a group portrait (sometimes 'with lady' accompanied by, e.g., common sense, reason, understanding or faith) are encountered largely in literature, especially in poetry and drama. The subject also features prominently in the graphic art of the period. Here, it is noticeable that, with the onset of the Renaissance, the familiar and constantly varied iconographical motif begins to acquire new narrative elements drawn from the Bible and classical literature (mainly Ovid). This is the epoch when, in the words of the historian of science Werner Kutschmann, the senses become 'metaphors of the correlative feelings or sentiments of the human individual'.[18] The use of the five external senses is represented largely by means of a corresponding action or activity on the part of the persons represented. The result is that the allegorical content no longer emerges so clearly, since the foreground is now occupied by the 'realistic' representation of human behaviour.

One of the first to depict all five senses in a group was the Dutchman Adam van Noort (1562–1641), who taught Peter Paul Rubens. The accompanying engraving was the work of Adriaen Collaert (1560–1618). In it, we see five half-naked women standing in a circle round a table and offering worldly pleasures to a man, who is also scantily dressed and crowned with a laurel wreath in the manner of a classical hero. 'Touch' declares herself by insinuating herself into the man's embrace. 'Sight' dispenses light by illuminating the scene with a torch. 'Hearing' plays for him on a lute. 'Taste' (the only clothed figure) offers him exquisite fruit. 'Smell' offers the hero a second, and presumably fragrant, laurel wreath. In the background, we see four dancing children, bearing the attributes of the elements. Just in case we are left in any doubt as to the meaning of these colourful goings-on, the engraving is inscribed with a motto in Latin which, as so often in allegories of the five senses, urges a cautious approach to the use of the senses: 'Accipe et oblatis prudentius utere donis' ('take the gifts offered, and use them with prudence'). In this picture, we can already observe the change from sensory symbolism to images of bourgeois society that was first described by the German art historian Hans Kaufmann in his pioneering study of the senses in Dutch art of the seventeenth century.[19]

This iconographical change is expressed most clearly in a painting known as *Lively Company*, or *The Return of the Prodigal Son*, which is attributed to the early seventeenth-century Antwerp artist Ludovicus Finsonius (see figure 4.4). Again, the centre of vision is occupied by a table, around which a group of fashionably dressed men and women is seated. Two of the female figures are playing music. A man on the left is drinking from a wineglass, whereas the man opposite him prefers the scent of a carnation to the taste of wine. At the centre of the picture is a couple who are engaged in intimate and ardent embrace. The scene is observed by an older woman. A young female figure with a deck of cards next to her is looking in another direction. Here, the traditional symbolic attributes of the senses (notably the

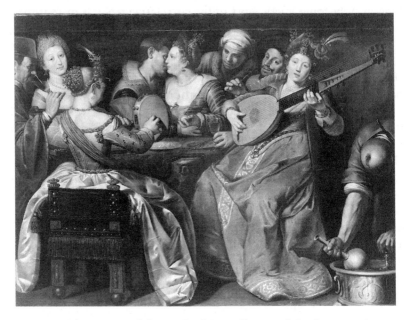

Figure 4.4   The Return of the Prodigal Son (allegory of the five senses); painting by Ludovicus Finsonius (seventeenth century)

animals) are missing. The picture is representative of a trend that can also be observed at roughly the same time in the Netherlands to the north. Take Esaias van den Velde (c.1591–1630), for example, who places five couples round a table outdoors; or Jan Steen (1626–1679), who in a painting now in The Hague mixes old and young round a table to create the 'polyphony of sensory stimuli' (Hans Kaufmann) so typical of these portraits of bourgeois society. The often static-looking grouping of five ideal types (men or women embodying the five senses) gives way to more ambitious and less monotonous figural compositions, which, though they show human life in full bloom, by no means lack a moral-didactic purpose (social criticism, theme of *vanitas*). But at the same time, the allegorical finger-wagging has largely vanished; animal symbolism in particular loses importance. This new, deliberately restrained and allegorically unencumbered representation of the united senses found imitators in Germany, and to a lesser extent in France, Italy and Spain. The family portrait by the Nuremberg artist Daniel Preißler (1627–1665) is particularly worthy of note. In the year of his death (of all times to choose!), Preißler painted his family of five, assigning one of the traditional attributes of the senses to each of its members.

Typically, the classical allegorization of the five senses that drew upon a whole repertoire of obvious animal metaphors did not vanish entirely from early modern painting. Indeed, it even experienced something of a revival in the eighteenth century.

Another genre of the early modern period in which the five senses were presented as an ensemble was the still life. The popularity of this topic is attested by the fact that, in his *Great Book of Painting* (1707), Gerard de Lairesse (1640–1711) more or less classified the subjects suited to still life in accordance with their relations to the five senses. He even advised his fellow painters to portray the particular qualities of the senses as vividly as possible and, where necessary, to refer to well-known fables or allegorical figures in separate, so-called bas-reliefs. Jacques Linnard (1600–1645), Sebastian Stoskopff (1597–1657), Maria van Oosterwijck (1630–1693) and Giuseppe Recco (1634–1695) all produced works that followed his instructions to the letter.[20] The iconographical statement – often given away in their titles – of most of these still lifes concerns the *vanitas* of human life, which is a topic also encountered at the same time in the poetry, drama and prose of the baroque period. Johann Michael Moscherosch (1601–1669), Jakob Balde (1604–1668) and Barthold Heinrich Brockes (1680–1740) are among the prominent German authors who treated the five senses under the aspect of *vanitas*.[21]

The so-called showpiece confectionery that was so much in vogue in the seventeenth century was an altogether different type of art. This consisted of visually splendid, elaborately contrived and extravagantly laid dining tables, which were not so much a critique of the senses as expressions of the pure joy of life and delight in its pleasures. Georg Philipp Harsdörffer (1607–1658) commented on this type of symbolism: 'Not only are the ears entertained by melodious and heart-warming music, poetic eulogies and songs, and the brain invigorated by fragrant water and incense, the mouth delighted by the daintiest food and sweet drinks, the hands occupied with selecting the choicest morsels, but that most excellent of the senses, the eye, is treated to a display of subtly allusive dishes that is the perfect stimulant to good conversation.' And the poet goes on to explain that 'these feasts for the eyes were not intended merely to embellish the table, but were also dedicated to the glory and memory of the invited guests.'[22] In time, sensuous and extravagant table decorations and lavish courses of dishes such as these went out of fashion. Nonetheless, this type of aristocratic representation of wealth and *joie de vivre* was remembered into the eighteenth century.

Visual imagery

Individual scenes or cycles of images involving the choice and symbolic interpretation of one particular sense occur more frequently than all-embracing allegorizations. Biblical exegesis follows a similar procedure, dwelling now on the eye, now on the ear and occasionally on another sense as sign or symbol.

The visual sense is undoubtedly the richest source of imagery, and to this day the eye is the sense organ most frequently used as a symbol. So what we offer here can only be a representative selection of visual allegories.[23]

Dark and light eyes

The image of the luminescent eye derives from Empedocles, Plato, Theophrastus and other Greek natural philosophers, who thought that the sense of sight was by nature incandescent. Augustine, too, considers the eye to be a luminous body. This led to the idea that the visual organ supplied light to the whole body, which was often supported by references to passages in the Bible (e.g., Luke 11: 34; Matt. 6: 22). This light metaphor is expressed most succinctly in Hugo von Trimberg's *Der Renner* (The Groom) (1290/1300): 'The eye bears light to the body, / The light of the soul is intelligence.' We encounter a similar example several centuries later in Goethe's *Theory of Colour*: 'As the creature of light, the eye does everything of which light itself is capable. It mirrors the world from the outside and man from within.'[24] In Assyrian-Babylonian representations and medieval texts, the luminous, bright eye betokens perfect vision and above all life.

The connection between the eye and light further allows the eye to be equated with knowledge, as for instance in Augustine: 'Without light there is no knowledge, and even perfect eyes cannot see in the dark.' Equations of the eye with the knowledge of God are correspondingly numerous. The allegorical interpretation of Matthew 6: 23 ('If therefore the light that is in thee be darkness, how great is that darkness') by Church Fathers such as Ambrose and Gregory the Great are examples of this kind of reading.

Healthy and keen eyes

'Provided his eyes are pure and completely clear, the gaze of the soul is very strongly expressed by the eyes of such a person, because the soul dwells powerfully in his body', writes Hildegard of Bingen. However, in her interpretation, healthy eyes are not automatically equated with sharp eyes. According to Johann Agricola (1494?–1566), the common figure of speech 'he has sharp sight' could be just another way of saying that he was a robber or thief. On the other hand, the sharp-sighted roe in the Song of Songs (2: 7) could also be interpreted as an allusion to Christ. Other animals, such as the lynx or the eagle, have also been praised for their keenness of vision since ancient times, and have proved their usefulness in literary and artistic allegorizations of sight requiring easily comprehensible attributes and symbols of vision borrowed from the natural world.

Open and closed eyes

According to Heinrich von Seuse (*c*.1295–1366) and other medieval authors, open eyes are signs of divine grace. The opening of the eyes is also often a way of imaging the way in which man acquires knowledge. Thus, Christ first has to open the eyes of the people of Emmaus (Luke 24: 31) before they can see him as the resurrected Christ. However, the open eyes of sleeping animals such as lions and hares are symbols of vigilance. Since Boetius (470–524), the opening and closing of the eyes has been used as a symbol of life as such. To the German mystics of the Middle Ages, on the other hand, closed eyes implied genuine contemplation of God. The closing of the eyes is also read as a sign that someone either does not recognize something, or refuses to understand it. Rudolf von Ems (*c*.1200–1254), for example, accuses the Jews of rejecting the Christian gospel of salvation 'with their eyes closed'. According to Gregory the Great (*c*.540–604), a predilection for sin closes the eyes of the soul to truth and opens them to vanity.

One eye and many eyes

There have been detailed accounts of one-eyed, fabulous beings (gorgons, cyclops, etc.) since before the time of Isidor of Seville (*c*.570–636). We need only recall Polyphemus in Homer's *Odyssey* (IX, 355ff.), whose eye was burned out by Odysseus in a scene which was also often represented in paintings. The subject was particularly popular in the symbolic art of the sixteenth and seventeenth centuries, where it expressed the triumph of intelligence over brute force.[25] The Church Father Hrabanus Maurus, mentioned above, interprets the monocularity of the Arimaspians, who are described in the *Lucidarius* (*c*.1190/95) as fabulous beings with one eye on their foreheads, as a humble striving (*simplex intentio*) for heaven. The non-religious image of multi-ocularity is chiefly derived from the story in Ovid's *Metamorphoses* (I, 623ff.) of hundred-eyed Argus, whom the goddess Juno ordered to watch over her rival, who had been turned into a heifer. The eyes of Argus – like the eyes on the peacock's tail – were connected with the astral myths of antiquity. Thus, in Georg Philipp Harsdörffer's *Poetischer Trichter* (Poetry Primer) (1647/53) we read of: 'The blue field of heaven with the flowers of a thousand stars. The Argus with hundreds of eyes who keeps watch over this earth.' The now proverbial eyes of Argus remind us how easy it is to deceive someone. The seven eyes of the lamb (Rev. 5: 6), on the other hand, are interpreted as the seven gifts of the Holy Ghost, in compliance with the Christian doctrine of salvation. Other many-eyed beings in the Bible (Rev. 4: 6; Ezek. 1: 18; Ezek. 10: 12) are thought to be emblems of clarity, knowledge, illumination or election. Pseudo-Dionysius (second half of the fifth century) sees the many eyes of the cherubim as signs of the ability of these angelic beings to see and recognize God.

Beautiful and ugly eyes

Beautiful eyes are frequently associated with positive characteristics, for perception has been explained according to the principle of like for like since antiquity. Only beautiful eyes, therefore, can recognize the beauty of the sun or creation. Medieval authors make a special point of stressing the beauty of the eyes of God, Jesus or the Virgin Mary and interpreting them as beacons of salvation. But beautiful eyes (notably those of women) are also symbolically significant in the secular context. For they are the attributes of *Minne* or courtly love, as preserved in the modern expression 'making eyes at someone'. Ugly eyes (deep-set, red, fiery) are usually attributes of infernal beings or villains. In the words of Konrad von Megenberg: 'The form and colour of the eyes are a mirror of the good or evil disposition of their possessor.' But ugly eyes do not automatically invest their owner with the power of the 'evil eye'. The destructive powers of the *ayin ha-ra*, or evil eye, which are mentioned in many passages of the Old Testament (e.g., Prov. 28: 22), were also familiar to other cultures. And there are still many people in modern Europe who will try to ward off the evil of this magic by making protective signs.[26]

Pure and sinful eyes

According to a view that is hardly confined to the Western cultural region, the eyes are also mirrors of positive characteristics and dispositions. In the Christian tradition, Mary the Mother of God is often represented as the 'eye of chastity'. In the opinion of the late medieval mystic David of Augsburg (*d.* 1272), the prospective follower of Christ must be 'chaste of visage'. Lowered eyes are a sign of chastity, as well as shame and humility. 'To the earth she lowered her face, / she looked at her feet and no other place', says Wernher's twelfth-century *Life of Mary*. But, according to the Bible, the eye of man may also reflect negative characteristics and moods, such as pride, envy, anger and, above all, lustfulness. Thus Albrecht von Halberstadt (*c.*1200) describes the envious eye as crooked and squinting. Walther von der Vogelweide (*c.*1170–*c.*1230) and Mechthild von Magdeburg (thirteenth century) use the term 'sinful eye' as a pars pro toto for sinful humanity. Biblical exegetes accuse David of unchaste looks when his gaze dwells on Bathsheba as she washes herself (2 Sam. 11: 2). In medieval sermons and penitential books, unchaste eyes are stigmatized as sinful on the authority of Matthew 5: 28 ('Whosoever looketh on a woman to lust after her hath committed adultery with her already in his heart'). According to the Church Father Jerome (*c*.348–420), *impudici oculi*, or lustful eyes, see only the beauty of the body, never that of the soul. Expressions for particular kinds of gazes, such as 'loose looks' (Heinrich Frauenlob, *d*. 1318) and 'playful eyes' (Berthold von Regensburg, *c*.1210–1272), imply shamelessness. The backward look of Lot's wife (Gen. 19: 26) is interpreted by medieval religious texts as a lustful contemplation of the world that can only play into the hands of the Devil. The image of sinful eyes continued in use for several centuries and played a significant role in the emblematic works of the baroque. One of these images shows a whip, which is being swung over the globe of the earth, a horse and a piece of clothing. A pair of eyes can be made out on the ground. The accompanying epigram expounds the moral theology binding on every Christian: 'This globe here shows you the world, which is round like a sphere, always moving, never still. By this globe you see a horse, a garment, and two eyes lying on the ground. Now what our dear Lord Christ teaches us is this: may everything in the world that delights the sinful flesh – lustful looks, pride and fornication – be forever accurst.'[27] All of which leaves us in no doubt that man and his senses could not simply be left to their own devices. The proper use of the senses was thus the foundation of all the various Christian regimes and essential to the entire order of state and society. It is therefore hardly a coincidence that Thomas Hobbes's celebrated and much-quoted classic of modern political theory *Leviathan* (1651) begins with the words: 'For there is no conception in a man's mind, which hath not, totally, or by parts, been begotten upon the organs of Sense.'[28]

Imagery of the sense of hearing

An image in Johannes Sambucus's popular handbook *Emblemata* (2nd edn, 1566) shows a man holding his ear to the ground in order to hear the thunder of distant canonfire more clearly.[29] The Latin motto ('non sufficit ad singula sensus') explains the artist's meaning: one sense alone is not enough. The appended Latin text tells us that success hinges on the combined operation of all the powers and senses. Nonetheless, hearing often appears on its own as a metaphor of the ensemble of the human powers, without references to other senses.

As in the case of the eye, figurative meanings are attached to the representation of the ear as one or many (as well as to the natural duplication of these organs).[30] 'I hear with a thousand ears', writes Friedrich Schiller (1759–1805), by way of implying that he is listening with particular intensity. The ear always appears in the singular in descriptions of its physiology. In the poem on the senses already mentioned above, the Hamburg poet Brockes writes: 'The ear is a tool with which to make out / sounds that come to us from without.' Rabbi Löw (1525–1609), a Jewish scholar from Prague, also refers to the ear in the singular when he compares it to a gate. The late medieval writer Konrad von Megenberg uses the same image. By way of indicating that its function goes beyond the mere perception of sound, he describes the ear as the 'gateway to the soul'. Earlessness, on the other hand, implies obstinacy and insensitivity. Luther glosses Matthew 11: 15 and Revelation 2: 7 as: 'He that hath ears to hear, let him hear, and he that doth not, let him be left behind: earless, unhearing, deaf.' Augustine believed that the congenitally deaf and dumb were paying for the sins of their parents, which touches on the topos of illness as a punishment for human failings that is not peculiar to Christianity.[31]

A good deal of aural imagery focuses on the external shape of the ear. Large ears and small ears carry different meanings. Konrad von Megenberg thought that someone with big ears was stupid but gifted with longevity, an opinion already espoused by the Persian physician Rhazes, or Ar-razi (c.865–925), in his *Liber ad Almansorem*. Paracelsus (1493?–1541), on the other hand, considered this physiognomic feature to be a sign of both good hearing and good memory. He was also not alone in regarding small ears as a 'a bad sign, for they usually imply that a person is evil, spiteful and unjust.'[32] When attached to a woman, however, small ears were considered beautiful, in the Middle Ages as well as in other periods. Even thick and thin ears are associated with human character traits. Johann Agricola's collection of proverbs contains the example of the slender ears 'that are quick to . . . understand'. Thinness is equated with sensitivity and sensibility, and its counter-image is the proverbial pair of 'thick' ears typical of those who refuse to listen.

Chaste and unchaste ears are not identified by their external form, but inferred indirectly from the way people behave. In Grimmelshausen's *Simplicissimus* (1668), for instance, 'chaste ears' are 'forced to hear this shameless word.' A contemporary of Grimmelshausen, the voluble Viennese preacher Abraham a Santa Clara (1644–1709), also uses the expression figuratively to illustrate the chaste disposition of a girl. On the other hand, the ears are often used to signify lasciviousness, as for example in the famous *Garden of Delights* by Hieronymus Bosch (*c*.1450–1516), which features a pair of cleanly severed human ears amid completely naked men and women. In ancient Egypt, ears were sometimes associated with the female genitalia. Indian mythology contains the story of a virgin called Kunti, who, when the sun god blatantly tries to extract a love tribute from her, pleads exemption on the grounds of her chastity, whereupon the god suggests making love to her ear. The Orthodox church propagated the idea that Mary conceived the Saviour through her ear. Having initially rejected this doctrine, the Western church later embraced it, and it duly began to appear in late medieval panel paintings. A *conceptio per aurem* of this type can be seen in the *Altar of the Passion* at the former Cistercian convent church in Marienthal zu Netze. The picture shows the child Jesus and the Holy Ghost in the shape of a dove emerging from the mouth of God on a sheaf of rays that glides towards Mary's ear. Here the ear, whose natural function is the reception of sound waves, is enlisted in the struggle for the soul's salvation as the organ 'of Mary's Immaculate Conception'.[33] The Annunciation is another subject that was treated by numerous artists in the sixteenth and seventeenth centuries. In these pictures this scene from the life of Mary often features allegorized animals (hare, bull, stag, boar) and symbolic musical instruments (harp, lute, lyre, violin). The idea of the ear as an organ of reception and conception is just a short step away from the notion that the organ of hearing is also capable of giving birth. Aural birth first appears in classical mythology (the legend of Athena). The most striking example in the art of the Middle Ages may still be seen on the tomb of Landgrave Henry I, grandson of St Elisabeth of Thuringia, in the church of St Elisabeth at Marburg an der Lahn. This tomb sculpture was completed in 1320, and depicts the landgrave on his deathbed. From his left ear an angel is 'delivering' the dead man of his soul in the shape of the *eidolon*, or miniature image of the man, which according to Homer (*Odyssey*, XI, 222) leaves the body after death to take up a shadow existence in Hades.

The copious portrayals of sermon scenes in the religious art of the Middle Ages and the early modern era suggest that the God-fearing persons who commissioned them were not merely trying to put a dampener on the 'pleasures of the ear' (Paracelsus). For the ear was at the same time regarded as the most suitable 'instrumentum disciplinae' in the project of securing submission to the church through religious instruction and correction. The central role of listening in a Christian society committed to living according to God's commandments is nowhere more clearly evident than in an illustrated manuscript at Utrecht (Codex 32, f. 28r), which turns Psalm 48: 2 ('Great is the Lord, and greatly to be praised in the city of our God') into a scene of public instruction in Holy Scripture.[34] A group of men and women arranged in a semicircle gaze towards three people standing on a hill above them. One of them is holding a psaltery (symbolizing the exaltation of the Lord in the Bible) and is turned towards the Psalmist, who stands on the ledge of a cliff. The second person is brandishing a rod of chastisement, while the third is holding a flail (symbol of manual labour) and a book (signifying study and learning). It is not hard to interpret this scene, for we have all at one time heard the expression: 'If you won't listen, you'll have to learn the hard way.'

Olfactory imagery

The symbolic vocabulary of the sense of smell can refer both to the organ itself, the nose, and to the object of its perceptions, namely smell. The range is impressive. Indeed, the palette of metaphors covers everything from the medieval scented garden to the baroque baby's bottom.[35]

In the Bible, the sense of smell occurs largely in association with fragrance. In early modern visual representations of the five senses (e.g., those by the Dutch painter Marten de Vos, 1532–1603) we find treatments of the scene in which God breathes soul into Adam

(Gen. 1: 7) or where Mary Magdalene anoints the feet of Jesus ('the house was filled with the odour of the ointment', John 12: 3). These two passages reveal how breath and fragrance were considered symbolic of divine proximity or presence. Hrabanus Maurus makes a point of stressing that Jesus was sweet-smelling, a reading for which there is plenty of support in the New Testament: 'Now thanks be unto God, which always causeth us to triumph in Christ, and maketh manifest the savour of his knowledge by us in every place. For we are unto God a sweet savour of Christ, in them that are saved, and in them that perish' (2 Cor. 2: 14–15). This also explains why the French founder of the Salesian order, Francis of Sales (1567–1622), uses images such as *odeur*, *onguents* or *parfums* in his vocabulary of devoutness.[36] Fragrance can also be a sign of paradise, particularly in medieval cults of saints and relics.[37] It would be possible in addition to cite numerous examples of the fragrance of the sacred in non-Christian cultures.[38]

In view of the figurative meanings attached to pleasant smells in the religious context, it is hardly surprising that in the Middle Ages scent was considered a sign of power and status. The medieval poet Rudolf von Ems (*c*.1200–1245) writes: 'He ordered the roads to be strewn with pure and pleasant-smelling things in honour of his rule.'[39]

Besides the sphere of power, smell was also read as symbolic of the dark realm of sexuality, the best-known example being a passage in the Old Testament: 'The mandrakes give a smell, and at our gates are all manner of pleasant fruits' (Song of Solomon 7: 13). Similar sexual imagery (flowers, fruit) appears in medieval and early modern representations of smell. Take, for instance, the five-senses cycle comprising the *Lady with the Unicorn* at the Musée de Cluny in Paris, or Jan Breughel's *Smell* (now in the Prado Museum in Madrid), which is part of a series of this kind.

Bad or evil smells can betoken the approach of death (2 Cor. 2: 14). According to the Viennese court chaplain Abraham a Santa Clara, they are also signs of imminent plague. Apart from this, images of stench were used to stigmatize strangers and outsiders – particularly Jews – until well into the modern era. The *foetor judaicus*, a stench allegedly peculiar to Jews and a reminder of their proximity to the Devil, notoriously persists as a stereotype into the twentieth century.[40] But supposedly 'typical' smells or stenches were used not just to expose and isolate Jews, prostitutes and witches. The association of certain – usually unpleasant – smells with such purely social categories as sex, age and nationality continues to this day.[41]

The physical configuration of the olfactory sense itself is fraught with allegorical potential. The Kabbalists believed the triangular shape of the nose represented the first letter (שׁ = Schin) of one of the Hebrew names of God (*Schaddai*). As David Kaufmann – one of the great figures of Jewish studies in the latter part of the nineteenth century – notes in his book on the senses in the Jewish Middle Ages, many Jews saw the nose as 'the seal of God set on our faces'.[42] But the practice of attaching human characteristics and behavioural dispositions to specific nasal shapes was not confined to Judaism. The physiognomic works of the Neapolitan scholar Giovanni Battista della Porta (1543–1615) contain a profusion of relevant examples. Porta interprets a whole series of typical 'nasal forms' by means of quotations from classical literature.[43] Aristotle is his main authority for the then widespread notion that a long nose reaching down to the mouth was a sign of boldness and bravery. Porta construes the nose that is bent like the beak of a crow as a sign of greed, whereas a hooked or aquiline nose betokens courage. A big-nosed individual, on the other hand, is typically one who judges others too severely and is interested only in his own concerns. However, as a reference to Polemon (315–266/5 BC) suggests, the big nose can also be a sign of bravery. Polemon is again Porta's source for the idea that the owner of a small nose is politically unreliable (*mutabilis consilii vir*). Albertus Magnus is summoned in support of his interpretation of the pointed nose as a sign of moral laxity, while his diagnosis of the flat or ape-like nose as a symptom of voluptuousness again rests on the authority of Aristotle. This latter preconception has, of course, been with us for a long time. Late in the nineteenth century, Wilhelm Fließ, a colleague and correspondent of Freud (1856–1939), speculated about the connections between the size of the nose and the length of the penis.[44] The so-called nasal reflex theory, which posited an interaction between the nose and the genital apparatus, enjoyed widespread support in the medical circles of the time. People often had operations on their noses for quite non-cosmetic reasons. On a final, legal-historical, note it is perhaps worth mentioning here that, a hundred years before Porta's time, the amputation of the nose by the local executioner was performed in token of atonement for sexual transgressions.[45]

The imagery of taste

In comparison to other areas of sense perception, the sense of taste crops up far less often in graphic representations. This is particularly true of the sense organ itself, the tongue. The tongue appears much more often as a symbol of the human power of speech than as a sign denoting the faculty of taste. This is undoubtedly connected with the fact that the taste buds on the surface of the tongue were not discovered until relatively late. Nonetheless, the role of the tongue in the sense of taste was common medical knowledge by the end of the Middle Ages at the latest, as can be seen from a popular text entitled *Proplemata Aristotilis teütsch* (1492): 'They that have the cold sickness [one-day fever with bouts of shivering] find all drinks bitter to the tongue.'[46]

Since pictorial descriptions of the tongue are usually derived from its function as the instrument of language rather than the organ of taste, this part of the body does not, like the other senses, lend itself to figurative combinations with the word 'pleasure'. When Paracelsus writes of the 'pleasures of the tongue' he simply means a predilection for 'good victuals, good wine': the word refers merely to the enjoyment of food. In his *Physicalische und moralische Gedichte* (Physical and Moral Poems, 1721–48), Barthold Heinrich Brockes writes:

> It is a pity that we neither heed nor measure
> What God puts into food to give us pleasure.
> Taste is an astonishing work of creation,
> Astonishing too the tongue's powers of sensation.

Here again, the significance of the organ of taste is confined to the realm of the concrete: the more or less enjoyable consumption of food. It is only in the older physiognomies that the tongue has a symbolic function not primarily connected with eating and drinking.[47] Here the form of the tongue supposedly tells us something about the person concerned. Witches and spirits, for instance, have withered or rough tongues.

There is an extensive range of imagery relating to passages in the Bible in which the word 'taste' is used in its original meaning. The water that is changed into wine at the marriage feast of Cana, for instance, is tasted by the governor of the feast (John 2: 9). Similarly, the feeding of the five thousand with loaves and fishes, another famous New Testament meal scene, is used to symbolize the sense of taste in early modern representations. Take, for instance, the series of pictures by the Dutch painter Marten de Vos, which were etched by Adriaen Collaert. In Jewish biblical exegesis, taste was identified with Jacob's son Issachar (Heb. reward), because it was the sense that was commonly regarded as the most rewarding.[48] A New Testament passage dealing with the Eucharist (1 Peter 2: 3) and Psalm 34: 8 ('O taste and see that the Lord is good') are interpreted Christologically as referring to the ingestion of spiritual nourishment via the senses. The expression 'to taste death' appears in several places in the Bible (Matt. 9: 1; John 8: 52; Heb. 2: 9) and is, of course, already consciously figurative.

In the Bible taste is not least a sense that plays a central role in the collective memory of the Jewish people. One expression of this gustatory symbolism is the *Seder* plate containing the bitter herb (*maror*), along with other items of food commemorating the Exodus. This symbolic food, with its lingering aftertaste, is an excellent 'mnemonic'.

Before the sixteenth century, the concept of 'taste' was rarely used figuratively outside religious contexts. Most cases are found in philosophical, literary and theoretical texts that drew attention to the resemblances between writing and the tasting of food and drink, in the sense that both were concerned with qualities of taste. In the celebrated and widely read *Essays* (1580) of Michel de Montaigne (1533–1592) metaphors of taste are used to symbolize literary production and aesthetic judgement.[49] This figurative use of the term 'taste' then becomes widespread in the eighteenth century. For most of the seventeenth century, however, sensationalistic interpretations of *gusto* are relatively rare in aesthetics, since the traditional location of the faculty of judgement in the intellect continues to hold sway.

On the other hand, the moral tracts of sixteenth-century Italian and Spanish authors do contain occasional applications of the term 'taste' to non-literary contexts, notably social behaviour.[50] These are concerned mainly with behaviour at court where, according to Norbert Elias, it was vital to offer a daily demonstration of 'correct' or 'superior' taste in order to preserve one's status in the corporative hierarchy. There is even some evidence that taste was used by the bourgeoisie as a yardstick of human strengths and weaknesses, one example being a verse by Hans Sachs (1494–1576) written in 1553. The poem deals with the subject of how to behave in marriage:

> In the medical books we find
> That the tastes are nine in kind.
> Nine tastes daily pulling to and fro,
> Making married life difficult for high and low.
> The taste of sweetness will only begin to tell
> If the tastes will agree to marry as well.

Here the sense of taste is used in simple graphic illustration of a basic rule for living that anyone will understand.

So it is perhaps not surprising that the idea of taste came to be shaped more and more by imagery and that the physiology of taste declined in importance. This historical conceptual development reached its climax in the age of German and French classicism. 'People used to have one taste. Now there are several tastes. / But tell me, where is the taste of these tastes?', asked Goethe and Schiller in one of the epigrams in their joint collection *Xenia* (1796).

Tactile imagery

Aristotle had assigned no specific organ to the sense of touch and insisted that haptic perception was distributed all over the body. Nevertheless, if it was to be represented at all it had to be positioned somewhere in the body. The obvious organ was the hand, with which the human being feels, holds and 'grasps' in the metaphorical sense.[51] The Hebrew word *jad* (hand) appears in almost 2000 places in the Old Testament, making it one of the most frequently used nouns in the Bible.[52]

Haptic sense perception initially appears in the Bible in the real-life context of substitution for sight. Blind Samson gropes for the pillars supporting the hall (Judg. 16: 26). But we probably immediately think of the groping hands of blind Tobias in Rembrandt's masterpiece, or the remarkable drawing by Peter Paul Rubens (1577–1640) of a blind man feeling his way forward with outstretched arms.[53]

In the biblical scenes which were used to adorn sixteenth-century allegories of touch this normally fifth and last sense is represented by various forms of hand-touching. In the five-senses cycle of the Dutch artist Marten de Vos mentioned above, we find it first in the scene depicting the miraculous draught of fish, in which a chastened Peter falls down at the feet of Christ, who reaches out his hand to him, saying, 'Fear not; from henceforth thou shalt catch men' (Luke 5: 10). A second picture shows Adam and Eve being expelled from the Garden of Eden by the angel after Eve has plucked the apple from the tree of knowledge that God had expressly forbidden her to touch (Gen. 3: 24). Taken together the biblical passages used in these allegories symbolize the ambivalence of the tactile sense: on the one hand it is the source of salvation and on the other the cause of doom.

Following Aristotle's praise of the relative reliability of touch in situations where the other senses may be deceived, it is not surprising that, in the Bible, touching and feeling are the most effective ways of convincing ourselves of the real existence of a thing or phenomenon. The texts attributed to Hermes Trismegistos, which date back in part to the first century BC, describe the knowledge of God as a matter of seeing him and touching him with our hands.[54] In the New Testament, the knowledge of God is similarly 'hands-on'. Thus, the astonished disciples touch the hands and feet of the risen Christ to convince themselves that he is not a ghost (Luke 24: 38–9), and the sceptical Thomas touches the wounds and inserts his hand into the side of the Saviour and Redeemer when he appears before him and the other disciples in a room with locked doors (John 20: 27). Touching consequently becomes the simplest and most basic form of communion with the sacred. This plastic idea was not least a factor in the formation of the medieval cult of relics, in which a large role is played by the touching of the bodily remains of saints or items of their clothing (e.g., the holy gown).

According to the American medical and cultural historian Sander Gilman, many medieval pictorial representations of sensory perception, for which the term 'feeling' first appears in German at a very late date, refer to pleasure, and particularly to sexual lust.[55] Indeed, there can be little doubt that tactile experience had sexual connotations until well into the early modern era. When the characters of the decidedly earthy Shrovetide plays spoke of liking to 'feel a woman', they had more in mind than the fondling of breasts and the various other forms of sexual harassment. Most of the pictorial representations of this time that show a man reaching into a woman's décolletage

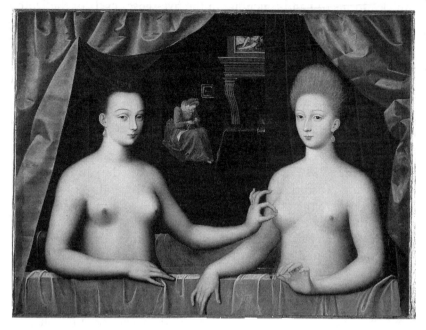

Figure 4.5   Gabrielle d'Estrées and her sister in the bath; anonymous painting (*c.*1592), school of Fontainebleau

are unambiguous iconographic symbols of sexual intercourse.[56] The lascivious touching of the female breast is the subject of what is surely one of the most erotic works of Renaissance art. This picture shows a pretty young woman delicately fingering one of the nipples of Gabrielle d'Estrées, mistress of the French King Henry IV (see figure 4.5). Along with their indirect allusions to the Fall, the numerous representations of Eve are also plainly intended as allegories of the moral perils of touching.[57]

On the other hand, the emblematic art of the sixteenth and seventeenth centuries is understandably more concerned with the relation between sensation and sickness and pain. Dürer's famous self-portrait, in which he depicts himself holding a finger to the place on his abdomen that is hurting, is only marginally symbolic, since the artist is clearly aiming at a straightforwardly naturalistic account of his own experience of pain.[58] However, in the Dutch art of this period, notably in the work of Jan Molenaer (1654–after 1690), David Teniers (1610–1690) and Adriaen Brouwer (c.1605/6–1638), we come upon indisputably allegorical representations of the sense of touch centred on the theme of pain during sickness and treatment.[59] A painting by Caravaggio, depicting the pain-wracked face of a little boy bitten by a lizard, is essentially a representation of sensation under the aspect of pain.[60] The interpretation of the tactile sense as a medium of pain and other unpleasant physical experiences was largely influenced by Cesare Ripa's *Iconologia* (1593), a standard work on iconography for artists in which the sense of touch is almost exclusively associated with pain. This book forms the basis of an iconographic tradition extending from the baroque period to mannerism and the rococo.

— 5 —
Practices: The Senses and their Ailments

Neither of these two things [physical and mental health] can be preserved unless the limbs of the senses are in a healthy condition, so they must be protected against injury and debility, for otherwise we will lose them.

Zedler's Universal Lexicon (1743)

Sensory diagnosis and therapy

The physicians and healers of the major cultures of antiquity were already fully concerned with keeping the external senses in a healthy condition. In addition to magic formulas against colds – supposedly responsible for 'the sicknesses of the seven apertures of the head' – ancient Egyptian papyri contain prescriptions under headings such as 'strengthening of the eyesight', as well as advice for the treatment of hardness of hearing. The physical decline of the senses that accompanied the ageing process was familiar enough to the ancient Egyptians, as witness the famous dictum of the sage Ptahhotep:

For at the end of life the eyes are small, the ears deaf . . . the mouth is silent and can no longer speak, the heart becomes forgetful and can no longer remember yesterday . . . the ability to taste passes away . . . the nose is blocked and can no longer smell . . . the arms grow weak and the legs have ceased to obey the commands of a heart that has grown tired.[1]

The main focus of attention was naturally the two sense organs whose perceptual functions were prized the most: the eyes and the ears. But the acuteness of all five senses also played a large part in medical diagnosis and therapy, and not only in the medicine of antiquity.

Galen, the most celebrated physician of Graeco-Roman antiquity after Hippocrates, did not merely restrict sense perception to a diagnostic function in medicine, but also assigned it a central role in drug therapy. In his view, a doctor required the senses of touch, smell, sight and taste to help him determine the general and specific properties of pharmacological remedies, which would enable him to assess their effectiveness and decide how they should be administered at the sick bed. Thus, doctors were advised to begin developing their taste perception by concentrating on a single, unmistakable quality of taste (e.g., pungent), a practice which might involve chewing onions or a clove of garlic over a long period of time.[2]

The modern pharmacologist does not necessarily require a good nose when assessing the therapeutic value of a substance, merely the appropriate gauges and laboratory procedures. But in chemistry and pharmacy, this gauging was performed by the senses of smell and sight until well into the eighteenth century. The centuries-old hegemony of sense perception in early forms and precursors of experimental and applied science is aptly termed 'sensuous technology' by the American historian of science Lissa Roberts.[3]

Sense perception maintained its traditional role in medical diagnosis for almost as long, if not longer. In one of the Hippocratic texts (*The Surgery*) we come upon the following recommendation: '[Examination: look for] what is like or unlike the normal, beginning with the most marked signs and those easiest to recognise, open to all kinds of investigation, which can be seen, touched and heard, which are open to all our senses, sight, touch, hearing, the nose, the tongue and the understanding, which can be known by all sources of knowledge.'[4] Hippocrates' advice to doctors to use all five senses when investigating symptoms reappears in a similar form in an influential work by Samuel Gottlieb Vogel (1750–1837) entitled *Kranken-Examen* (Examining the Sick, 1797), which contains a lengthy discussion of the diagnostic value of the individual senses. On the subject of taste, he writes: 'Asking the patient about the way he is tasting is essential to the preliminary investigation of almost any illness.'[5] According to this Rostock professor, a doctor should not only take into account the patient's subjective descriptions, but also confirm his opinion by scrutinizing and, if necessary, feeling the patient's tongue. It was only when nineteenth-century medicine began to abandon traditional symptomatology for scientific diagnosis[6] that 'historical semiology', which was defined by the Jena doctor David Grau (1729–1768) as 'knowledge of the altered condition of the sick as observed by the senses', finally disappeared.[7] Grau distinguished this theory of signs from 'philosophical semiotics', which attempted to identify the causes of the changes taking place in the patient's body by means of rational or logical deduction.

Yet empirical medicine, which was dominated from antiquity to the early nineteenth century by the Hippocratic and Galenic theory of the four humours, was not the only context in which the five senses were regarded as important. Consider, for instance, the early Christian practice of the anointing of the sick, known since the twelfth century as 'the last rites'.[8] In Catholic tradition, the anointing of the sick is a sacrament instituted by Christ and preached by St James. This teaching was raised to the status of dogma by decision of the Council of Trent in 1551, and was one of several questions on which the Council of Trent drew a firm line between the church and the doctrines of Luther. The doctrine of *extrema unctio* is embodied in canon law (*Codex Iuris Canonici*, ch. 937–947) and the *Rituale Romanum* (1614),[9] which regulate every detail of the ceremonial order of liturgical observances in the Roman Catholic Church. One of the earliest descriptions is provided by Bishop Henry I of Breslau (r. 1302–19), whose book of ritual embodies the basic elements of the liturgical instruction later prescribed in the *Rituale Romanum*.[10]

In Catholic pastoral practice, the sacrament of extreme unction is still usually administered as follows: the summoned priest enters the house of the sick with the greeting 'peace unto this house!' Prayers and psalms are recited by those present, followed by penance and absolution. Only then does the priest put on his stole and proceed to administer the sacrament of extreme unction to the sick person. *Zedler's Universal Lexicon* of 1740 gives the following description of the solemn and ceremonial rite: 'The seven parts of the body are then anointed. These are the eyes, ears, nose, mouth and hands comprising the five senses; the kidneys, which are the seat of sinful desires and, finally, the feet, which have trodden the path of evil.'[11] The author of the entry notes that the anointing of the kidneys, which represented the sexual organs, is normally performed only on men.

The practice of anointing the kidneys had been discontinued by the nineteenth century at the latest, although it is still preserved in the liturgical texts.[12] The anointing of the five sense organs, on the other hand, remains obligatory to this day. Priests must anoint the eyes, ears, nose, mouth and hands, even if one of these organs has never functioned or is missing. When the medical enlightenment of the late eighteenth century finally began to reach the priesthood, the manuals of pastoral medicine stated expressly that when administering this sacrament the priest had to overcome any feelings of disgust, and not be afraid of open wounds and running sores, for a 'thorough washing of the hands after the act will suffice to remove any really suspicious germs.'[13] In a period that was still entirely dominated by the notion of the 'miasma', or the fear of pathogenic vapours rising from the earth, and which lacked any detailed knowledge of sources of infection and bacterial agents of disease, such considerations obviously played a lesser role than in the bacteriological age that began towards the end of the nineteenth century with the discoveries of Robert Koch (1843–1919) and Louis Pasteur (1822–1895). The choice of the five senses for anointment had less to do with their physiological importance and central position in the human body than with the idea that they were the gateways of the soul and therefore the places at which the latter was vulnerable to attack by sin. The Strasbourg preacher Geiler von Kaysersberg (1445–1510) goes to the heart of the matter at the end of the fifteenth century: 'And then take note of the sins of the five senses: listening to evil talk; looking at things that raise thoughts of sin; smelling and tasting the vapours of the body; touching in a way that pollutes the soul; knowingly consuming the fruits of crime.'[14] Nevertheless, the mortally ill rested and continue to rest their hopes on this form of religious medicine. In this sacrament, they perceive not merely a path to spiritual redemption, but above all a remedy that may come to their aid when medicine seems to have reached the end of its wisdom.[15]

This stubborn reinterpretation of a religious ritual originally aimed at the immortal soul rather than the ephemeral body was a thorn in the side of Luther and his disciples. The reformers abolished the anointing of the sick and instead recommended repentance and spiritual self-examination to the terminally ill. In the Lutheran church, spiritual support in times of mortal danger from now on consisted simply of communal prayer and the administration of communion. Zachäus Faber, for instance, who was a Protestant minister and superintendent in Chemnitz at the beginning of the seventeenth century, poked fun at the papists, claiming that they had developed all kinds of medicines for death, such as the anointing of eyes, ears, nose and so forth, in the belief that these last rites would not only redeem them from their sins but also restore them to health.[16] A contemporary of Luther, the humanist Erasmus of Rotterdam (1469?– 1536), had demonstrated his scepticism towards the supposed restorative effects of anointing the sick in his famous *Colloquia* (1519). One of these satirical dialogues, *Two Kinds of Deathbed*, portrays the ridiculous struggle of doctors, priests and religious orders for possession of the body and soul of the dying and, more importantly, their property.

The health and sensitivity of all five senses played a not insignificant part in the debate surrounding the so-called vicariousness of the senses. Immanuel Kant took this to mean 'the use of one sense as a substitute for another',[17] the issue being whether, in the case of the total or partial failure of one sense or sense organ, its functions could be compensated, if not replaced, by another. This problem was the subject of an intense and copiously illustrated debate among natural philosophers and physicians that continued until well into the modern era. A popular medical work of the early eighteenth century contains a description of the adaptability of the human sense organs: 'If one of the human senses is damaged or weakened, the strength of another increases and becomes dominant. Many blind people have such a subtle sense of smell or refinement of touch that they can distinguish one colour from another by relying on these senses alone.'[18] In his *Observationes*, Felix Platter (1536–1614), who was the health officer of Basel, cites the case of a blind man whose sense of touch was so well developed that he was able to distinguish between several different kinds of wood and to earn his living as an organbuilder.[19] The English physician John Bulwer, who invented a sign language, showed how deaf and dumb people could develop comparable abilities in his copiously illustrated *Philocopus, or The Deafe and Dumbe Mans Friends* (1648). Metaphorical expressions such as 'seeing with one's ears' and 'hearing with one's eyes' have their roots in the idea of a 'vicariate of the senses' that has a long tradition in Western literature – we need look no further than Shakespeare's famous lines, 'A man may see how this world goes with no eyes. Look with thine ears' (*King Lear*, IV: 6). One of the earliest instances of this topos is a place in Cicero's *Tusculan Disputations* (AD 45), where we find the following piece of advice: 'as a little while ago we diverted the blind to the pleasure of hearing, so we may divert the deaf to the pleasure of sight.'[20] The claim that blind people can, in fact, possess superior hearing has meanwhile been confirmed by modern sensory-physiological research, as reported in the German weekly newspaper *Die Zeit* (8 July 1999) under the headline 'The blind hear better in space', which referred to a report in the respected scientific journal *Nature*.

Defective vision

'Seeing and hearing are the most prized of the senses',[21] is the succinct reply of *Zedler's Universal Lexicon* (1743) to the question of the sensory restriction that people experience most keenly, and the sense organs that are therefore most in need of special care and maintenance. The ensuing survey of the most frequently occurring sensory defects and their prevention and treatment begins, therefore, with vision, before proceeding to hearing and then the other senses in their traditional order.

The meaning of the loss of vision is conveyed by none other than Leonardo da Vinci in his *Treatise on Painting*: 'who loses his eyes leaves his soul in a dark prison, without hope of ever again seeing the sun, the light of the world.'[22] Exactly how many people suffered this fate before the nineteenth century is unknown, since the relevant statistics begin only in the nineteenth century. They tell us, for instance, that around 1871, in the Grand Duchy of Baden, there were 5.3 blind persons for every 10,000 inhabitants.[23] The figure for the Netherlands at roughly the same period is only slightly lower. There are again no statistics concerning the most frequent causes of blindness until the close of the nineteenth century.[24] Barely 5 per cent of the people listed as blind had been so from birth. Over 45 per cent had lost their sight through infections such as trachoma, scarlet fever, smallpox and syphilis. Glaucoma was the cause of blindness in 9 per cent of all cases. Eye injuries resulting from violence (e.g., wars or accidents) were somewhat more numerous.

The ophthalmology of the period from antiquity to the eighteenth century distinguishes very few disease groups as causes of blindness or impaired vision:[25] 1) thick dense whitish corneal scars, or leucoma; 2) weakened vision with no visible cause, though conspicuously black pupils (amaurosis); 3) various types of inflammation; 4) acute sepsis of the cornea; 5) clouding of the lens (cataracts), whose cause was thought to be the discharge of bad mucus descending from the brain to the lens and pupil; 6) glaucoma, which is today understood as permanent damage to the retina and optic nerve due to abnormally high internal pressure in the eye. Some of these causes of blindness such as trachoma are no longer of significance in the industrialized countries of the West, whereas others, such as glaucoma, still account for most cases of blindness in the aged.

Even modern ophthalmology is rarely able to give people back their eyesight, although the possibility of preventing blindness by means of surgery and medication has been greatly enhanced. Right up to modern times, only a miracle, or in rare cases a 'cataract couching' performed by a bold and skilful operator, could preserve, or sometimes restore, the sight of the eye. The Roman author Celsus first described an operation of this kind in the seventh book of his celebrated *De medicina*, which treats the subject of cataracts:

> Thereupon a needle is to be taken pointed enough to penetrate, yet not too fine; and this is to be inserted straight through the two outer tunics at a spot intermediate between the pupil of the eye and the angle adjacent to the temple, away from the middle of the cataract, in such a way that no vein is wounded. The needle should not be entered timidly, however, for it passes through empty space; and when this is reached even a man of moderate experience cannot be mistaken, for then there is no resistance to pressure. When the spot is reached, the needle is to be sloped against the suffusion itself and should gently rotate there and little by little guide it below the region of the pupil; when the cataract has passed below the pupil it is pressed upon more firmly in order that it may settle below. If it sticks there the cure is accomplished.[26]

Apart from one or two minor improvements, this was the way cataract operations were performed until well into the nineteenth century.

But cataracts were, of course, just one cause of blindness among many, so the cataract couching, which was known and successfully performed since antiquity, only ever prevented a handful of people from going blind. Miraculous cures were therefore very much in demand, as witness the host of biblical representations on the theme of 'Christ healing the blind'.[27] The passages in question were familiar to everyone in both word and image: Matt. 9: 27–30; 20: 30–4; Mark 8: 22–5; John 9: 1–7. The frequent mention of the healing of blindness in the Gospels made it suitable for use as the iconographic sign of the sense of sight, as for instance in the five-senses cycle (*c.*1575) by Marten de Vos, in the background of which we see the New Testament scene of Christ healing a blind man with a touch of his hand. The late medieval and early modern cult of saints likewise evinces the deep longing of many blind people to receive back their sight from God. The legend of St Ottilie, who was blind from birth and then reputedly healed the blind after her own miraculous cure, was a frequent subject of pictorial representation, in which her emblem is a pair of eyes.[28] Another saint said to have cured the blind was St Lucy, who put out her own eyes.[29] In the pre-modern world, the frequency and expectations with which the blind travelled to places of pilgrimage in search of a cure is not only attested by the large number of preserved votive gifts with eye motifs. It also emerges in more recent studies of surviving miracle books. On their evidence, the number of blind pilgrims whose fervent prayers were supposedly heard varied from 6.4 to 19.5 per cent, depending on the place of pilgrimage.[30] One of these many spontaneous and miraculous cures is described in the *Miracula Sancte Elyzabet* (1233–5):

> When Bezela was still lying in, a few days after her delivery a ghost appeared one night by her bed, next to which there was a fire burning. It took the form of a boy sitting in the fire, and after a little while it disappeared. She was so shocked, that she immediately lost the sight of her right and left eyes, and was blind for seven years. She received back the light when a small piece of skin fell from her eye and her eyesight was completely restored.[31]

Miraculous cures abound in other traditions besides the Christian. The votive offerings in the temples of antiquity and the accounts of Greek and Roman writers bear witness to such miraculous cures.[32] The best known is perhaps the story of the Egyptian king Pheron, recorded by Herodotus (II, 111). This ruler was punished with blindness after he had arrogantly cast a spear into the Nile while it was in flood. He was sightless for ten years. An oracle then advised him to wash his eyes in the urine of his faithful wife. According to the report, this immediately restored the king's eyesight and in gratitude he donated two obelisks to the shrine of Helios, the god of light.

'Thou shalt not curse the deaf, nor put a stumblingblock before the blind' (Lev. 19: 14): this biblical commandment shows that recovery from blindness was an exception to the norm of a life blighted by sickness. There is ample evidence that in the major cultures of antiquity, and particularly in early Christianity, the blind were not solely dependent upon the charity of their fellow creatures, but were often able to earn a living and, in rare cases, even to hold high public office.[33] In ancient Egypt, we encounter the blind as doorkeepers, harpists and bards. Roman law did not require the blind to have legal guardians, so they could largely take care of their own legal affairs. State provision for the blind is a modern phenomenon, although the first institution for the blind was opened as long ago as 1260 in Paris. It was a pious foundation created by the French king Louis IX, following a failed crusade, and was intended to help three hundred crusaders who had been blinded during the venture.[34]

Before modern times, dealings with the blind were coloured by moral and religious attitudes. Christian thought regarded blindness in particular as a heavy trial and affliction placed upon the sufferer by God. On the other hand, responses to blindness were also influenced by a distinction that had been made by Aristotle: 'No one will offend the feelings of a blind man who was born that way, or who fell ill or suffered an accident . . . though everyone will blame the man who has gone blind through drunkenness or other forms of excess' (*Nicomachean Ethics*, III, 1114a).

Persons whose eyes had been put out as a punishment or an act of revenge were in a special category. The gouging of the eyes is a relatively frequent theme in the Bible and in the legends surrounding saints in late medieval *exempla*.[35] In art and painting, blinding was a popular motif until well into the baroque era.

Regardless of whether someone's eyes have been gouged out or the empty eye-sockets are the result of some other kind of violence, the sight of such a person is capable to this day of arousing horror, or even spreading fear and terror. In ancient Egypt, artificial eyes, made of metal or precious stones, were placed on mummies to preserve the human appearance of the dead. The artificial eye first appears in medical literature in the writings of the French surgeon Ambrose Paré (*c.*1510–1590): 'It is very skilfully fashioned from gold or silver and made to look like a natural eye by an artist or by firing [the process for enamel].'[36] By the eighteenth century, this technique was standard practice in ophthalmology, as Lorenz Heister (1683–1758) explains in his famous manual of surgery (1763): 'If the patient has had to have an eye removed, or has lost an eye through injury or sepsis resulting from smallpox and other diseases, it is customary to insert an artificial eye exactly resembling the good one to conceal the great disfigurement.'[37] This surgeon, who taught in Helmstedt, also gives practical hints for the care of these false eyes (regular washing, removal before sleep, etc.) and describes a method for keeping them supple.

Although both Aristotle and natural philosophers who succeeded him had dealt with the perception of individual colours, colour-blindness remained undiscovered as a visual deficiency until the end of the eighteenth century. The first description of a case of colour-blindness was completed in 1777 by the English physicist and philosopher Joseph Priestley (1733–1804). In a contribution to the *Philosophical Transactions of the Royal Society of London*, Priestley described the strange visual defect of a cobbler named Harris: 'He observed also that, when young, other children could discern cherries on a tree by some pretended difference of colour, though he could only distinguish them from the leaves by their difference of size and shape.'[38] Priestley quickly learned from his enquiries that two of Harris's siblings suffered from the same defect. In a later contribution to the distinguished journal, he confirmed that this defect of colour perception was inheritable. Priestley's findings were corroborated by the experiments that the English chemist and physicist John Dalton (1766–1844) performed on himself and wrote up in the *Edinburgh Journal of Sciences* in 1798. For a long time after this, colour-blindness was known as Daltonism. A firm supporter of the mechanistic conception of the body, Dalton bequeathed his eyes to science in the hope that anatomical dissection might reveal the presence of a corresponding colour filter.[39]

Short-sightedness and long-sightedness are, to this day, the most widespread visual deficiencies. According to recent estimates, between 15 and 20 per cent of the population of the Western world is short-sighted enough to require visual aids. Precisely when, where and by whom spectacles were invented is unknown, but there is no doubt that this form of visual assistance is a medieval invention. One of the first references to spectacles is found in a work by the Arab physician Ibn Al-Haytham, known as Alhazen, dating from around the year

1000, which mentions certain spherical segments made of glass that make an object appear larger. The English scholar Roger Bacon gives a more detailed description of the production of these magnifying glasses in his *Opus majus* (1267):

> If a man looks at letters or other small objects through the medium of a crystal or of glass or of some other transparent body placed above the letters, and it is the smaller part of a sphere whose convexity is towards the eye, and the eye is in the air, he will see the letters much better and they will appear larger to him . . . Therefore this instrument is useful to the aged and to those with weak eyes.[40]

The first spectacles were probably made in Italy. Around 1300, the city council of Venice issued quality-control regulations for the production of spectacles. In the fourteenth century, several leading physicians of the time, including the French surgeon Guy de Chauliac (*d.* 1368), recommended the use of glasses in preference to a variety of eye-fortifying preparations of dubious efficacy. Two centuries later, the famous Dresden ophthalmologist Georg Bartisch (1535–1606/7) was recommending precisely the opposite.

The earliest wearers of spectacles left very few accounts of their problems and the way they coped with weak vision, so the remarks on the subject in the unpublished notebooks of the Cologne councillor Hermann Weinsberg (1518–1597) are worth quoting in some detail here.[41] At quite an early stage of his life, this chronicler noticed signs of short- and long-sightedness that grew more pronounced with the passage of time. Weinsberg was just thirty-three when he began to complain of 'something slightly wrong with my sight'. By the time he had passed fifty, his vision had become so bad that he could no longer read writing or make out the position of the hands on a clock without spectacles, and also had difficulty in recognizing anyone further away from him than forty 'Cologne feet' (about 11.5 metres). The older he grew, the more he was afraid that he would one day be completely blind. Blindness was much more common among the aged in those times than it is today. Relatives of Weinsberg, as well as people in his circle of acquaintances among the citizens of Cologne, had gone blind in old age and become completely dependent on the help of others. It was no doubt largely due to this fear that his deteriorating vision gradually began to affect his social behaviour. At first,

Weinsberg found it difficult to come to terms with the fact that his sight was getting worse as he grew older. He wore glasses all the time, and occasionally swallowed 'head pills' (a remedy for head ailments), no doubt because he thought they would improve his sight. When he reached sixty, he finally accepted a failure of vision that was making it impossible for him to read and write by candlelight, and also becoming a barrier to social contacts. Weinsberg certainly had the good fortune to be living the retired life of a pensioner by this time, and was only occasionally taking on cases as a lawyer. After the death of his second wife, his health made it impossible to entertain further hopes of the great political career that was perhaps still open to him as an alderman and solicitor. He now admitted that he harboured no further political ambitions, 'because I am old, and memory and sight grow weaker daily'. The year before, he had noted in his journal that: 'To begin studying, giving advice and practising the law again at my advanced age would be burdensome. I am old and my eyes are dim. I stare at the paper so long that I am afraid I shall grow dizzy.' Even though Weinsberg was essentially resigned to his poor sight in old age, the attendant inconveniences distressed him. Having survived his seventieth year, he ruefully noted that his poor sight also prevented him from recognizing friends and acquaintances on the other side of the street, so he could not acknowledge them; and that they, who often did not know of his acute short sight, thought he was doing it on purpose and took offence accordingly.

Hermann Weinsberg probably owned just one pair of glasses that ceased to served its purpose as his eyesight deteriorated. A century later, however, the glasses of spectacles were quite commonly re-ground and adjusted to changes within the wearer's eye. However, those who could actually afford this found it very tiresome. That inveterate letter-writer Elisabeth Charlotte von der Pfalz (1652–1722), sister-in-law of Louis XIV, was one: 'If we had spectacles that lasted for ever that would be fine; but once they have served one well for several years, they have to be altered again, which I find very bothersome.'[42] Spectacles were also a status symbol. Since they were initially worn mainly by scholars and clerics in the Middle Ages, this particular type of visual aid became a symbol of intelligence, as well as sly cunning. Spectacles came into fashion in the Spain of Philip II under the motto 'the larger the glasses, the more elevated the wearer.'[43] It was not until the eighteenth century that spectacles became a mass-produced article and a modish accessory of the educated bourgeoisie, causing Goethe to fear that the 'armed gaze' of the bespectacled would penetrate 'the innermost secrets of his being'.[44]

Hearing problems

According to a survey conducted by the German Green Cross, 11.3 million Germans suffer from defective hearing, although hardly a tenth wear a hearing aid. The ratio of congenital to acquired deafness is given as 1:1 in surveys made in the late nineteenth century.[45]

Loss of hearing is still considered a great misfortune today. Kant could imagine no greater deprivation, for a person stricken with deafness was 'condemned to loneliness even in the midst of company'.[46] The pre-modern perception of deafness, as opposed to blindness, is described by Petrarch in *De remediis utriusque fortunae* (Remedies for Fortune Fair and Foul), which is probably his best-known book: 'Which of the two is proportionately more or less bothersome is hard to say, save for the fact that blindness is more hazardous, and deafness more ludicrous; wherefore those hard of hearing are usually viewed as imbeciles, while the blind are considered as much more wretched – and humans harass the deaf with their laughter and the blind with their pity.'[47] But were the hard of hearing really mocked and regarded as deranged, as Petrarch claims? In the absence of other sources, it is difficult to give an answer. The association of deaf with 'foolish or simple-minded' is mainly literary. The Middle High German *Buch der Rügen* (Book of Rebukes), for example, contains the phrase 'he is deaf in all his senses.'[48] Wolfram von Eschenbach uses a similar expression in his epic *Parzival* (475: 6): 'sô was ich an den witzen toup' ('so my wits were deaf'). Here, the loss of hearing is equated with the incapacitation of all the senses, including the ability to think.

On the other hand, we are better informed about the legal status of deaf mutes. In contrast to the blind, deaf mutes needed a guardian to represent their legal interests under Roman law.[49] Under canon law, they were allowed to marry. Luther's explicit affirmation of their right to participate in holy communion says a lot about the religious restrictions with which deaf mutes had to contend at that time.[50] If their participation had been taken for granted, there would have been no need for the reformer's intervention.

Precisely how hardness of hearing was experienced by the deaf themselves before the invention of the ear trumpet (not before the second half of the seventeenth century), to say nothing of the transistorized hearing aids of the second half of the twentieth century, is known only from stylized literary testimony, such as the poem on deafness by Jonathan Swift (1667–1745).[51] The autobiographical notes of Hermann Weinsberg also reflect this experience. Weinsberg was long past fifty when he first detected a weakening of his faculty of hearing. The loss of hearing that typically accompanies the ageing process and, according to the most recent research, affects almost a third of those over sixty-five got worse for him in the course of time. In the self-description he wrote at the age of sixty, we read: 'My hearing is now also beginning to get weaker, I feel a buzzing and ringing in my head. I don't know if there is some substance there that causes it. Yes, as the body ages with the passage of the years, the five senses of man also get old. When people speak loudly and clearly I can hear very well.' What Weinsberg is describing as a layman are the typical symptoms of presbyacusis, or progressive deafness in the aged, which begins in the inner ear. The drastic reduction of the capacity to register higher sound frequencies is manifested by the affected person's tendency to hear male voices better than female voices, and to have perceptual difficulties in company, or in speech contexts in which there is a lot of background noise. The phenomenon of so-called ringing in the ears is a symptom of tinnitus, a noise in the ears that often occurs in the second half of life.

The psychological study of ageing has meanwhile examined the effect of hardness of hearing on the psychology and social behaviour of older people. One of the most important symptoms is undoubtedly the feeling of insecurity arising from the difficulty of understanding communication. As the case of Hermann Weinsberg shows, deafness leads to social isolation, for the aurally disadvantaged individual avoids difficult speech situations and social contacts that might cause frustration. Furthermore, the reduction of communicative ability that accompanies hardness of hearing could, and still does, compel a person to retreat from public life, as the biography of the Cologne councillor once again demonstrates so clearly.

The oldest medical-historical sources show that hearing disabilities were familiar to early physicians.[52] The famous Egyptian *Ebers Papyrus* (*c.*1550 BC) describes a remedy for hardness of hearing. Among the various causes of illness listed in the Hippocratic texts, wind and weather feature among the main causes of hearing problems; and the same source also contains a reference to a case of deafness following injury to the skull. The Roman author Celsus, whose *De medicina* we quoted above, actually provides a highly differentiated aetiology for hardness of hearing, including the blockage of the outer acoustic meatus by earwax, foreign bodies and ulcers. His renowned Greek contemporary Galen distinguished between an injury to the organ of hearing and a lesion of the cochlear nerve, but, since the existence of the inner ear was unsuspected at the time, he was unable to point to concrete, classificatory characteristics. The functional separation of blocked sound conduction from defective sound reception was the work of the Italian physician Hieronymus Capivacco (*d.* 1589). Capivacco connected one end of an iron rod to a zither and the other to the teeth of a partially deaf patient. If the latter could hear the sound of the plucked strings, it followed that the problem was the acoustic meatus and not the insensitivity of the cochlear nerve. With this method, the Paduan teacher of medicine laid the foundation of modern techniques of deafness diagnosis. The first physician to use a prototype of the tuning fork ('furca qua ad cibos utimur') for diagnostic purposes was Günther Christoph Schelhammer (1649–1712).

And what of therapies for defective hearing? Therapeutic measures such as ear flushing were practised in antiquity. But as the Byzantine physician Alexander von Tralles (525–605) informs us, other more drastic measures might also be employed: 'Many physicians not only prescribe all imaginable forms of internal treatment, but also perform an arteriotomy [opening of an artery] afterwards, and then take a trumpet, place it against the acoustic meatus and blow down it. Others create a cacophonous noise with bells, while others again have used instruments invented by themselves.'[53] A gentler form of auditory training, involving the stimulation of the cochlear nerve by soft sounds ('cum subtilibus vocibus incitare'), was recommended by the medieval surgeon Lanfranc of Milan (*c.*1245–before 1306). His colleague Arnaldus de Villanova (1235–1312?) induced his patients to sneeze while holding them firmly by the nose. Among antiquity's famous deaf was the Emperor Hadrian (76–138), who had the habit of cupping his hand behind his ear in order to amplify sound, the efficacy of which was later confirmed by Marcus Aurelius's future personal physician, Galen, in his theory of the function of the outer

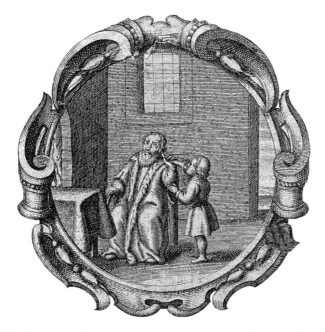

Figure 5.1   Listening through an ear-trumpet (seventeenth century)

ear as a receiver of sound (see figure 5.1). But the numerous miraculous cures of deafness witnessed in the Gospels, the aural motifs of ancient votive offerings and the medieval miracle books demonstrate just how little medicine was able to do in cases of total deafness before the twentieth century.

Deaf mutism proved particularly difficult to treat. For a long period of time, it was considered to be merely an anatomical problem deriving from simultaneous damage to the faculty of hearing and the nerve responsible for the tongue. Thus, well into the early modern era midwives would tear the frenulum linguae of a newborn baby, for fear that the child might otherwise become a deaf mute. Until the sixteenth century, deaf mutes were hardly treated at all, merely encouraged to concentrate on strengthening their other senses. As Augustine notes in the *Liber de magistro*, deaf mutes communicated by means of gestures: 'Have you not seen men when they discourse, so to speak, by means of gestures with those who are deaf, the deaf likewise using gestures? Do they not question and reply and teach and indicate everything they wish or at least a great many things? When they use gestures they do not merely indicate visible things, but also sounds and tastes.'[54] The first reference to systematic instruction in gestural phonetics occurs in the work of the English chronicler and Church Father the Venerable Bede (672–735). In sixteenth-century Spain, the conspicuously frequent incidence of deaf mutism among the aristocracy stimulated new ideas on the teaching of deaf mutes. One person deserving of special mention in this context is the Spanish schoolmaster Ramirez de Carrión (1579–1652), who incorporated the then already familiar semaphore alphabet into his innovative and successful system of teaching the deaf and dumb. By the seventeenth century, the publication of books on the teaching of phonetic language to deaf mutes was no longer a Spanish speciality. Perhaps the best-known work on the subject is the *Philocopus* (1648) of the English physician John Bulwer, which contains numerous illustrations of how, with patience and skill, deaf mutes could be taught sign language, lip-reading and phonetic script. All the same, his proposal for the establishment of a 'schola mutorum ac sudorum', or school for deaf mutes, which was similar in form to that of the Swiss pedagogue Johannes Lavater (1624–1695), found little support in the seventeenth century.[55]

Loss of the sense of smell

The popular book by Petrarch (1304–1374) on the right 'spiritual medicine' for good times and bad typically bemoans deafness and hardness of hearing, but has nothing to say about loss of the sense of smell. Instead, there is a chapter entitled 'On sweet and agreeable smells' (I, 22). The total or partial loss of the olfactory sense was evidently not considered to be as serious a loss as deafness or blindness. Unlike Christianity, Judaism attached ritual significance to the ability to distinguish smells, notably in the *Havdala* ceremony that concluded the Sabbath. When Rabbi Jacob Reischer (*d.* 1733), one of the leading rabbinical authorities of the modern era, was asked whether a man with no sense of smell was entitled to pronounce the prescribed benediction over the sweet spices at the end of the Sabbath, he replied that it was permitted because, although he might be incapable of physically savouring the fragrance, such a man was nonetheless capable of spiritual delectation.[56]

Zedler's Universal Lexicon (1735) provides an early example of the occasional interest of the medical community in this physiological problem. The headword 'Smell, loss of' is itself an indication that the science of medicine was rather at a loss with cases of this kind: 'Those who lose their sense of smell are unlikely to recover it, particularly if they are old. The most useful treatment in these cases is marjoram, which may be applied in any way.'[57] The author of this relatively short entry also recommends rosemary, anime resin and amber as stimulants for weakened olfactory nerves. In his *Neues Arzneibuch* (New Pharmacopoeia, 1568), Christoph Wirsung (1500–1571) was similarly sceptical of the possibility of treatment: 'This is a by no means minor defect of the human body, and the learned say it cannot be remedied if we have been born with it or have grown old. And even if it [the sense of smell] could be restored, this could not be achieved without a great deal of time and effort.'[58] In those times, only the temporary loss of smell brought on by heavy colds and the like could be treated more or less quickly with various kinds of expectorants and fragrant substances.[59]

Although of inferior rank, the sense of smell was nonetheless conceded a certain importance in everyday life, and was by no means left out of account in preventative health care. On reaching sixty, Hermann Weinsberg confided to his journal that: 'sense of smell good, exercise it often when I am sitting or thinking, I smell lavender, rosemary, flowers and herbs.'

Aromatic substances have played a part in the treatment of a host of illnesses since antiquity and are today back with a vengeance in the form of aromatherapy. One of the main proponents of this type of therapy was Caelius Aurelianus, who practised in Rome in the third century AD and dispensed strong-smelling substances such as vinegar, rose oil and castoreum to epileptics.[60] This Roman physician was also able to distinguish between loss of smell due to paralysis and the similar symptoms of ozaena, a disorder of the nose which renders the patient insensitive to a foul-smelling nasal discharge. The opposite case of an extremely sensitive nose has scarcely ever been seen as problematic by doctors. Nevertheless, this particular medical phenomenon stimulated the novelist Patrick Süßkind to write his best-seller *Perfume* (1985), and has also been a source of inspiration to several other writers.[61]

Poor sense of taste

The temporary or permanent loss of the sense of taste is again treated rather cursorily by medical literature until well into the modern era. We are hardly surprised by Wilhelm Sternberg's conclusion to his *Physiologische Untersuchungen über den Geschmackssinn* (Physiological Investigations of the Sense of Taste, 1906): 'Hitherto, we have failed to consider that many people are tasteless and indifferent with regard to the sense of taste, and that in the realm of taste, as elsewhere, the dull and feeble-minded greatly outnumber the acute.'[62] We find an early note on this deficiency in *Zedler's Universal Lexicon* of 1735: '*Gustus depravatus* is caused by an excessive flow of bile into the stomach, and from there into the blood, so that the mouth tastes nothing but bitterness. The sense of taste is particularly affected by colds.'[63] Without sensitivity to taste, the sensuous enjoyment of food and drink is impossible. This is confirmed not only by the discussion of the dangers of artificial or strange tastes in Petrarch's little book of consolation (I, 22). We also find the sixty-year-old chronicler Weinsberg taking heart from the fact that that his sense of taste had scarcely deteriorated with the passing of the years: 'still enjoy the taste of good wine, food and drink.'

Numbness and paralysis

Before the advent of modern diagnostic techniques (e.g., X-ray images, ultrasound, computer tomography), the loss of physical sensation (*tactus imminutus*) was interpreted either as a localized injury to the part of the body in question, or as a symptom or side effect of a serious illness such as leprosy or a stroke. Doctors became interested in loss of sensation at a fairly early date. Albucasis (*d. c.*1010), who was the personal physician of Caliph Hakam II in Córdoba, touched on the loss of feeling in a work that became one of the founding texts of early Western surgery: 'and note that the sufferer cannot feel burning heat like a healthy person because he is in fact suffering from *hidr* [numbness].'[64] The correctness of Albucasis's observation that a part of the body that has been cauterized will become numb was expressly confirmed by other medieval authors, such as the Salerno physician Roger Frugardi (before 1140–*c.*1195).

—— 120 ——

When examining people for leprosy, which was a practice that continued into the early modern period, physicians looked not only for tell-tale changes to the surface of the skin but also tested its sensitivity by inserting a needle into the calf or middle finger. Any numbness in the suspected patient was regarded as *signa univoca*, a clear symptom of the dreaded disease.[65] However, as Hermann Weinsberg's journal shows, you did not necessarily have to be suffering from an unusual illness to be concerned about the state of your sensation: 'I soon discover that there's nothing wrong with my sensation when the fleas begin to bite' – a fleabite being hardly a rare event in those days.

Although local anaesthetics were not introduced into surgery until towards the end of the nineteenth century, the pain-numbing effects of certain substances had been known since antiquity. These substances had narcotic as well as anaesthetizing effects, however, and were rarely used to make the body completely insensitive to pain. It was difficult to calculate the correct dosage, and many experienced surgeons considered the risk that the patient might not wake up from this artfully induced unconsciousness to be too high. Galen, for instance, cautioned against the irresponsible use of narcotic medicaments such as opium, mandrake root and hyoscyamus seeds. If a surgeon wanted to treat a disease properly, he had to refrain from using numbing narcotics.[66] Fantasies of painless surgical incision were widespread before the anaesthetic triumphs of the nineteenth century, as may be judged from the commentary on Genesis by the medieval theologian Peter Abaelardus (1097–1142), where we read that God made Adam 'insensibilem' in order to ensure that the creation of Eve from his rib would be painless ('nullam doloris').[67] On the other hand, cutaneous hypersensitivity, a condition in which the skin reacts to the slightest stimulus in the manner of an ornamental mimosa, does not appear in medical literature until the beginning of the nineteenth century. However, botanists had long been familiar with the so-called touch-me-not plant ('noli me tangere') that had generated all kinds of speculation concerning the metaphorical relations between plant life and human behaviour. The known tendency of the seed-heads of certain plants to burst at a touch suggested the following image to *Zedler's Universal Lexicon*: 'This is why the above-mentioned *herba sensitiva* (sometimes called *Pudica casta*, and known to the Portuguese as *Vergonhada*, i.e. *Verecunda*) is about as chaste and modest as a whore on heat who, if the expression be permitted, is unable to hold in her waters at the touch or the sight of a man.'[68] The common association of touch with sexuality has no doubt influenced interpretations of the risen Christ's words to Mary Magdalene ('Noli me tangere'; John 20: 17).[69] In more recent translations of the Bible, the word 'tangere' has been translated as 'hold', so the original allusion has been lost.

Loss of sensation was considered treatable by some and incurable by others: 'Loss of sensation due to rage, madness, *soporosis adfectibus* [a condition resembling deep sleep], *Apoplexia* [stroke] and similar disorders can be cured without difficulty, for if the main complaint has been dealt with, the other parts of the body learn to feel again by themselves' – or so *Zedler's Universal Lexicon* claims.[70] However, the same source also states that the art of medicine was usually at a loss in cases of 'blocked nerves', or damaged neural tissue. The Basel physician Felix Platter reports a case of this type in his *Observationes* (1614): 'The arm of a stone mason who had slept on his elbow during the night was so numbed that it became dead and limp. Despite trying various remedies, the man only recovered his sense of touch and the use of his arm two years later.'[71] If therapy failed to restore sensation in one or several parts of the body, the only remaining hope was a miracle. The medieval miracle books are full of alleged cures of numbness and recoveries from paralysis at the intercession of saints. The Marburg *Miracula Sancte Elyzabet* (1232/5), for example, chronicles the case of a certain Henricus from the diocese of Trier, who suffered from a huge swelling of the leg that turned it completely numb ('it was as though dead'). After two visits to the tomb of St Elisabeth of Thuringia, he was finally restored to health and, as two witnesses confirmed, was able to 'return home on his own two feet, completely restored'.[72] A similarly spectacular case that occurred during the Thirty Years' War is reported in the records of the monastery at Eberhardsklausen, which was a popular place of pilgrimage in the Rhineland. A bed-ridden and paralysed nun from Cologne had apparently already sought relief in various medicines, and immersion in the waters at Aachen. When these therapies failed to produce results, she sent someone to make an offering to the image of the Mother of God at Eberhardsklausen. Immediately after this, the nun experienced an improvement: 'At first she felt a little pain and sensation in her legs, which had been wizened, numb and insensitive, but once she had set out on the promised pilgrimage, the miraculous help and intercession of Mary Mother of God, was wonderfully apparent to all.'[73]

It is evident from this miraculous story, which was confirmed by several eye-witnesses, and from comparable cases reported in other late medieval and early modern miracle books, that long-lasting or permanent loss of sensation in the body and limbs, particularly when accompanied by paralysis, was perceived as a serious deprivation. People turned to all kinds of remedies, beginning with surgery and medication. 'Religious medicines' (prayers of petition, pilgrimages, etc.) were resorted to only after the latter had failed to work. And today, more than three centuries later, many people whom neuro- and micro-surgery have failed to help, despite all the intervening progress, still make the pilgrimage to Kevelaer, Lourdes or Fatima in the hope of once more being able to feel their numbed and paralysed limbs.

— Part III —

From the World of the Senses to the World of Reason (Eighteenth and Nineteenth Centuries)

— 6 —

Philosophical Sensualism
in the Age of Sensibility

> We are all sensualists today, we of the present and future of philosophy;
> not in theory, but in practice; as practitioners.
>
> Friedrich Nietzsche, *Beyond Good and Evil* (1886)

Sensualistic theories of perception

The language teacher, journalist and doctor Jean Paul Marat (1743–
1793) was one of the symbolic figures of the French Revolution and
also one of its most radical representatives. In 1773, he published
first in English a now forgotten medical and anthropological essay
entitled 'On Man'. The work, which was later published in French
in Amsterdam, contains a detailed treatment of the five senses and
their functions. Marat the revolutionary, whose fate is the subject
of numerous books and paintings, is undoubtedly better known than
Marat the medical author, which is perhaps a good reason for taking
a fresh look at this early piece, which irritated Voltaire and led him
to make disparaging remarks about its then still obscure author. The
fifth section of the first book contains a systematic application to
the five senses of the theory of the body as a machine propagated
by the French physician Julien Offray de La Mettrie (1709–1751), in
his influential *L'Homme machine: A Study in the Origins of an Idea*
(1748):

> As the general organ of sensation, the body is simply a machine con-
> sisting of nerves and nervous processes. With regard to the individual
> organs of sensation, it is a very elaborately constructed mechanism, in
> which the senses are the parts that impinge on objects: the meninges,
> the supporting tissue and the nerves, which are the channels that con-
> vey to the mind the impressions they receive.[1]

While Marat's book is hardly the work of an original thinker, his chapter on the senses contains a hint – largely ignored by recent research – that the phenomenon of colour-blindness was already quite familiar to the medical and scientific community some years before Joseph Priestley's pioneering discovery in 1777. As far as general sensory physiology is concerned, Marat's thought bears the imprint of French sensualistic thought. The 'sensualist philosophers', as Immanuel Kant (1724–1804) called them, derived all knowledge from the passive reception of sense data, in contrast to the 'intellectualist philosophers', who stressed the function of reason in the process of perception.[2]

The spiritual fathers of French philosophical sensualism included René Descartes, in whose dualistic theory of the body there is no longer a place for the Aristotelian tradition of thought. Descartes' reduction of the inner senses to purely physical mechanical functionality was just one expression of this. However, the English philosopher John Locke (1632–1704) proved to be a more lastingly influential figure than Descartes. In his major work *An Essay Concerning Human Understanding* (1690), Locke emerges as both the staunch champion of empiricism and a vehement opponent of the Platonic theory of innate ideas.[3] Locke, who practised as a doctor all his life, claimed that all experience derived from just two sources: *sensations* and *reflections*: 'This great Source, of most of the *Ideas* we have, depending wholly upon our Senses, and derived by them to the Understanding, I call SENSATION.'[4] Starting out from his theory of sense perception and the idea that the human mind was like a blank sheet of paper, Locke proceeded to develop his theory of perception, reflection, memory and volition.

Locke's thought, which quickly became the foundation of the sensualistic school of philosophy that was to become so dominant in the eighteenth century, spread rapidly and gathered many supporters, both in England and in other countries. The first figure to be mentioned here is the Irish philosopher and theologian George Berkeley (1685–1753), whose theory of perception was, as we shall see, discussed at great length by the French *encyclopédistes*, notably by Etienne Bonnot de Condillac (1715–1780). In his *An Essay Towards a New Theory of Vision* (1709), Berkeley had already challenged Locke's sensualistic approach by pointing to space as an example of a perception that did not simply take place by means of the senses.[5]

Taking the motor activity of the eye ('sensations arising from the turn of the eyes') as his principal model, Berkeley posited a reciprocal relationship between sensory and motor functions. He gave a more radical twist to this empirico-realistic idea of sense perception in his major work *Treatise Concerning the Principles of Human Knowledge* (1710). Here, the existence of things is grounded in the fact that they are perceived ('esse est percipi'). But it does not follow from this that things do not exist prior to their actual perception by the five senses, for, according to Berkeley, who was not for nothing a theologian, there is still such a thing as a divine being, and therefore an objective reality beyond the bounds of human knowledge. Thus, the human mind perceives only representations or ideas conveyed by the senses, which do not originate in the mind itself, but are communicated to it by God.

In his *A Treatise of Human Nature* (1739–1740), the Scottish philosopher David Hume (1711–1776) likewise maintains that human knowledge is derived from sensory perceptions: 'To hate, to love, to think, to feel, to see; all this is nothing but to perceive.'[6] In Hume's view, therefore, vice and virtue are not properties of objects, but subjective sense perceptions. He separates the contents of human consciousness into 'impressions', 'representations' and 'ideas'. Impressions are immediate, living sense data. Ideas are merely the pale copies of them created by the memory or imagination. In addition to them, Hume distinguishes three separate kinds of sense impressions: primary and secondary impressions, and impressions that are the expression of pleasure and pain.[7] Recent writers have perceived a connection between Hume's fervent advocacy of the senses and his personal life. His nervous breakdown in the spring of 1730 altered the course of his life and made him realize that thinking could not be disconnected from sense impressions, and that sense impressions were rooted in the body. 'His nervous breakdown', wrote the English medical historian Roy Porter, 'no doubt taught Hume that his philosophical project of solving the problem of identity by examining sense impressions led to precisely the morbid introspection that was making him ill.'[8]

In France, it was Locke who made the greatest impact on the *encyclopédistes*. The introduction to the *Encyclopédie* by Jean Le Rond d'Alembert (1717–1783) shows just how familiar sensualistic ideas already were to French philosophers and doctors by the mid-eighteenth century. It contains the programmatic statement that is taken up and elaborated again and again in other contributions to the famous reference work: 'All our immediate knowledge consists simply of what we receive through our senses; from which it follows that we owe all our ideas to our sensations.'[9] The dominant sensualism is, however, less pronounced in the contribution *Sens* (*Métaphysique*) by Louis Chevalier de Jaucourt (1704–1779) than in the article on *sensibilité* by the doctor Henri Fouquet (1727–1806), who taught at Montpellier. Here, the concept of 'sensibility' which became so important in the late eighteenth century, and nowhere more so than in the works of Jean-Jacques Rousseau (1712–1778), is defined as follows: 'Sensibility is the capacity of certain parts of the living body to perceive impressions [*impressions*] of external objects and to generate reactions [*mouvements*] corresponding to their intensity.'[10]

This concise definition is largely in agreement with John Locke's understanding of 'sensations', namely the stimuli produced on our sense organs by the external world. However, Fouquet's article already foreshadows the later development and extension of the objects to which the term applied, as is particularly evident in his detailed exposition of the differences between sensibility and motility, and the dependence of *sensibilité* upon climate, age and gender.

Awakening the senses of statues and machines

The French *Encylopédie*, which had to battle constantly against censorship, was edited by Denis Diderot (1713–1784). Its team of collaborators included Voltaire, d'Alembert, Montesquieu, Buffon, Turgot, Helvétius and Etienne Bonnot de Condillac. With his much discussed *Traité des sensations* (Treatise on the Sensations, 1754), Condillac was one of the founders of philosophical sensualism. He strongly criticized Locke's assumption of two independent sources of knowledge (sensation and reflection) and questioned the latter's autonomy: 'Judgement, reflection, desire and passion are nothing more than sensation itself.'[11] Condillac's main purpose was to show that 'all knowledge derives from the senses, above all the sense of touch.'[12] The image of the marble statue (*homme-statue*) which he uses to illustrate his theory has become famous. This statue is gradually 'brought to life' in a series of stages, in the course of which it receives the five senses in the order of smell, hearing, taste, sight and touch.

Once in possession of the sense of smell, the statue becomes capable of attentiveness, but is as yet unable to form an idea of the various changes taking place around it. The same applies to the other senses, which are capable of only limited perceptions when operating in isolation. It is not until it receives the sense of touch that the statue acquires the idea of space and extension. General ideas, on the other hand, depend on the collaborative effort of all the senses: 'If we now assume that it [the statue] reflects on these bodies, and considers their qualities without reference to the five ways in which they are affecting its organs, it will form the general idea of "sensation". That is to say, it will conflate all the impressions it receives from the bodies around it into one single class.'[13] This combination of sense impressions is performed under the direction of the sense of touch. Once the sense of touch begins to co-operate with the other senses, the statue, which, up to this point, has processed the sense data purely passively, acquires the capacity either to expose itself completely to the impressions streaming towards it from the outside world, or to withdraw from them.

At roughly the same time, though quite independently of Condillac, the Genevan naturalist Charles Bonnet (1720–1793) also chose the image of bringing a statue to life as a way of exemplifying the central role of the sense organs and sensations in human perception. It is surely no accident that philosophers should turn so quickly for inspiration to the myth of Pygmalion (in which a sculptor falls in love with his own ivory statue of a woman and asks the goddess Aphrodite to breathe life into her).[14] Condillac, for instance, was obliged to admit that Diderot had already used an idea similar to this in his *Lettre sur les sourds et muets* (Letter on the Deaf and Dumb, 1751), as had Georges-Louis Leclerc Buffon (1707–1788) in his *Natural History* (begun 1749). However, Condillac was probably simply exploiting a visual motif that was very popular in the second half of the eighteenth century. We need think only of the use of the Pygmalion myth by painters such as François Boucher (1703–1770) and Charles André van Loo (1705–1765). There are also striking parallels between these mythical revisions and the version by Johann Jakob Bodmer (1698–1783) in his story *Pygmalion and Elise* (1747), which was based on an anonymously published narrative by the Frenchman

André François Boureau-Deslandes (1690–1757). In this tale, the awakening of the marble statue is described as follows: 'The beloved statue suddenly received light which arose within her; she acquired the power of movement; her senses combined to render the objects about her intelligible and she gradually began to distinguish between them.'[15] Condillac describes basically the same event: 'Among the colours that spread into the depths of her eye in that first moment, there may be one that she distinguishes in a particular way, and sees as though separately.'[16] Both texts, then, are concerned with the very first use of the visual sense and the gradual ordering of the numerous impressions of colour flowing into the eye. A few decades later in Germany, Moses Mendelssohn (1729–1786) fashioned the statue motif into a 'psychological-allegorical dream vision'.[17]

A 'philosophical sensualist' such as Condillac would also have been fascinated by the world-famous 'Flute Player' (1738) produced in the workshop of the brilliant French mechanic and automator Jacques Vaucanson (1709–1782). This wooden figure was almost life-size and played just like a human being. The movements of its lips, fingers and tongue were astonishingly life-like and it was capable of playing twelve different tunes on a transverse flute. Contrary to what might have been expected, it was not built round a musical box, but instead contained a complicated system of bellows operated by gears that generated air, which was then converted into musical notes by the flute. This work of art was undoubtedly one of the inspirations behind La Mettrie's famous *L'Homme machine: A Study in the Origins of an Idea* (1748). Inventive eighteenth-century clock-makers and makers of automata were inspired in turn by La Mettrie's book to perfect the mechanical human being. 'The Writer', a widely acclaimed automaton made by Pierre Jaquet-Droz (1721–1790), is one example of the craft; another is a masterpiece of ingenuity called 'The Chess-Playing Turk' by the mechanical engineer Wolfgang von Kempelen (1734–1804) – though this figure had a real person concealed inside it.[18]

This 'automata-mania' was not without its critics and debunkers. The German novelist Johann Friedrich Richter (1763–1825), better known as Jean Paul, poked fun at these fake 'human beings' and the naïve curiosity of the astonished public. In 1789, he published a satire describing the gradual animation of 'a most agreeable new woman made of pure wood, whom I recently invented and married.' The story was published along with an equally hilarious humoresque called the *Machine-Man,* in which this prolix German storyteller pours scorn on all such 'follies':

> But now I shall amuse myself by imagining that human beings have advanced to a higher level of machinality and, having allowed myself that, I will proceed to imagine that they have reached the highest level possible, and that instead of five senses they now have five machines [. . .]. I will next fancy that they have gone even further and are now even able to answer the call of nature by means of an hydraulic device. They will not even keep their own selves, but have new selves carved for them by the materialists, although this seems rather unlikely – even animals will cease to exist, for since Archytas, Regiomontan, Vaucanson have already given us artificial pigeons, eagles, flies and ducks, all the remaining fauna will be petrified and ossified too, and whole menageries, containing neither life nor fodder, will be left unlocked, and clever people who have read their Spener will fancy the Day of Judgement is either at hand or has already been and gone – the whole thing will be quite appalling and *natura naturans* will pass away, leaving only *natura naturata* and machines with no one to mind them.[19]

One wonders what Jean Paul would have written had he had any idea of the metamorphoses that lay in store for his fanciful patent 'wooden woman'. Today, we not only have scientific names for fetishists who are sexually aroused by the feel of a statue or a wax doll (pygmalionists), but also mass-produced, 'sensually' erotic automata made of rubber or plastic – available either by mail order or from any of the usual outlets.

While the radically materialist aspect of sensualism is revealed in the elaborate construction of robots and literary treatments of the Pygmalion myth, the experimental aspect of this type of thought surfaces in areas we would nowadays consider as belonging to the domain of psychology, namely the study of living people, especially those who have only gradually acquired the full use of all their five senses. It is first seen in a question put to John Locke by the English physicist William Molyneux (1656–1698) in a letter dated 7 July 1688. Molyneux wanted to know whether a person blind from birth who suddenly received his eyesight would immediately be able to tell the difference between a cube and a sphere by means of what would, in his case, be the unfamiliar sense of sight.[20] Locke initially ignored this question and did not address it in detail until the second edition of his *Essay Concerning Human Understanding* (1694). But the scientific community of the day was not entirely persuaded by his thoughts on the matter. The problem was only deemed to have been solved after the publication of Denis Diderot's celebrated *Lettre sur les aveugles* (Letter on the Blind, 1749). One of the most important contributions to the debate was a report by the English surgeon William Cheselden (1688–1752), which had first appeared in 1729 in the *Philosophical Transactions of the Royal Society*. There, Cheselden described how a young man blind since birth had suddenly received his sight, following an operation on his eyes. Initially, the patient had been unable either to assess the size of objects correctly or to distinguish between various shapes. For a short period after the operation, he had also found it very difficult to see in perspective. Although a similar study by an ophthalmologist named Grant had been reported in the English periodical *The Tatler* in 1709, Cheselden's detailed description had the greater impact, since his reputation as a surgeon was by then already established in England and abroad.[21] Condillac, for instance, specifically mentioned Cheselden's publication, which he regarded as proof of the co-ordinating function, and hence the superiority, of the sense of touch, which he himself had tried to demonstrate in his description of the statue's progressive acquisition of the five senses in the *Treatise on the Sensations*.

Sensory-psychological experiments

In their attempts to prove the correctness of their theories of sense perception, the philosophical sensualists did not confine their enquiries to the blind or deaf-mutes. News of strange foundlings also aroused their curiosity. The first 'wolf-child' to attract the interest of the contemporary scientific community was a boy who had been discovered in 1694 in the forests of Lithuania, where he been living for a long time with bears. As Condillac informs us, the boy 'displayed no signs of rational behaviour, walked on all fours, had no knowledge of language and produced sounds that bore no relation to anything human.'[22] A little more than a century later, the inhabitants of the small French village of Aveyron discovered in a wood a boy aged about twelve, who had apparently spent half his life in the wilderness.[23] Once the report of this discovery reached Paris, doctors and

—— 133 ——

scientists immediately hastened to examine the 'wild' boy. One of the doctors was no less a figure than the psychiatrist Philippe Pinel (1745–1826). Pinel noted that the boy's sense of touch was undeveloped. Pierre-Joseph Bonnaterre (1751–1804) also examined him and came to the same conclusion: 'Thus we have the order of the senses as nature seems to have established them in the wild boy who is the object of these observations: the sense of smell is first and most perfected; taste is second, or rather these two senses are but one; vision occupies the position of third importance, hearing the fourth, and touch the last.'[24] The continuing influence of Condillac's privileging of the sense of touch is underlined by the fact that the majority of the medical experts who rushed off to examine him considered the wild boy to be undeveloped and mentally retarded on the grounds of the unusual character of his sensory hierarchy.

While the story of the wolf-child of Aveyron is now no more than a marginal note in the history of science, the life and death of Kaspar Hauser (1812?–1833) continues to be the stuff of novels, films, plays and non-fiction. Medical science has also returned to the case on numerous occasions. In the present context, we are interested above all in the curious sensory perceptions of this 'child of Europe', as Johannes Mayer has called him. The Bavarian lawyer and councillor of state Anselm von Feuerbach (1775–1833), who was a contemporary witness, has left us the following description: 'Not only his mind but many of his senses seemed at first to be entirely paralysed and only slowly opened to receive external impressions. Several days elapsed before he became aware of the striking of the church clock and the peals of the bells, which plunged him into amazement.'[25] But, after just a few days of adjustment to his new surroundings, the doctors who were examining Kaspar noticed the extreme acuteness of his senses. The Royal Bavarian municipal court doctor Paul Sigmund Karl Preu (1774–1832) noted in his report that, 'compared to those of other people, his senses are still strikingly acute, although they have become progressively less so since he became used to eating meat. At first . . . he was able to smell things like decomposing animal matter and dried bones from some considerable distance.'[26]

Kaspar Hauser also soon became a showpiece guinea pig of homeopathic medicine, which was at that time already a subject of heated controversy. Homeopathic doctors realized that his phenomenal sense of smell presented them with a golden opportunity to conduct trials of their medications with a healthy person. The afore-mentioned Dr Preu wrote a report of one of these experiments for the *Archiv für homöopathische Heilkunst* (Archive of Homeopathic Medicine, 1832): 'When he held the small glass containing a concentrate of a millionth of sulphur at arm's length, a strong, pungent, alumic smell penetrated his nose and head, and the place where the small blister had healed began to flare up again.'[27] Other homeopathic drugs were tried out on Kaspar in solutions of varying dilutions and concentrations. In all cases, the extreme sensitivity to smell that had struck the doctors and teachers the moment they first met him in May 1828 was confirmed anew.

In addition to accounting for the cause of his death (a stab wound to the heart), the forensic autopsy performed after Kaspar's mysterious murder remarked on other striking features which, according to the prevailing wisdom, shed light on his unusual sensory acuteness: 'The large commissure of the cerebrum was developed very prominently. The thalami were also large and excellently formed.'[28]

When he came to explain Kaspar Hauser's extreme sensitivity, which had lessened as he gradually adjusted to the conditions of ordinary life, Dr Preu, who acted as an expert witness, drew on the theory of tellurism developed by the Jena professor Dietrich Georg Kieser (1779–1862). Tellurism was influenced by the thought of Friedrich Wilhelm Joseph Schelling (1775–1854), whose philosophy of nature assumes the presence of a universal polarity. It draws a distinction between the telluric and solar forces that influence the life of man. If the telluric force of the moon is predominant, then according to this notion, which was widely accepted in medical circles, the outcome may be somnambulance or clairvoyance. One of the signs of such 'locally sensitive somnambulism', as Kieser called the phenomenon, was a noticeable intensification of hearing, taste and smell.

So it is hardly astonishing that Justinus Kerner (1786–1862) should compare his observations of his patient Friederike Hauffe, the famous *Seherin von Prevorst* (Clairvoyant of Prevorst), with those in the case of Kaspar Hauser. It supported his hypothesis that there was a 'night side of nature' and therefore a genuinely real world of spirits.[29] Like Kaspar Hauser, this most celebrated 'clairvoyant' of literary history became the 'willing' subject of sensory-physiological experiments which were based upon an amalgam of contemporary mesmerism and sensualistic notions and ideas. The Swabian doctor and poet tested the effect of various plants and fruits on his patient by giving her bunches of grapes, which she was not supposed to eat but just feel with her hands. Another sensibility test was devised for her faculty of hearing. For this he used a Jew's harp to observe the effects of musical rhythms on her 'nervous spirit'.[30]

Justinus Kerner was not, in fact, the first to observe that, when put into an artificial state of somnambulism (e.g., by being stroked with a magnetic rod), the subject became more receptive to sensory impressions (particularly when they were aural or tactile). The earliest reference is found in a report published in 1788 by the Zurich doctor Johann Heinrich Rahn (1749–1812). Phenomena of this kind fascinated not only the physicians of German Romanticism. Clemens von Brentano (1778–1842), the compiler of the famous collection of German folk songs *Des Knaben Wunderhorn* (The Boy's Magic Horn), tells of a stigmatic nun from Dülmen named Katharina Emmerick, who was reputedly able to recognize the relics of saints and persons consecrated by the Catholic Church from the way they felt to her touch.[31]

The sensitivity of the female sex

On 17 February 1829, just a few months after the publication of Justinus Kerner's most controversial and certainly best-known book (*Die Seherin von Prevorst*), Johann Wolfgang von Goethe and Johann Peter Eckermann were discussing the various philosophical currents of the day, when the conversation turned to sensualism. With reference to the *Critique of Pure Reason*, in which Kant draws the distinction between 'sensualist philosophers' and 'intellectual philosophers' mentioned above, Goethe remarked that: 'The time has come for some distinguished and capable thinker to produce a critique of the senses and the human understanding, and if this were to be done properly the task of German philosophy would be complete.'[32] Exactly twenty years earlier, an influential work by the French doctor and physiologist Pierre-Jean Georges Cabanis (1757–1808) had appeared under the title *Rapports du physique et du morale de l'homme* (On the Connection between the Physical and the Moral in Mankind). Cabanis countered Condillac's sensationalism and its overemphasis of external sense impressions with more recent scientific observations. He too, however, insisted that sense perception was the absolute precondition of all human ideas, feelings, needs and volitions. In this context, he suggested a famous comparison: the brain processed sense impressions in the way that the stomach digested food. But along with the sense impressions produced by the external world, Cabanis also acknowledged the presence of inner drives which were independent of external influences. Nonetheless, most of this two-volume study is devoted to the 'sensations', as Cabanis, following Locke and Condillac, calls perception by means of the five senses. He devotes two long chapters to the 'physiological history of the sensations', laying particular emphasis on influential factors such as age, gender, temperament, illness, diet and climate. Here, Cabanis adopts a subdivision similar to the one already used in the *Encyclopédie* article on *sensibilité* mentioned above.

The category of gender undoubtedly had the greatest impact, for in the age of sentimentality gender served time and again to justify the division of roles and discrimination against women. By tying the process of knowledge to elementary sensations, and by largely abnegating the role of reason in the making of distinctions, sensualism did much to legitimize the different roles of men and women in society by grounding them in biology. In 1754, Dorothea von Erxleben, née Leporin (1715–1762), the first woman in Germany to qualify as a doctor of medicine, published her famous apologia. Here she summarized the reasons that prevented the female sex from embarking on formal study, and confronted the preconception that women were less rational than men.

The argument that, as more sensitive beings, women were unsuited to study, and certainly unsuited to medicine, does not crop up in learned circles until the end of the eighteenth century. This is probably why Dorothea von Erxleben mentions only the 'affects' or emotions and not the senses. Women were allegedly more prone to emotion than men, and this notion was used repeatedly to buttress the idea that women were incapable of learned pursuits.[33] Yet Poullain de la Barre (1647–1725), a former Jesuit priest, disciple of Descartes and early supporter of higher education for women, had already maintained categorically that sexual difference was essentially confined to the genitalia, and that men and women were equipped with exactly the same sense organs. He was therefore unable to find any significant differences of sense perception.[34]

—— 137 ——

In philosophical sensualism, the thesis that the external senses of women were more sensitive than those of men first appears in Henri Fouquet's article on *sensibilité* for the *Encyclopédie*, which appeared in 1765. Fouquet maintained that the more acute sensitivity of women was due mainly to the fact that they had wombs, which, according to the medical wisdom of the times, were a source of rising *vapeurs* (vapours). This is virtually all that Fouquet has to say on the subject. Just a few years later, however, two works appeared in France that dealt with the sensory-physiological peculiarities of women exhaustively: Antoine Léonard Thomas's *Essai sur le caractère, les moeurs et l'esprit des femmes dans les differents siècles* (Historical Essay on the Character, Manners and Minds of Women; Paris, 1772), and Pierre Roussel's *Système physique et moral de la femme, ou Tableau philosophique de la constitution, de l'état organique, du tempérament, des moeurs, & des fonctions propres au sexe* (Physical and Moral System of Woman, or Philosophical Tableau of the Constitution, Organic Condition, Character, Manners and Duties of the Sex; Paris, 1775).[35] Thomas believed that, if the traditional relations between the sexes were to be understood correctly, the relative strengths and weaknesses of the individual physical organs, including the sense organs, would need to be taken into account. He attributed the supposedly superior imaginative powers of women to the 'mobility' of their senses, which were directed at all objects indiscriminately and capable of keeping the impressions received in a kind of permanent storage. His explanation of the then widespread preconception that women were quick to grasp things, but apparently incapable of fathoming them, was likewise based on sensory physiological premises. The reason lay partly in the sheer variety and abundance of their sense impressions, wrote Thomas, although it was precisely this disadvantage that made their sex so appealing.

Pierre Roussel comes to similar conclusions in his book on the sensuality of women. The enduring influence of this markedly sensualistic treatise on sexuality and morality was not confined to France. In Roussel's view, women's organs were naturally softer and more flexible than men's, which explained their greater nervous sensitivity and emotional susceptibility. With no prospect of shaking off the 'tyranny' of sense impressions, women were incapable of thinking abstractly and proceeding to profounder knowledge.

A treatise by the Bordeaux physician Paul-Victor de Sèze (1760–1830), entitled *Recherches physiologiques et philosophiques sur la sensibilité des femmes, ou La Vie animale* (A Physiological and Philosophical Enquiry into the Sensibility of Women, or Animal Life; Paris, 1786), underlines the importance of these sensualistic and moral-philosophical doctrines of feminine sensibility as a means of rationalizing the existing social roles of women, and justifying their restriction to the vocation of maternity. The title itself suffices to tell us where the author is coming from. Sèze maintains, for instance, that a woman needs more natural sensory acuteness than a man in order to hear her child crying and to go and attend to it immediately – and if the latest sensory-physiological research is anything to go by, his argument would appear to be not entirely wide of the mark (see *Frankfurter Allgemeine Zeitung*, 21 October 1998). A few years later, one of Mirabeau's supporters, the above-mentioned doctor and philosopher Cabanis, produced a treatise on the physique and morality of humanity which pegged the traditional restriction of the wife to the household to her organically conditioned *sensibilité* and its concomitant physical frailty.[36]

The German physicians and physiologists of the period were likewise looking to ground their gender-specific interpretative models in empirical science. The Dresden professor of obstetrics and physician to the Saxon royal family, Carl Gustav Carus (1789–1869), was one. In 1853, for instance, he was still contending that:

a body with a noticeably hard and heavy bone structure (whether biologically male or female) is invariably a sign of male mental characteristics – strength, will-power, decisiveness and generally superior powers of comprehension – whereas a body with a soft, light and fragile skeleton (again regardless of gender) is always the sign of an essentially feminine mind, characterized accordingly by lower will-power, a softer temperament and rather more sensibility than intellectual vigour.[37]

The image of sexual characteristics projected by these French and German physiologists and empirical sensualists is thus one of paired opposites. Where man is a person of reason, woman is a creature of the senses. The potency of these ideas may be seen in the sensualistically coloured images of woman in the writings of the

German Romantics. Novalis, for instance, declares in no uncertain terms that 'reason dwells in man, feeling in woman . . . Man will therefore desire the *sensual* in a *rational* form, and woman the *rational* in a *sensual* form.'[38] His fellow poet Friedrich Schlegel delivers himself of the following instructive remark: 'Woman is outwardly magnetic and inwardly elastic. Her hands and feet are the fragile organs of her feelings, as are her nose, her mouth, her eyes and her ears.'[39] The masculine mind, on the other hand, rather resembles the eye and the ear, and sometimes even 'the less noble senses' – an allusion to both the sense of touch and the male sex organ.

The celebrated French gastronomer Brillat-Savarin (1755–1826) has some consoling words for a sex that seems otherwise left in the lurch by nature. In his opinion, unlike men, women have a 'natural' gift for the pleasures of the table: 'Gourmandism is far from unbecoming to the ladies: it agrees with the delicacy of their organs, and acts as compensation for certain pleasures which they must deny themselves, and certain ills to which nature seems to have condemned them.'[40]

Together, these examples illustrate the extent to which the 'sensual philosophers', with their interests in sensory physiology and the natural history of the senses, contributed to the polarization of gender roles in the nineteenth century. The supposed physical and mental differences between men and women were explained for the most part by the different structure of the female physique and the greater or lesser sensitivity of the sense organs that followed from it. This blending of physiological and psychological characteristics with moral-philosophical ideas stands in sharp contrast to the attempts of some early modern writers (Luther, for example) to phrase the traditional division of roles in terms of rights, duties and activities as opposed to peculiarities of character.[41]

The sense and credibility of these attempts to derive sexual characteristics from the uses of the senses were only rarely questioned at the end of the eighteenth and beginning of the nineteenth century. Jean Paul was one of the few writers who poured scorn from the beginning on the ragbag of biology, determinism and essentialism with which Roussel, de Sèze, Cabanis and other sensualistic writers of the time attempted to underpin sexual identities. In his comic fictional biography of the 'woman made of wood' based on the Pygmalion theme, Jean Paul asks rhetorically: 'If the blind Blacklock (according to Monboddo's account) could produce brilliant descriptions of visible objects that he had never seen, why should it be any more difficult for my wife to produce comparable, or even superior, poetic representations of sense impressions, feelings or thoughts with which she has no previous personal acquaintance?'[42] Jean Paul's delicious persiflage raises another of the hotly debated issues of the time, namely the specific contribution of the senses to aesthetics.

7

The Senses and Aesthetics

> To be an orator, scholar, poet or philosopher you need to feel, but you are
> not a philosopher, poet, orator or scholar merely because you feel.
>
> Denis Diderot, *Continuing Refutation*
> *of Helvétius' Work 'On Man'* (1773–4)

The sensory perception of the beautiful

In 1734, the Englishman George Stubbes (*fl.* 1697–1737) published a
dialogue in the style of Plato which dealt, among other things, with
the old issue of whether we grasp the beautiful by means of the
senses or the understanding.[1] Stubbes's fictional Socrates holds firmly
to the view that 'The Perception of Beauty is then only to be attributed to the Understanding.' His interlocutor Philebus, who is already
familiar to us from the Platonic dialogue of the same name, disputes
this: 'If the senses are not sufficient, you must at least allow them to
be necessary, to the Perception of Beauty.' But Socrates stands by his
opinion and, as usual, has the last word: 'The Mind needs not the
Assistance of the Senses in the Discovery of Intellectual Beauty.' With
regard to the pleasure we experience when contemplating a work of
art, he adds: 'It is evident that the Beauties of this Kind are only
discoverable by an Intellectual Perception; since the Taste of the elegant
Pleasures they inspire, depends on knowledge.'

At almost the same time that Stubbes was attempting to defend
the rule of reason over the fine arts, the champions of an empirical-
sensualistic concept of beauty were already beginning to make
themselves heard. In England, the leading advocate of this tendency
was Francis Hutcheson (1694–1746), with his *An Inquiry into the
Original of our Ideas of Beauty and Virtue* (1725). With reference
to Anthony Ashley Cooper Shaftesbury (1671–1713), who believed
that beauty could not be grasped by the senses but only experienced

immediately by means of some inner feeling, Hutcheson proposes a distinction between a moral faculty of judgement and a feeling of aesthetic value. His principal criterion of the aesthetically beautiful is what he calls a harmonious relationship between unity and diversity, which is perceived by the senses. Sensory perception and the pleasures associated with it originate in a natural 'sense of beauty' which is related in turn to a 'moral sense'.

The concept of taste employed by David Hume in his essay *Of the Standard of Taste* (1757) is also grounded in empirical-sensualistic experience.[2] Beauty, writes Hume, is perceived by taste ('mental taste'). He too does not regard beauty as a quality of things, though he concedes that objects may possess natural characteristics which evoke feelings of beauty. 'Beauty' is therefore defined here as a kind of correspondence or agreement between objects and sense impressions and their organs.

We encounter similar theories of the beautiful in the works of the French writers of the period who came under the influence of philosophical sensualism. Foremost among them was Charles Batteux (1713–1780), for whom the essence of art was embodied in the purely empirical imitation of natural beauty. He too regarded beauty as a kind of perfection, characterized by order, proportion and harmony. His definition is well known: 'Beauty is perfection recognized by the senses.'[3] The good and the beautiful are one and the same thing, for both 'find entry to our hearts through the senses alone.' So for him it was hardly coincidental that poetry was 'simultaneously the most sensuous expression of the good and the beautiful'.[4]

Denis Diderot also treated the sensory perception of beauty at some length in his article entitled '*Beau*' in the *Encyclopédie*: 'So when I say that something is beautiful because of the relations [*rapports*] I observe in it, I am speaking not of intellectual relations, nor of imaginary relations supplied by our fantasy, but of real, tangibly present relations perceived by our understanding [*entendement*] with the aid of the senses.'[5] Diderot draws a distinction between real beauty (*beauté réel*), which is relatively independent of the subject, and a perceived beauty (*beauté aperçu*), which exists only in relation to the person observing it. He therefore explicitly excludes the idea of absolute beauty. Thus, Diderot was not the only writer to find himself facing the question whether the blind, for example, were capable of experiencing something as beautiful. In his *Lettre sur les aveugles*

—— 143 ——

(1749), he tries to show that blind people are able to apprehend beauty by means of the sense of touch: 'The blind man learns to apply the concept of beauty correctly by examining by touch the particular arrangement we require of the parts forming a whole, if that whole is to merit the name of beauty. But when he says "that is beautiful", he is not pronouncing his own judgement, but merely repeating the judgement of those who can see.'[6] As Diderot explains in greater detail in his *Continuing Refutation of Helvétius' Work 'On Man'* (1773–4), this implies that the artist must possess perfect senses if he is to create something genuinely beautiful. A short-sighted person could never be as competent a painter, sculptor, or judge of a work of art as someone with excellent vision. The plausibility and persuasiveness of this sensualistic form of argumentation may be judged from the fact that, as late as the second half of the nineteenth century, art critics were still crediting the deaf with only very limited artistic abilities. It was thought that, though they were good copyists, their work lacked perfection. The art critic Juan Antonio Ceán Bermúdez, who was a contemporary of Francisco Goya (1746–1828), had made out a similar case. He thought that Goya's deafness was the key to an understanding of his striking painterly style (boldness of execution and dark melancholy colours).[7]

But it was not just individuals that were classified as more or less 'insensitive', and therefore poorly equipped for original artistic creation or true artistic enjoyment. As the French doctor and professor of surgery Pierre Fabre (1716–1793) claimed in his *Essai sur les facultés de l'âme, considérées dans leur rapport avec la sensibilité et l'irritabilité de nos organes* (Essay on the Faculties of the Mind, Considered in Relation to the Sensibility and Excitability of our Organs, 1785), even nations and peoples had to learn to improve their sensitivities if they were to become capable of the highest achievements in literature or drama. A beginning had been made in France by Corneille. He had been followed by Racine, whose faculty of sensation was, in Fabre's view, even greater and more highly differentiated than Corneille's. Finally, the truly great had arrived on the scene: 'Pascal, Molière, La Fontaine, Despréaux, Fénelon, Bossuet, Bourdaloue, Massilon and so on contrived to excite through their diverse productions the most intense sensations in the sensible organs of the French people, according to the various modifications of their sensible system.'[8] This sensualistically influenced doctor and philosopher suddenly surfaces as a literary critic, brandishing the sensorium as his yardstick.

Empirical theories of beauty, in which beauty was primarily attributed to nature, also developed in Germany in the first half of the eighteenth century. There are lines of connection between them and French sensualism which, as we have seen, held that nature was the *fons et origo* of beauty. Friedrich Christian Baumeister (1709–1785), who had been taught by the philosopher Christian Wolff (1679–1754), contended that beauty was perceived by means of the senses. The Swiss poetic theorist Johann Jacob Breitinger (1701–1776), on the other hand, drew upon Wolff's distinction between immaterial and material beauty during the 'literary war' in which he and his colleague Johann Jakob Bodmer (1698–1783) were ranged against Johann Christoph Gottsched (1700–1766). In his *Critische Dichtkunst* (Critical Poetics, 1740), Breitinger defines poetic beauty as 'the brightly shining ray of truth which penetrates so deeply into the senses and emotions that we are unable to prevent ourselves . . . from feeling it.'[9] Not surprisingly, Breitinger differed from Gottsched in holding that literature should engage the feelings rather than the intellect.

The birth of aesthetics

The first epistemological turning point in the contemplation of the beautiful occurs with the writings of Alexander Gottlieb Baumgarten (1714–1762). In his major philosophical work *Aesthetica* (written in Latin, 1750–8), the beautiful becomes the object of a theory of sensorial cognition, or aesthetics.[10] Under the influence of Wolff, Baumgarten assigns aesthetics to a sphere in which 'the laws of sensible and living knowledge' and the 'logic of the lower faculty of knowledge' – already touched upon by Gottfried Wilhelm Leibniz (1646–1716) – find a point of mediation. Baumgarten believed that the perfection in a work of art depended on the comprehensive organization of all the sensory powers. He distinguishes between different types of sensory ideas: perceptions and sensations (*repraesentationes sensuales*), illusions (*phantasmata*) and inventions (*figmenta vera et heterocosmica*). He agrees with Leibniz that, compared to rational or logical insights, which are derived from reason, sensory perception appears 'confused'. However, he is convinced of the existence of a 'logica facultatis cognoscitivae inferioris', or logic of the senses, and that it is one of the central objects of aesthetics. In the 'metaphysics of the beautiful', as Baumgarten once called it, beauty is defined as a perfected whole, consisting of a correspondence between the parts and the whole, which we apprehend with our senses. In this way, sensory knowledge, which is no longer reducible to logic, is incorporated into the system of philosophy under the name of aesthetics: 'Aesthetica nostra sicuti nostra logica' (§13; 'Our aesthetics is a form of logic'). The 'aesthetic horizon' assumes its proper place alongside the 'logical horizon' (§119) in the theory of perception, i.e., epistemology.

In addition to theoretical reflections of this kind, the second part of *Aesthetica* attempts to classify and categorize poetic art according to the new aesthetic criteria. However, Baumgarten does not manage to produce more than the beginnings of the 'empirical aesthetics' he had called for earlier in his *Philosophical Letters from Aletheophilus* (1704). Referring to the scientific work of Francis Bacon and Robert Boyle (1627–1691), he appealed for greater attention to the 'weaponry of the senses' and their tools ('magnifying glasses and telescopes, artificial ears . . . barometers, thermometers').[11] But his cry passed largely unheard. It was not until the twentieth century that Walter Benjamin systematically incorporated technology and technological progress into aesthetics in his celebrated essay *The Work of Art in the Age of Mechanical Reproduction* (1936). In this much-quoted work, Benjamin argues that modern techniques of reproduction have not only affected art externally, but also fundamentally altered its very nature, as a result of which eighteenth-century aesthetic concepts such as 'creativity and genius, eternal value and mystery'[12] are no longer relevant. In Germany, as we have seen, Baumgarten's *Aesthetica* marks the beginning of a turn towards subjectivity in theories of the beautiful which later acquires its definitive form in Kant's *Critique of Judgement* (1790). The Jewish philosopher and 'Aufklärer' Moses Mendelssohn, for instance, takes up Baumgarten's definitional statement that beauty consists of the recognition of sensuous perfection: 'The word [beautiful] may only be applied to things that impinge upon our senses suddenly and with great clarity.'[13] In his treatise *Briefe über die Empfindungen* (Letters on the Feelings, 1775) Mendelssohn goes on to argue that beauty is not manifold but whole and unified: 'Sameness and unity within diversity are the properties of beautiful objects. They must represent a kind of order or perfection that impacts upon our senses without any effort on our part.' Beauty also means, and at the same time dispenses, sensual pleasure: 'When we feel the desire for beauty, our mind wants to enjoy it at leisure, so to speak. Beauty must first captivate our senses and then spread to our reason.'[14] Mendelssohn's treatise on the feelings attempts to combine traditional metaphysics with sensualistic aesthetics. Thus, beauty is more than just something we grasp with our senses. It aims at a 'heavenly' perfection that can be grasped only by the reason, and not by the senses.

The very title of the programmatic work of poetic theory *Aesthetica in nuce* (Aesthetics in a Nutshell, 1762) by Johann Georg Hamann (1733–1788) establishes a connection with Baumgarten's pioneering work. According to Hamann, pure reason is a construction, for all knowledge depends on the senses. This means that the creation of humanity is also a 'sensory revelation' through which God expresses his glory. Hamann believed that the entire stock of human knowledge and happiness consisted of images: 'The senses and passions speak and understand nothing but images.'[15] He regarded poetry as 'the mother tongue of the human race' whose task was to 'purge the natural use of the senses of the unnatural use of abstractions.' The poet addresses the senses directly for, as 'the old foster-parents of beautiful nature', they have long been repressed under the harsh regime of reason and rationalistic philosophy: 'Nature operates through the senses and passions. If you mutilate their tools, how are you then supposed to experience feeling?'[16]

The *Sturm und Drang* period regarded poetry as a necessary antidote to the philosophy of the Enlightenment. To a writer such as Johann Gottfried Herder (1744–1803), who was strongly influenced by Hamann, it was the original, buried entrance to genuine life. Herder saw the poet as 'the bearer of nature to the soul and heart of his fellow men'.[17] He not only reckoned beauty to be a 'phenomenon of truth' but also thought that aesthetics had been insufficiently considered from the perspective of 'beautiful sensuousness' and that, until it was, there could be no 'fruitful theory of the beautiful in any of the arts'.[18]

Herder's contemporary Gotthold Ephraim Lessing (1729–1781) chose the example of unpleasant feelings as his way of demonstrating that there were only minor differences between poetry and painting.

He also clarified the role of the senses in the perception of the opposite of the 'beautiful' or 'pleasant'. In chapter 25 of his aesthetic treatise *Laokoon, oder Über die Grenzen der Malerei und Poesie* (Laocoon, or On the Limits of Painting and Poetry, 1766), the natural feeling of disgust is attributed to the involvement of the sense of sight along with the 'lower senses' (smell, taste and touch):

> A port-wine stain on a face, a hare-lip, a flattened nose with prominent nostrils or a complete lack of eyebrows are all ugly disfigurations which are incapable of offending the senses of smell, taste or touch. However, we certainly feel something in their presence that is much more akin to disgust than anything we might experience at the sight of other physical malformations, such as a misshapen foot or a hunched back.[19]

Turning to the purpose of this kind of sensory experience, he continues: 'But painting is not interested in portraying revolting subjects for their own sake; like poetry, it seeks to enhance our sense of the ridiculous and the terrible.'[20]

It is also worth noting in this context that Lessing's philosophical writings include a short piece with the intriguing title *Daß mehr als fünf Sinne für den Menschen sein können* (That There May be More than Five Human Senses), in which he argues that the senses determine the limits of the mind's ideas and that the senses are material in nature. This marks Lessing as an exponent of the sensualistic ideas that had already gained a foothold in Germany. On the other hand, Lessing's preface to his edition of Karl Wilhelm Jerusalem's *Philosophische Aufsätze* (Philosophical Essays, 1776) reveals how much his theory of sensuous knowledge of the beautiful owed to his friend Moses Mendelssohn. For here he quotes with approval a remark in the latter's *Briefe über die Empfindungen* to the effect that sensual pleasure is something other than a feeling of greater physical well-being, and that the connections between the body and the mind would be accompanied by feelings of mental harmony.

With the work of Johann Joachim Winckelmann (1717–1768) the restriction of aesthetic theory to sensations and feelings as practised by Hamann and his successors comes to an end. In his *History of the Art of Antiquity* (1764), this connoisseur of art, who perished in such tragic circumstances in Rome, argues the need for both a philosophical theory of beauty and a precise knowledge of the historical manifestations of art: 'In the large and lavish works describing old statues that have appeared so far, we search in vain for a proper analysis and knowledge of art. The description of a statue should demonstrate the reasons for its beauty and tell us about the peculiarities of the style of this art.'[21] Here, and for the first time, aesthetics calls for the assistance of the history of art. In his study of Greek art, Winckelmann was concerned to show the ways in which antiquity thought about beauty, and noted that 'our ideas of beauty in general are vague.'[22] The perception of beauty varied from one individual to another. Here, then, we observe the first signs of the turn to subjectivity that became Kant's guiding principle. Winckelmann saw beauty as a relative term, and this was owing not least to the fact that 'beauty is experienced by the senses, but understood by the mind.'[23] The distribution of these accomplishments simply varied from one individual or nation to another: 'The instrument of this sensation is the external sense, and its seat is the inner sense; the former must function properly and the latter must be subtle and sensitive. Many people lack the gift of good eyesight, just as there are many who are hard of hearing or have a poor sense of smell.'[24] According to Winckelmann, who was familiar with Montesquieu's ideas, climatic influences (and, at this time, the word 'climate' meant more than just the weather conditions of a country) also played a significant part in shaping the aesthetic sensibility. For this reason, 'our concepts of beauty and those of the Greeks are more correct than those accessible to peoples whose . . . view of the image of their creator is half blocked.'[25]

Thus, with Winckelmann, aesthetics takes on a new dimension. Sensations and feelings are no longer the exclusive focus of attention and begin to make way for a more historical and philosophical approach. This new approach to the aesthetically beautiful became mandatory for Lessing and Herder, as it was later for Hegel. Schelling on the other hand noted that precisely the 'historical aspect'[26] was the most crucial and difficult part of the project of the philosophy of art, although this did not deter scholars and critics from following the path marked out by Winckelmann.

By 1800, it was becoming difficult to keep track of aesthetic theories, causing Jean Paul to remark that 'we are living in an age when the aestheticians outnumber everyone else.'[27] However, this did not discourage him from producing his own *Vorschule der Ästhetik*

(Primer of Aesthetics, 1804). By this time, the idea that beauty consisted of the sensuous unity of the manifold was considered *passé*, as Jean Paul himself points out. The appearance of Kant's *Critique of Judgement* (1790) was the decisive factor in this development, for Kant systematically rejected the traditional foundations and replaced them with the principles of subjectivity and purposefulness.[28] According to Kant: 'Beautiful is what, without a concept, is liked universally' (§9, B32). From this it follows that aesthetic perception can only be subjective: 'apart from a reference to the subject's feeling, beauty is nothing by itself' (§9, B30). A science of beauty of the kind envisaged by Baumgarten was therefore impossible. Critical enquiry could only stake out the boundaries of aesthetic judgement. Aesthetics was, thus, just one more manifestation of Kant's *a priori* principles of judgement. Kant also considered the concept of usefulness to be important in aesthetic judgement. He took beauty to be 'an object's form of *purposiveness* insofar as it is perceived in the object *without the presentation of a purpose*' (§17, B61). This remarkably paradoxical notion of beauty as 'purposiveness without purpose' was later the target of much comment and criticism.

The 'analytic of beauty' to which Kant devotes the entire first section of the *Critique of Judgement* cuts the ground from under the feet of empirical and psychological methods of analysis. Not unexpectedly, his doctrine of autonomous aesthetic judgement ran into criticism from Herder, whose aesthetics were, as we have seen, strongly tinged by philosophical sensualism. Georg Wilhelm Friedrich Hegel (1770–1831) also had problems with Kant's critique of aesthetic judgement, albeit for quite different reasons. Nevertheless, he considered it 'the starting point of any true conception of the beauty of art'.[29] But notwithstanding the Kantian revolution, Hegel, like so many philosophers before him, could not refrain from devoting at least a few words of his *Philosophy of Fine Art* (1835–8) to what he saw as the restricted role of the senses in aesthetic perception. Here, it is noticeable that Hegel carefully positions the sense of smell at the bottom of the sensory hierarchy, and would probably have preferred to exclude it altogether from the purview of aesthetics.

By the time of Kant at the latest, the theory of sensuous knowledge had ceased to be an influence in aesthetics. But it was not consigned to oblivion entirely, for even neo-classical writers such as Friedrich Schiller, who thought of themselves as disciples of Kant, continued to believe that beauty was the sensible form of truth. Note also Hegel's comment that his own preferred idea of beauty as 'conformative unification (*Ineinsbildung*) of the rational and the sensuous'[30] had already been fleshed out by Schiller.

Aesthetic practice

As originally conceived by Baumgarten, that is as the science of sensuous knowledge, aesthetics was not without influence on the practice of the arts. In the age of sentiment[31] at the close of the eighteenth century, subjects and representational forms that touched the senses and feelings were increasingly a source of inspiration to artists. In his *Anthropologie für Ärzte und Weltweise* (Anthropology for Doctors and Philosophers, 1772), Ernst Platner (1744–1818) notes that, 'because of their nature and constitution', it is above all 'pleasant subjects . . . that attract the attention by stimulating the circulation of the nervous juices.' His examples are 'attractive views, beautiful paintings, finely proportioned and simple things, gleaming, cheerful, gay, sumptuous objects, certain kinds of music, spiritual and energizing drinks and smells, and so forth.'[32]

So it is not surprising that theatre, and above all musical theatre, increased in popularity during the eighteenth century. As the theatre historian Jörg Krämer has pointed out, the art of this period changed from a 'primarily representational to a fully autonomous system of sensory production, to which the multi-media form of music theatre was particularly well adapted.'[33] In the eighteenth century, the pronounced differences between visual and acoustic perception, which today's opera- and operetta-goers can still experience for themselves, were also a continual reminder of the need to discriminate between correct and incorrect perception.[34] In this connection, we might consider the controversy surrounding opera buffa, the new Italian style of music that found prominent supporters and opponents in France towards the end of the *ancien régime*.

At that time, the label 'buffonist' was synonymous with 'republican' or 'materialist', and this was hardly fortuitous. For the latter designation implied that the admirers of this unaffected and popular form of operatic music were influenced by sensualistic materialism. Inspired by Giovanni Battista Pergolesi's famous opera buffa *La serva padrona* (The Maid as Mistress), whose premiere in 1752 had divided the French audience into two camps, Jean-Jacques Rousseau wrote a comic opera entitled *Le devin du village* (The Village Sorcerer). It was first performed on 18 October 1752 at the palace of Fontainebleau. Although Rousseau thought the piece had been badly acted, the effect was 'unequalled', as he later wrote in his autobiographical *Confessions* (1782–8).[35] The music and singing were simply overwhelming and the audience was moved to tears, which confirmed Rousseau's theory that 'music acts more intimately on us, arousing through one sense affections similar to those roused through another.' 'The musician', continues the Geneva philosopher, 'will churn up the sea, fan the flames of a conflagration, cause streams to flow, rain to fall and rivers to swell. . . . However, he does not present these things immediately, but awakens within us the sensations we feel at the sight of them.'[36]

The influence of sensualistic philosophy was also evident in another, more profane and prosaic art form, namely the 'showpiece confectionery' familiar since the sixteenth century. These had always been something of a pageant of the senses, but in the eighteenth century they were 'constructed with even greater ingenuity',[37] according to the author of a standard work on court etiquette. Although now less common, they were much more lavishly and exquisitely designed than previously, and the sensual pleasures that accompanied them were intensified accordingly. It should be noted that, towards the end of the *ancien régime*, culinary aestheticism was linked very closely to the art of cooking. This meant, for instance, that the colour of a dish was only considered beautiful if it expressed its gastronomic quality.[38]

The new concept of taste

'Just as bad taste in the physical realm involves the stimulation of the palate with flavours that are too spicy and overrefined, so bad taste in the realm of art consists in taking more pleasure in artificial ornamentation than the beauty of nature',[39] wrote Voltaire in the *Dictionnaire philosophique* (1764). He is alluding to the so-called Quarrel of the Ancients and Moderns that had dominated the intellectual life of France and other countries since the end of the seventeenth century. 'Taste', which was originally a purely sensory-physiological concept, soon began to be introduced into discussions of correct social conduct (*honnêteté*). It then went on to acquire a wide range of meanings in the debate surrounding the use of classical literature as a model of literary style, which numbered Jean de La Bruyère (1645–1696) among its distinguished French exponents. According to La Bruyère, who sided with the 'Ancients', or classicists, it was the possession of (literary) taste that enabled us to recognize aesthetic excellence. The decisive moment of this process was the 'point of perfection', which, according to the literary historian Hans Robert Jauss, is reached when 'taste experiences the work of art's agreement or lack of agreement with its own ideal, the correspondence or non-correspondence of the beauty perceived with the most perfect beauty imaginable.'[40] La Bruyère's adversary Charles de Saint-Evremond (*c.*1616–1703), on the other hand, argued that judgements of taste were temporal and therefore changeable: 'The tastes of earlier centuries have no monopoly on truth . . . , the genius of our own century is entirely contrary to the spirit of fables and false mysteries.'[41]

Charles Perrault (1628–1703), who was the most prominent representative of modernity, appealed not least to taste in his campaign against the domination of art by classical rules. He rejected the law of mimesis and embraced the view that aesthetic judgements could only ever be subjective. The only guideline for artistic and literary creation was the 'goust de ce siecle', 'the taste of the present age'.[42] Readers and audiences may once have preferred classical literature, but tastes had changed in the meantime, so this was no longer the case. Perrault also emerges as a believer in progress. In his view, it was the privilege of the modernists of any age to add their contribution to the perfection of taste. Thus, while the 'Moderns' propagated a relativistic concept of taste (*beau relatif*), which did not preclude a gradual refinement of artistic and literary quality, the 'Ancients' clung to the principle of imitation and proclaimed the tastes of classical antiquity as absolute standards of judgement.

In both the rationalistic and sensualistic schools of enlightened thought, the concept of taste is a key term in the philosophical quest for criteria of aesthetic judgement. Rationalists such as Jean-Pierre de Crousaz (1663–1750) believed that reason decided taste and was fully capable of arbitrating doubtful cases correctly. But reason could also be refined by taste. Taste was assigned largely to nature and the world of feelings or sentiments (*sentiments*), whereas judgement was credited with powers of reflection. As we have already seen, the French sensualists thought that the purpose of a work of art was to release feelings and to produce pleasure by awakening the senses. One of their most prominent representatives on the terrain of aesthetics was Jean-Baptiste Dubos (1670–1742), whose *Réflexions critiques sur la poésie et la peinture* (Critical Reflections on Poetry and Painting, 1719) influenced not only Diderot, Voltaire and other *encyclopédistes* but also leading German-speaking aesthetic theorists (Bodmer, Breitinger, Lessing). Dubos declared that, 'since the primary purpose of poetry and painting is to move us, poems and paintings are only meritorious to the extent that they touch us and appeal to us.' This was a radical rejection of rationalistic epistemology, which had equated art with reason. To express the immediacy and spontaneity of judgements of taste, Dubos resorted to his famous comparison of art to cooking in the domain of physiological taste: 'We possess a sense that enables us to tell whether a chef has followed the rules of his art correctly. I do not need to be acquainted with these rules in order to judge his ragout. I simply know if the ragout is good.'[43] According to Dubos, all human beings possess an innate 'sixth' sense that enables them to pronounce aesthetic judgements.

The debate on the concept of taste in eighteenth-century France shows how the conceptual range of taste was being redefined and expanded. Philosophers, artists and men of letters were no longer interested primarily in the moral aspects of taste. Although still clearly based on the physiological sense of taste, the figurative use of the term henceforth subserved rationalistic or sensationalistic distinctions between good and bad art or literature.

The same applies to the German-speaking world, where French theories of taste had found followers at a fairly early stage. One of the major German works on the subject was the *Untersuchung von dem guten Geschmack* (Enquiry Concerning Good Taste, 1727) by Johann Ulrich König (1668–1744), where we find the following definition: 'Taste is the sensation which is born in the common sense from the impressions received by our sense organs. As Dubos has stated, it is the sense that judges the value of all things.'[44] The author, who was a court poet at Dresden, distinguishes in detail between a 'moral' taste, which regulates social behaviour, and a 'sentient' taste, which plays a vital role in aesthetics. König's most important achievement was undoubtedly his introduction of French theories of taste to Germany, which paved the way for Baumgarten's empirical-sensualistic aesthetics.

With Kant's *Critique of Judgement*, the debate on the concept of taste reaches a turning point which may also be regarded as a terminus. Given the conflict of opinion among sensationalists and rationalists, it was necessary to find a way of doing justice to the sensorial aspect of judgements of taste, while at the same time guaranteeing their general validity and intersubjectivity. Kant manages to accommodate these two very different demands by, on the one hand, stressing the subjectivity of the cognitive faculty and, on the other hand, by explicitly confirming the aprioristic general validity of aesthetic judgement:

> The principle of taste is the subjective principle of the power of judgment as such. A judgment of taste differs from logical judgment in that a logical judgment subsumes a presentation under concepts of the object, whereas a judgment of taste does not subsume it under any concept at all, since otherwise the necessary universal approval could be [obtained] by compelling [people to give it]. But a judgment of taste does resemble a logical judgment inasmuch as it alleges a universality and necessity, though a universality and necessity that is not governed by concepts of the object and hence is merely subjective. (§35, B145)

With this, taste becomes a transcendental concept, leaving no room for further arguments about the role of aesthetic judgement.

After Kant's historical-philosophical break, it is only in contexts where the concept of taste is used in its original, physiological sense, namely regarding the consumption of food, that opinion may continue to be divided. While nineteenth-century Germany witnessed 'an elevation of the fine arts at the expense of the culinary arts'[45] – with the latter being banished to the level of the lower senses (notably by Hegel) – developments in France took a somewhat different course. There, Jean Anthelme Brillat-Savarin published his (initially anonymous) *Physiology of Taste* (1826), whose basic affirmation of sensualism was, in fact, only apparently at odds with Kantian theory. According to Brillat-Savarin, the taste judgements of the genuine epicure will differ from those of a person to whom 'nature has denied either an organic delicacy or a power of concentration, without which the most delicious dishes can pass them by unnoticed.'[46] But it is also perfectly possible for taste to be acquired. This was demonstrated not least by the pedagogical attempts to train the supposedly undeveloped or retarded gustatory senses of children such as the wild boy of Aveyron and Kaspar Hauser, who had grown up either in total isolation or out in the wilderness, by allowing them to sample different kinds of food. At a more elevated level, Brillat-Savarin's gastronomical treatise may be read as a scientific introduction to the pleasures of the table, and as such it found many imitators in France (e.g., Alexandre Balthazar-Laurent Grimond de la Reynière, Alexandre Dumas).[47] Unlike in France, however, gastronomy failed to develop into a subject of general interest on the other side of the Rhine. Consider, for example, the first edition of *Gastrosophie, oder Die Lehre von den Freuden der Tafel* (Gastrosophy, or The Science of the Pleasures of the Table, 1852) by a German gourmet and amateur of the taste buds named Friedrich Christian Eugen von Vaerst (1792–1855). This was still not sold out in 1918, whereas Brillat-Savarin's book went through several editions within a few years of publication.

— 8 —

The Education of the Senses

To train the senses it is not enough merely to use them; we must learn to
judge by their means, to learn to feel, so to speak; for we cannot touch,
see, or hear, except as we have been taught.
Jean-Jacques Rousseau, *Emile, or Education* (1762)

The training of the senses

With Augustine leading the way, the early Church Fathers had castig-
ated the moral failings of the senses and called for the disciplining
of covetous looks and pleasure-seeking eavesdropping – to say nothing of the lascivious fondling of one's own or someone else's body.
Yet throughout the Middle Ages and into the modern era, the attitudes of ecclesiastical writers to this subject were marked by a certain
ambivalence. For their strictures were aimed not at sensory perception as such, but merely at the undisciplined or unseemly use of the
sense organs. For all that they preached the dangers and sinfulness of
the senses, they were hardly in a position to deny their spiritual or
religious use value. The English writer and clergyman Thomas Adams
(*c*.1590–1653/5) is an exemplary figure in this tradition of 'sensory
ambivalence' (Ludwig Schrader). In one of his popular sermons he
preaches the chastisement of the senses, while at the same time crediting Christianity with actual victory in the struggle against unbridled
sensuality. 'The eye, the ear, the foote, the hand, though wild and
unruly enough, have been tamed.'[1]

The notion that vice, with which every single one of the senses has
some association, may also be enlisted in the service of God-pleasing
virtue is nowhere more clearly expressed than in the writings of
Ignatius of Loyola (1491–1556), who tenders the following piece of
advice to a young Jesuit who was complaining that the 'constant
suppression of his sensuality' was depriving him of his energies:

'For the sake of always having one's powers available for the service of God, it is often more meritorious to allow the senses some kind of respectable diversion, rather than to suppress them.'[2] The suppression of the senses was precisely the purpose of the 'application of the senses' preached by Loyola in his famous *Spiritual Exercises*. Written in 1548, this highly influential religious-didactic tract contained rules and instructions for the noviciates of the Society of Jesus and became one of the most formative documents of the Counter-Reformation. The aim of the exercises was to purify the soul and temper the passions, and in this context Loyola's main concern was the five senses: 'If anyone wishes to imitate Christ our Lord in the use of the senses, he should recommend himself to His Divine Majesty, and after the consideration of each sense say a *Hail Mary* or an *Our Father*' (*Exercises*, no. 248). Loyola is speaking quite specifically about the sensorial experience of God in line with the medieval tradition of the *imitatio Christi*. He also urges the reader to contemplate the fires of hell and to concentrate his thoughts on the depravity that is often the companion of sense perception, and on the punishment that awaits it in the world to come:

> See in imagination the vast fires, and the souls enclosed, as it were, in bodies of fire . . . hear the wailing, the howling, cries, and blasphemies against Christ our Lord and all His saints . . . with the sense of smell, perceive the smoke, the sulphur, the filth, and corruption. . . . taste the bitterness of tears, sadness, and remorse of conscience . . . with the sense of touch feel the flames which envelop and burn the souls. (*Exercises*, nos. 66–70)

The counterpart to this decidedly sensorial evocation of the torments of hell is the use of the senses at the end of the first day of the second week of the exercises, when senses such as smell and taste are given the much more agreeable task of savouring the infinite sweetness and loveliness of God (*Exercises*, nos. 122–5).[3] This particular form of 'coming to one's senses' may be interpreted either as a form of mystical contemplation or simply as an unusually intense form of prayer. It is anyhow clear from his instructions that Ignatius of Loyola's spiritual exercises gave central importance to the sensuous experience of faith.

In its struggle for human souls, the Counter-Reformation owed much of its success to its exploitation of the five senses, for this helped to turn faith into something that could be experienced directly by the senses, whereas Protestantism preferred on the whole to rely on the power of the written and spoken word. The same considerations apply by and large to Anglicanism, which, although not as moralistic and ascetic as Protestantism, is not known to be particularly full of the joys of life. It is all the more surprising, therefore, to find the senses featured as the topic of a nineteenth-century Anglican service for children. In a sermon given at the church of St James the Less, London, the Reverend Joseph Maskell asked the congregation of children and young persons: 'Is it not a reproach to those who have all their senses and yet use them so ill, to think of what others far less favoured have done?'[4] Maskell was referring less to sins committed with the senses than to the manifest unreasonableness of this alleged misuse of the sense organs. He believed that the senses were the tools of reason, and that they therefore needed to be treated carefully and used with prudence. It followed that: 'Every sense may be trained if it be used with perseverance and judgement. We must indeed avoid *over use* of any sense, for that is most truly an abuse of it.'[5] The Anglican clergyman supplied his young audience with plenty of concrete examples, warning them, for instance, against overstraining their eyes by reading for long periods at night by artificial light. The central preoccupation of this remarkable sermon (which was printed in 1888) was thus not so much spiritual salvation as the potential damage to the body from the improper use of the senses. Instead of religious instruction in the avoidance of evil, the children received a lesson in the correct, i.e., rational, use of their senses. The Reverend Maskell thus stands apart from the tradition of the spiritual writers of the Middle Ages and early modern era, with their continuous denunciations of the depravity of the senses. He turns out to be a proponent of the modern educational ideas that had shaped the discourse of the senses since the appearance of Rousseau's *Emile, or Education* (1762).

The French sensualists had already insisted that the perfection of the human being hinged on the refinement of the senses. Rousseau adopted sensory education as the programme of the Enlightenment and the movement for educational reform. *Emile*, for instance, contains the story of a soldier who in younger years was taken by his father to a hospital for venereal diseases. 'This hideous and revolting spectacle sickened the young man.'[6] According to Rousseau, this

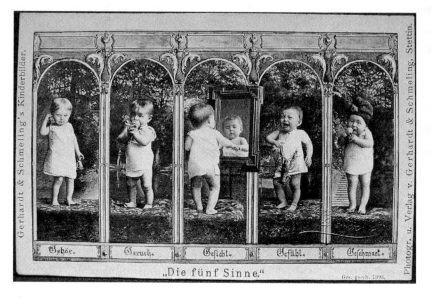

Figure 8.1   Training the senses in infancy: allegory of the five senses; photograph (1893)

drastic piece of visual instruction had later restrained the young man from involvement in amorous adventures. But the education of the senses was not confined to the period of adolescence. As Rousseau insists, it was vital for the senses to receive proper training from early infancy: 'The senses are the first of our faculties to mature; they are those most frequently overlooked or neglected.'[7]

A few decades later, this was all a thing of the past. Rousseau's words had fallen on fertile ground. In 1785, the German educationalist and publisher Johann Heinrich Campe (1746–1818) introduced a training programme for the five senses which was intended primarily for children up to the age of two. Johann Heinrich Pestalozzi (1746–1827) declared that, in their natural state, the senses were similar to those of animals: 'Mother! The brutal impressions of things that enter your child through the senses lie inside that child in a state of confusion, disorder and darkness.'[8] The Swiss educationalist insisted that this chaos of sense impressions could only be reduced to order by early training. Johann Christoph Gutsmuths (1759–1839), who is hardly remembered today, expressly included the schooling of the senses in his *Anweisung zur Leibesübung* (Instructions for Physical Exercise, 1793), laying special emphasis on the training of the sense of touch. One of the exercises involved blindfolding pupils and placing various gold and silver coins in their hands, which they then had to identify by touch. Friedrich Wilhelm August Fröbel (1782–1852), whose name is still associated with the introduction of the kindergarten, devised all kinds of 'games for the limbs and senses', which were intended to 'eradicate sensual impulses and thoughtlessness in any shape or form.'[9]

A conduct book published in Tübingen in 1834 reveals that physical training in the widest sense of the word was not the sole purpose of the painstakingly constructed courses in sensory education that appeared in the wake of Rousseau. With reference to the sense of touch, the author of the book, the writer, painter and poet Carl Friedrich von Rumohr (1785–1845), writes that: 'A soft skin and supple wrist movements are also required for touching, stroking and pointing at objects, for actions of this kind play an important part in polite conduct.'[10] The doctor and author Daniel J. Schreber (1808–1861), who had campaigned since the 1840s for the creation of the garden allotments that were subsequently named after him,* urged educators to encourage young people 'thoroughly to grasp the fine details of things perceptible to the senses'[11] and to include in their curricula exercises aimed at the sharpening of the senses. British and American educational advisers of the period made similar recommendations. A little book by Horace Grant (1865–1944), entitled *Exercises for the Improvement of the Senses for Young Children* (1886), contained tips such as identifying flowers by sniffing their scent through a handkerchief, or blindfolding little children and have them feel for pencils, paper and pebbles. Even ordinary writing lessons were turned into opportunities for sensory training. The German clergyman and pedagogue Johann Heinrich Schöne (1804–?), who invented the so-called *Taktschreibmethode* (isorhythmic typing method), saw the merits of his system in its capacity to discipline 'the eye, ear, hand, arm, indeed the whole body, including the intelligence'.[12]

As was only to be expected, one of the most popular health guides of the second half of the nineteenth century included medical

---

* Garden allotments are known as *Schrebergärten* in German.

—— 161 ——

advice on how to exercise the senses: 'Given that it is the senses that supply the brain with the intellectual nourishment necessary to the development and training of the human mind, they must be carefully trained and cared for if they are to serve their essential purpose.'[13] So the organ of smell should be cleaned regularly, and children should be told to avoid picking their noses for fear of damaging the sensitive mucous membrane. Yet for the best part of the nineteenth century the risk of nasal injury was a minor cause of concern compared to the amount of attention devoted to so-called self-pollution, or masturbation. In his famous book *L'Onanisme*, Samuel Auguste André David Tissot (1728–1797) had already argued against the arbitrary expenditure of semen, claiming that it dulled the senses, 'particularly sight and hearing'.[14]

Rousseau's theory of education was based on freedom rather than compulsion and envisaged punishment only as a means of last resort, although there was little evidence of this sublime ideal in the practices of schools. In the so-called disciplinary institutions, on the other hand, there was no conflict between education and punishment. Both the national armies, which laid greater stress on military drill and discipline after the eighteenth century, and the systems of criminal justice were looking more inquisitively at the 'teachable body' (Michel Foucault) and beginning to integrate it into a system of 'discipline and punishment'.

In contrast to the schools, which foregrounded the education of the senses, the prison was an eminently suitable place for the practice of 'sensory isolation'. This was the term used by the German doctor and author Ludwig Friedrich Froriep (1779–1847) to describe a scheme for prison reform which he touted as a humane form of punishment (see figure 8.2): 'Furthermore, I am convinced that the use of these methods of rendering prisoners temporarily blind, deaf and deaf-mute can easily be learned and practised by male and female prison guards, and that prison doctors and surgeons will be fully capable of advising and instructing them in their application.'[15] Froriep rejected accusations that the isolation of the senses by facial masks and leather ear flaps was a crueller form of punishment than solitary confinement, arguing that 'sensory isolation is, in actual fact, a far less severe measure than solitary confinement, for there are several ways of modifying these devices to make them more comfortable, without detriment to their main purpose of preventing communication,

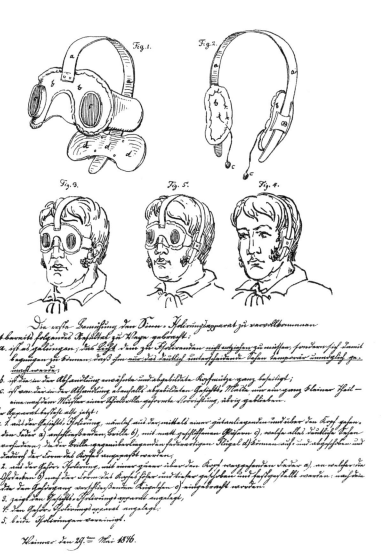

Figure 8.2 The isolation of vision and hearing according to L. F. Froriep (1846)

and, also, they need only be used for as long as it takes to achieve their purpose.'

Froriep tried to refute the second objection – that the implementation of his plan would present too many difficulties and jeopardize the prisoners' health – by referring his critics to the three medical authorities who had approved his suggestions. He also tried to rebut the criticism that, unlike the famous model penitentiary in Pennsylvania, his 'sensory isolation' did not guarantee total sensory deprivation. Quite the contrary. While Froriep's method did not absolutely exclude the possibility of physical contact between the prisoners on whom it was practised, it was of no consequence, for the prisoners concerned would be quite incapable of interpreting the meaning of such incidental bodily encounters.

But Froriep's clinching argument was undoubtedly the low costs involved in implementing his plan. A solitary confinement cell cost between 700 and 800 talers; his sensory deprivation system cost practically nothing. It could also be used in communal dormitories. The prisoners need simply be assigned to rooms according to certain categories. Institutional regulations would naturally have to be amended in accordance with the requirements of sensory isolation. A second economic advantage was that the prisoners would be able to continue working, since in most cases only the sense of hearing would need to be closed off. A further advantage was that 'young criminals located in any part of the prison would be able to take part in communal religious and spiritual instruction with isolated eyes, and assemble for work and meals with isolated ears.'[16] Furthermore, Froriep's cost-effective model was particularly well adapted to the occasional transportation of prisoners, temporary police arrest and appearances before courts martial. The face mask and ear flaps had also been tested successfully on persons suffering from mental disorders such as maniacal fury.

However inhumane such proposals may appear today, they represent the crux of an infiltration of the penal system by pedagogic, psychological and medical practices that had been under way since the beginning of the nineteenth century. Froriep's ideas appear to have met with little response in Germany, but at the beginning of the 1840s a system similar to his was introduced at the famous, and infamous, Pentonville prison in London. There, the inmates were taken out of their cells in facial masks at eight in the morning and led off to morning service in the prison chapel, where the seats were divided from each other by side walls to forestall eye-contact between prisoners.[17]

The disciplining of the gaze

The training of vision takes up the lion's share of the space in the many conduct books and educational manuals published in the late eighteenth and early nineteenth century. But the 'disciplina oculorum' was not invented by the Enlightenment. It had a tradition reaching back to the Middle Ages. For a long period it was confined to certain social groups (the court elite and women). In the course of the evolution of civilization, which is by no means as linear as Norbert Elias assumes, the chaste look not only becomes binding on but is flanked by measures intended to sharpen the sense of vision. This process is accompanied by the emergence of what Michel Foucault has called the eyes that 'see without being seen'.[18] The symbol of this development was the 'panopticon', or centralized prison, presented in blueprint by the English philosopher and reformer Jeremy Bentham (1748–1832) in 1791. 'The concept of the panopticon was one of the first instances of the mechanical conditioning of the sense of sight', observes Marie-Anne Berr.[19]

This disciplining of the gaze applied to both seeing and being seen and could be implemented most effectively within the setting of institutional disciplinary regimes. Besides early nineteenth-century prisons, barracks and orphanages were also built in the form of a panopticon. At the end of the eighteenth century, the living quarters of the famous Ecole Militaire in Paris consisted of austerely furnished cells, where the cadets were locked up for the night and kept under observation through windows. Even the communal lavatories were constructed so as to allow the duty overseer to see the cadets' heads and feet. By no means all such 'total' institutions followed this example, however. When the Zurich orphanage was rebuilt in 1771, the authorities insisted on separating the lavatories from each other by 'modesty walls',[20] and providing them with doors that made it impossible for anyone to look directly into the 'secret closet', as the toilet was then called. From the second half of the nineteenth century onwards, screens and partitions of this kind were built into all types of mass accommodation and public toilet facilities. In tenement houses, where there was just one toilet to each floor, the 'visual field' was similarly restricted.[21]

'Great importance attaches to the decent government of the eyes', writes Julius Bernhard von Rohr in his *Einleitung zur Ceremoniel-Wissenschafft der Privat-Personen* (Introduction to the Science of Personal Decorum, 1728), which became one of the best-known conduct books of the eighteenth century. This pedagogical requisite is already in evidence in early modern writings on the subject of *civilité*, Erasmus of Rotterdam's *De civilitate morum puerilium* (1530) being one celebrated example. In 1826, almost three hundred years later, the idea received medical backing from the celebrated physiologist Johannes Müller (1801–1858): 'The eye must learn how to make full use of the wealth of movements at its disposal without descending into self-indulgence.'[22] This influential physician considered healthy sensuousness to be inconceivable without proper observation of the decencies. A few years later, Rumohr argued a similar case in his *Schule der Höflichkeit für Alt und Jung* (School of Etiquette for Old and Young, 1834): 'Few people fully understand the enormous value of good eyesight, which explains the complete neglect of the care and training of the eyes in both domestic instruction and public education.'[23] He advised people to spare their eyes by refraining from reading in half-light and by occasionally lifting their heads to look into the distance during periods of intensive reading. Another conduct book of the period recommended the cultivation of a serene gaze 'from which everything gloomy, morose and surly has been banished, so that our eyes become a mirror of the natural contentment of our soul.'[24]

In his essay on nature (1826), the American author Ralph Waldo Emerson (1803–1882) noted that the health of the eyes depended on keeping the horizon as the boundary of the gaze when looking at landscapes. Doctors who had read Emerson, and also the works of his colleague Henry David Thoreau (1817–1862), advised their patients to allow their gaze to wander over nature and enjoy the beauty of the landscape, which would also be good for their mental and physical well-being.[25] The Görlitz doctor Christian August Struve (1767–1807), who wrote popular health manuals, had already dispensed the same sort of advice. To strengthen the eyes he recommended 'carefully organized visual exercises',[26] regular excursions into the open countryside and the sight of fresh foliage. These sensory exercises recall Rousseau's recommendations for children and included accustoming the eyes to darkness and assessing distances while out walking.

Some late eighteenth- and early nineteenth-century writers thought that the eyesight needed protection against other sources of damage. Diderot's *Encyclopédie* contains a passing note to the effect that masturbation was bad for the eyes. A decade later, the medical consequences of this 'sin of the flesh' were the subject of the popular work by Tissot mentioned above. Tissot's book on masturbation went through numerous editions and was translated into many languages, and includes a quotation from a letter to the author from a patient who had allegedly contracted venereal disease from the practice. As a result of the infection, so the patient claimed, his eyes had become 'sunk and always weak'.[27]

Well into the nineteenth century, doctors and laymen continued to believe that masturbation weakened the eyes. With Friedrich Nietzsche in mind, Richard Wagner (1813–1883) was persuaded that masturbation led to blindness. A doctor of his acquaintance reassured the worried composer that onanism could be considered responsible for the manifestly poor eyesight of the author of *Thus Spake Zarathustra* only in a very general sense.[28] In those days, 'self-pollution' was considered essentially a problem for young males, but doctors and theologians also sometimes accused women and young girls of this 'sin'. Although otherwise difficult to detect, female masturbation was thought to be deducible from external signs such as weak eyesight and aversion to light. Perhaps this explains one of the instructions contained in the *Rules of Christian Decorum and Civility* (1703) by Jean-Baptiste de la Salle (1651–1719), which was one of the most famous French conduct books of the early eighteenth century: 'Decorum requires that you cover your body when going to bed and avoid giving it the slightest glance.'[29]

Training the ears

'All misery . . . comes from hearing',[30] proclaimed the voluble preacher Abraham a Santa Clara in a theological interpretation of the event of listening: Adam and Eve had heard God's commandment but had failed to pay attention to it, and mankind had fallen. A century and a half later, even Christian circles had adopted a somewhat less negative approach to the sense of hearing. A little English book with the revealing title *The Christian Physiologist* (1830) merely glosses the biblical passage to which the Viennese preacher had referred with a cautionary note on all too frivolous listening: 'I plead only for a measured and rational caution in the acquirement of information.'[31] In the sermons of Joseph Maskell, which appeared a few decades later, one finds none of the traditional references to the sense of hearing as a source of moral peril. Quite the reverse: 'Truly we ought to thank God for the gift of this wonderful sense, to cultivate it and to employ it in the best possible manner.'[32] According to Maskell, a Christian education should be concerned rather to protect the hearing against possible damage. Excessive smoking and alcohol consumption were among the bad habits likely to impair the sense, and Maskell concludes his warning to his juvenile congregation with the words: 'Thus keeping our senses morally and physically pure, they will always be sensitive to that which is good and quickly find out and avoid whatever is evil.'[33] It followed that the sense of hearing should not only be kept healthy but also be trained, and he thought that singing lessons were a suitable way of achieving this.

Johannes Amos Comenius (1592–1670), who was undoubtedly the most famous educational theorist of the seventeenth century, was not only responsible for introducing the practice of sitting quietly that is still so heartily detested by many of today's schoolchildren. He also recommended musical instruction from the age of four ('let them learn to whistle and tinkle away, let their ears be led to melodies of every kind').[34] The training of the sense of hearing enters pedagogy definitively with Rousseau. For Rousseau, however, singing and vocal training were just means to the end of refining the ear: 'We need a quick ear, and power to judge from the sensations experienced whether the body which causes them is large or small, far off or near, whether its movements are gentle or violent.'[35] Similar motives led Johann Peter Frank (1745–1821), the author of a work in several volumes entitled *System einer vollständigen medicinischen Policey* (System of Complete Medical Administration, 1779–1827), to declare the 'delectation of the common people by the musical art' a medical issue. In his opinion, public health authorities should 'provide good musicians to delight the ear of the listener and dispel the demons of sadness during melancholy hours.'[36]

What applied to singing also applied to the eighteenth-century theatre. In an essay entitled *Über das gegenwärtige deutsche Theater* (On the German Theatre of the Present Age) Friedrich Schiller complained that the poor dramatic diction of many actors was 'sickeningly tiring to the ears'.[37] This could hardly have applied to the Jesuit theatre of the time, for otherwise there would not have been so many complaints that these performances imposed too much of a strain on the eyes and ears.

But the training of the sense was not just a matter of making it more sensitive. To cope with the attacks of anxiety that he attributed to the oversensitivity of his auditory nerves, Goethe came up with his own desensitization therapy. During military tattoos, he would position himself close to the drummers, 'whose tumultuous rolls and beats would have shattered the heart in your breast.'[38] The philosopher Arthur Schopenhauer (1788–1860) later referred to Goethe's anecdote when commenting on his own acute sensitivity to noise: 'We will not be truly civilized until the ears cease to be fair game, and no one has the right to intrude upon the consciousness of every thinking being within a range of a thousand paces with his whistling, shouting, yelling, hammering, whip-cracking, barking etc.'[39]

The art of silence was an important element in the education of hearing from the very beginning. Had Schopenhauer lived in the immediate neighbourhood of a school, he would undoubtedly have been delighted with the lessons in keeping quiet that were a required part of the curriculum at the time, despite their limited practical success. *Die deutsche Volksschule* (The German Elementary School, 3rd edn, 1876), which was the standard pedagogical work of the time, only describes the ideal: 'The pupils are sitting glued to their seats; no one dares to make the slightest movement; everyone is looking straight at the teacher . . . , if the teacher were not speaking we would hear a pin drop.'[40] The sorely tried sense of hearing was also occasionally granted some small relief on the cacophonous factory floors of the nineteenth century. 'Singing, whistling and other disturbances of the peace'[41] of a private nature were expressly forbidden by the factory regulations of the time, on pain of punishment. Here, however, the health of the factory workers was a minor concern, for the main point of such measures was the maintenance of general discipline and order.

In prisons, which laid particular stress on institutional discipline, the imposition of silence had a quite different rationale. Its primary purpose was to prevent communication in the cells, corridors and exercise yards. The proposal of the German prison reformer Froriep to force prisoners to wear 'earmufflers' when not in the solitary confinement cells is a perfect expression of this intention. This item of prisonwear consisted of cotton-lined leather ear-flaps with small rubber cones fixed to them, which fitted into the opening of the ear. To do him justice, Froriep did consider it worth mentioning briefly that the human guinea pigs on whom he tried out this corrective apparatus complained of an unpleasant, albeit temporary, buzzing in their ears.

The refinement of smell

In literature dealing with the senses we occasionally encounter the assumption that, like the sense of taste, the sense of smell was largely spared the 'civilizing dressage of the body'.[42] The historical facts do not support this, although it is clearly apparent that the refinement of the sense of smell was not accorded the same priority as the perfection of vision and hearing. The crown witness is once again Rousseau. In his system of sensory education, the sense of smell is typically the lowest item on the agenda, the reason being the dwindling evolutionary importance of the sense of smell in the discovery of sources of nutrition: 'Indeed I believe that if children were trained to scent their dinner as a dog scents game, their sense of smell might be nearly as perfect; but I see no very real advantage to be derived from this sense, except by teaching the child to observe the relation between sense and smell.'[43] Rousseau therefore saw little purpose in training the sense of smell from infancy – which would, of course, have involved restoring the child to that original state of nature in which his disciples a few decades later fancied they had discovered the 'wild child' of Aveyron and Kaspar Hauser.

Rousseau was thus simply concerned not to allow the sense of smell to atrophy any further, and this then became the purpose of the enlightened health-care pedagogy pursued by educationalists after the end of the eighteenth century. In 1859, Dr Daniel Schreber, whom we mentioned above, recommended exercising the sense of smell by 'not only comparing (with closed eyes) thousands of differently scented blossoms, leaves and roots, but also the smells of various kinds of wood (both living and dead) and earth etc.'[44] Carl Ernst Bock's health manual (7th edn, 1890) cautioned against the continual overstimulation of the olfactory nerves with 'strong smells and invigorating kinds of air'.[45] At around the same time, towards the end of the 1880s, the Reverend Joseph Maskell was claiming that long periods of exposure to bad air were extremely harmful to the sense of smell.

The consensus of the times was that badly aired sick-rooms and foul-smelling lavatories were the principal sources of wear and tear on the olfactory nerves, for which the best antidote was frequent exposure to fresh air. So olfactory education on the one hand cultivated a sensitivity to pleasant, less overpowering odours, and on the other hand put its faith in the avoidance of places where dreadful stenches lurked. An example from the city of Zurich shows that this dual strategy enjoyed a certain success even in the nineteenth century. As part of the city's mid-nineteenth-century public hygiene programme, the majority of houses acquired new and relatively odourless flushing toilets in place of the old earth closets. A few years later, the city council was complaining of the lack of tolerance shown by the users of the new sanitary installations: 'Since the conversions, [many people] have become oblivious of the frightful conditions of the past and are suddenly very quick to criticize, and become very incensed if the privies – whose windows they often keep permanently closed, while carelessly leaving the seats up and allowing the bowls to become caked in excrement – are not exactly free of smells.'[46] According to a survey completed in 1896, only 20 per cent of households in the first district of Zurich, which was home to the wealthier middle classes, lacked water closets. On the other hand, the vast majority (90 per cent) had no toilet siphons to expel smells.

There can be no question about it: an investigation conducted in 1897 by the Frankfurt Tenants' Association demonstrates clearly that, as more and more city dwellers began to feel disturbed by the permanent presence of the smell of other people's excrement and urine, the purification of the air of living areas developed into one of the concrete utopias of the late nineteenth century. A now privately owned collection of eight phials dating from the rococo age, each bearing the inscription 'air des femmes' – airtight jars containing 'women's farts', in other words – would probably have struck people even then as the bizarre hobby of a smell fetishist.

As we have already indicated, even fragrant smells were thought to be harmful to the sense of smell, particularly when used to excess. Rousseau had already cautioned against the bewitching scents of the boudoir with their promise of erotic adventure, and praised the 'man of dull feelings' with no nose for seductive perfumes. The extremely ambivalent character of smell, particularly in the intimate realm, is demonstrated by the books of marital advice and related publications which appeared around 1800. In one of them, we encounter the informative observation that very few men regarded the 'anchovy-butter smell of the stinking whore'[47] as an aphrodisiac. In the context of the connection between smell perception and sexual behaviour, the theory of the now forgotten American surgeon John Noland Mackenzie (1853–1925) deserves a passing mention. According to Mackenzie, there were a number of correlations between a sensitive nose and the stimulation of the male and female genitals. This was a version of the nasal reflex theory mentioned in an earlier chapter. At the turn of the twentieth century, its adherents included such distinguished psychiatrists as Wilhelm Fließ, Sigmund Freud and Joseph Breuer.

The perfection of the sense of taste

The refinement of taste was the central preoccupation of the gastronomic literature that enjoyed such huge demand in France at the end of the eighteenth century. This kind of writing soon found imitators in a number of other countries, although books addressed to gourmets and would-be gourmets were of rather limited appeal in countries such as Germany and England.

Joseph Addison (1672–1719) had already poked fun at French gourmets in the pages of *The Tatler* at the beginning of the eighteenth century: 'They are not to approve any thing that is agreeable to ordinary palates; and nothing is to gratify their Senses, but what would offend those of their Inferiors.'[48] In his socio-critical study *The Condition of the Working Class in England* (1844), written a century later, Friedrich Engels (1790–1860) drew attention to the fact that the sophistication of the sense of taste differed not only from country to country but also between the classes within countries: 'But the poor, the working-people, to whom a couple of farthings are important, who must buy many things with little money, who cannot afford to inquire too closely into the quality of their purchases, and cannot do so in any case because they have had no opportunity of cultivating their taste – to their share fall all the adulterated, poisoned provisions.'[49] All the same, as anyone can tell from a glance at a nineteenth-century English cookery book, the social gulf between *haute cuisine* and plain cooking was nowhere near as wide in Victorian England as in a country such as France. Indeed, it is difficult to avoid the conclusion that the contemporaries of Queen Victoria 'were lacking in any sense of the *enjoyment* of food.'[50] The cultivation of taste was for a long time the preserve of the French, who were pioneers in the field of gastronomy and are still renowned for their culinary arts and temples of gourmandism.

The purpose of the education of the senses as propagated above all by Rousseau, and taken up by his European disciples in the late eighteenth and early nineteenth centuries, was largely hygienic and thus concerned only partially with the refinement of taste. The celebrated author of *Emile* believed that divine providence had taught man how to recognize healthy and wholesome food by means of his palate. For this reason, the natural sense of taste should not be refined and spoiled unnecessarily. A child who had grown up in France would not die of hunger in a foreign land if he did not take a French cook along. 'Fruit, milk, a piece of cake just a little better, and above all the art of dispensing these things prudently, by these means you may lead a host of children to the world's end, without on the one hand giving them a taste for strong flavours, nor on the other hand letting them get tired of their food', declared the philosopher from Geneva.[51] Rousseau's pedagogic maxim finds a late echo in the *Enzyklopädisches Handbuch der Pädagogik* (Encyclopedic Manual of Education, 1895–9), which comments on the effects of the appetite on health as follows:

The 'gormandizers and sweet tooths' embody the uncontrolled passion for the select foods called delicacies in its most fully developed form. The sister of this craving is the compulsive consumption of snacks; its seat is the tongue; its aim is sensual pleasure; its cause – besides seduction – is an overstimulated or jaded palate; its physical effect is fatal damage to the digestive organs and nerves; and its moral and psychological end product is bland indifference, with all the unnatural and irrational accompaniments thereof.[52]

Comments of this kind show that many of these authors and educators were concerned less to civilize taste than to tame the appetites in accordance with an ideal of temperance rooted in traditional Christian asceticism. This kind of hostility to the senses is already evident in a French lexicon published in 1771: 'Gormandizing is a vice, although it is not as shameful as gluttony.'[53] The author, interestingly enough, was a member of the Society of Jesus.

Leaving to one side the question of sophistication and refinement, the historian must now ask whether culinary tastes did in fact change in the eighteenth and nineteenth centuries, and, if so, why and how. The first observable change is undoubtedly the development of the taste for sweet foods. As we know, this predilection was encouraged by the fall of the price of cane sugar imported from European colonies. In the sixteenth and seventeenth centuries, sugar was still one of the status symbols of the social elite. Because the use of imported sugar carried so much prestige, the less privileged social strata were understandably eager to emulate it. Thus, the trend in favour of sweetness originally belongs in the context of the spread of the consumption of tea, coffee and cocoa to all sectors of the population from the late eighteenth century onwards. These products were all bitter-tasting beverages which were usually sweetened with liberal quantities of sugar. State intervention and attempts at regulation were unable to stem the increasing consumption of coffee. In his criticism of the long-term unenforcibility of the 1777 ban on coffee drinking, the Prussian diplomat Christian Wilhelm Dohm (1751–1820) – who was also the author of a well-known treatise on Jewish emancipation – commented that: 'The regulation of this sensory pleasure according to the agenda of the state has created two factions within the state: those who drink coffee and those who don't . . . Sensory pleasures should never be the privilege of a single class [but] simply the reward of achievement. They are the natural deserts of wealth, industry and earnings.'[54] So from the end of the eighteenth century onwards, more and more of those who could afford to do so treated themselves to cups of sugared mocha and drinking chocolate. The birth of the modern sugar industry and the meteoric rise of sugar consumption throughout Europe after the 1850s are the signs of the 'sweet power' that has lastingly altered our 'natural' taste. But that is not all. As the American historian Sidney W. Mintz has observed: 'The first sweetened cup of hot tea to be drunk by an English worker was a significant historical event, because it prefigured the transformation of an entire society, a total remaking of its economic and social basis.'[55]

The taming of touch

The education of the sense of touch offers a more ambivalent picture. On the one hand, Rousseau urges us not to allow the sense to atrophy. On the other hand, the touching of both our own and others' bodies has clearly become more and more subject to social taboos. It all depends on the context and the kind of touching involved.

Eighteenth-century pedagogues, for instance, regarded the tactile sensitivity of the blind as particularly worthy of emulation. Rousseau advised against allowing children to become too used to heavy manual work, since their hands would become calloused and lose their 'fineness of touch'. He thought it essential to preserve this sensitivity so they would be able, for example, to identify objects by their feel in conditions of darkness. Rousseau also recommended walking barefoot. This served the opposite purpose of desensitizing the soles of the feet, enabling a child to survive without shoes during winter, should the need arise. A century later, Daniel Schreber came up with a similar set of reflections. He suggested that teachers should get children to put their hands behind their backs and give them various objects to hold, which they would then try to identify by their feel. Johann Christoph Gutsmuths promoted a similar procedure, called simply 'Exercises in Feeling'.[56] In this context, we also find authors insisting that the hands should be kept meticulously clean in order to maintain the sense of touch in a healthy condition. Such at least was the view of our acquaintance the Reverend Joseph Maskell, and he said so emphatically in the printed versions of his sermons for children.

But children were not the only ones who needed to hone their tactile sense. Since the end of the eighteenth century it had been considered important for prospective doctors to receive instruction in the art of palpation. The distinguished Göttingen obstetrician Friedrich Benjamin Osiander (1759–1822), for instance, invented a device that looked rather like a leather cuff, with which students of medicine could practise inserting their hands skilfully into the vagina of a mother giving birth. Osiander, who was the head of a maternity hospital, thought that manual dexterity would usually suffice in the case of 'living dummies', which was the demeaning term he used for pregnant women in the presence of his students. The treatment of women from the upper strata of society on the other hand, however, called for a little more decorum. In nineteenth-century private practice, the doctor had to kneel before the female patient in a case requiring gynaecological examination. He would then carefully and decently grasp her under her skirt and slowly feel his way towards her genitals. Otherwise he would have been guilty of the most serious offence against a lady's natural sense of shame. If we bear in mind that, in eighteenth- and nineteenth-century English slang, 'touching' was understood as a euphemism for sexual contact between obstetrician and patient, we get some idea of the extreme delicacy of this procedure.[57]

'See with a feeling eye / grasp with a seeing hand.' These famous lines from Goethe's *Roman Elegies* are another erotic allusion, created from the combination of the highest with the lowest of the senses. The Swiss writer Ulrich Bräker (1735–1798) alludes to his temporary renunciation of sexual contact in the words: 'on the way home, I again managed not to stir a finger'[58] – which takes us back to the subject of masturbation.

Medicine has long abided by certain protocols in respect of the touching and grasping of another body. A barber-surgeon was normally permitted to touch all parts of a male or female patient's body – anywhere, that is, where it hurt. Thus, in 1759, the English surgeon Henry Thompson could declare, with a confidence born of years of professional experience, that: 'Wounds are distinguished by Sight – Touch – Smell.'[59] Qualified, i.e., academically trained, doctors, on the other hand, tended to rely on traditional pulse diagnosis. By the early nineteenth century, however, this practice was being supplemented increasingly by palpation (examination by touch) and percussion (tapping the surface of the body in order to infer the condition of the organs below it from the sound produced). Nevertheless, in the 1870s, the renowned physiologist Hermann von Helmholtz (1821–1894) still regarded pulse-taking as the doctor's most important diagnostic tool.

The examination of the body by listening to the sound made by knocking on it was introduced into medical diagnosis by Leopold von Auenbrugger (1722–1809) in 1761, although it was not initially based on physical contact. The Viennese clinician's most famous publication contains a set of instructions which may strike the modern reader as somewhat bizarre: 'The upper part of the body should be covered by a shirt or the hand of the percusser provided with a glove (made from any material except smooth leather). If the naked breast is tapped with the bare hand, the contact with the smooth surface produces an additional noise that obscures the sound that is supposed to be produced.'[60] Auenbrugger's reasons for having the doctor perform the percussion wearing a glove were thus purely pragmatic and had nothing to do with sparing the patient's blushes.

Recent cultural-historical investigations have claimed that, since the eighteenth century, 'bodily contact has been revalued as rare, exclusive and emotional',[61] and there is indeed something to this. There is a wealth of evidence to suggest that sleeping in a common bed declined steadily over this period. If people were forced to lie close together – during journeys, for example – they no longer slept naked, but wore night-shirts. As always, exceptions prove the rule. Doctors and educators feared that involuntary mutual touchings during sleep might encourage masturbation. In early modern times, even dancing, which was the only legitimate form of touching between unmarried men and women, began to run into more and more critical crossfire from the moral apostles of the various religions and the self- and sometimes church- and state-appointed guardians of decency.

The period was marked by a sort of hierarchy of intimacy covering various forms of physical contact. Holding a woman by the hand was frowned upon in France for most of the eighteenth century. Louis-Sébastien Mercier (1740–1814) left a description of French etiquette on the eve of the revolution: 'The man of delicate feelings abhors nothing so much as kissing a woman on the cheek in public. It is better to avoid even touching her hand or the hem of her gown than to have witnesses.'[62] In Germany, the old custom of hand-shaking fell into temporary discredit at roughly the same time – as Julius Bernhard Rohr, an acknowledged expert on complicated court ceremonial, observes in a popular conduct book for private individuals in 1728. Strangely enough, he announces this ruling immediately after scolding precisely those 'who never properly touch each other's hand, as though each were afraid that the other had scabies.'[63] In the middle of the nineteenth century, the German pupils of boys' and girls' schools in the United States were still being told to refrain from 'touching everything that strikes us as new or interesting with our hands', and only to offer their hands to people they knew well. Furthermore, 'we only offer our hand to a friend after removing our glove.'[64]

Since the seventeenth century, the sense of touch had also gradually been excluded from the act of eating. In the words of one cultural critic, 'cutlery becomes the sign and means of more than just the creation of new distances.'[65] Only bread continued to be eaten with the fingers in polite company. All other food required the use of a fork. The baroque poet Johann Michael Moscherosch (1601–1669) keenly appreciated the sensorial impoverishment that this involved: 'how can I taste my salad if I don't eat it with my fingers?'[66]

The slow but steady vindication of the fork as an eating utensil is attested by studies of the everyday culture of German cities in the early modern era. Ruth E. Mohrmann notes, for example, that in the first half of the seventeenth century 88 per cent of the Brunswick households whose inventories have been preserved still possessed no forks. One hundred and fifty years later, this figure had fallen to just 40 per cent. It was not until the late nineteenth century that the fork became part of the basic equipment of a lower-middle-class kitchen, while working-class families largely continued to eat with knives and spoons. They probably often used their hands as well. In this context, it is important to remember Norbert Elias's earlier golden rule – frequently overlooked by the disciples of his theory of civilization – that 'new standards do not arrive overnight.'[67]

So much for table manners. But what about the touching and caressing (already mentioned briefly above) that included everything from the simple handshake to the grabbing of breasts, bottoms and private parts? Here we might refer to Richard Sennett's largely unverified thesis that, in the cities at least, bodily contact had been on the decrease in the hustle and bustle of public life since the eighteenth century.[68] The changes in middle-class lifestyles observable during this period also tend to suggest that the distance between people had grown. Upright and easy chairs feature ever more prominently in surviving domestic inventories, suggesting that people were less likely to find themselves sitting immediately next to each other on a bench or sofa, leaving fewer opportunities for voluntary or involuntary physical contact.

Finally, we should bear in mind that touching the body of another (particularly one belonging to a member of the opposite sex) was not automatically taboo. It all depended on the situation and the intention, as the Catholic theologian Alphons Maria di Liguori (1696–1787) explains in detail in his *Theologia moralis* (1763): 'An unmarried person who lets herself be touched in a way which is still felt to be respectable, such as being fondled, embraced and kissed according to the customs of the country, is not committing a sin unless she is positively aware that the other is harbouring evil intentions.'[69] Besides the tricky matter of the precise intentions of the supposed 'seducer', the unequivocal endorsement of the physical contact as 'honourable', or entirely within the bounds of what was commonly considered customary or normal, was of decisive importance for the practical consequences and application of this kind of rule of moral behaviour. These fine distinctions were doubtless familiar to young Russian peasants who, according to nineteenth-century reports, were in the habit of grasping the breasts of young girls. However, they did so only when no one else was looking. The peasant girls who participated in this 'fun', which was known as 'touch-me-not' (*nedotroga*),[70] were expected to put up a show of resistance before finally allowing the boys to feel their breasts. This anecdote underlines the lesson that a German writer of the Biedermeier period sought to impress upon his readers in a conduct book addressed to young and old: 'Touching and stroking presuppose some familiarity with the person concerned, if it is to be accepted in good faith.'[71]

— 9 —

The Transformation of the Senses by Industrialization and Technology

We see how the history of *industry* and the developed objective existence of *industry* is the *open book* of the *essential powers of humanity*, its sensuously present human *psychology*, which has never been grasped in relation to the *essence* of humanity but only ever in terms of a relationship of external utility.

Karl Marx, *Economic and Philosophical Manuscripts* (1844)

Mutations of space–time consciousness

At the end of the 1880s, the Münsterland farmer Philipp Richter (1815–1890) concluded the chapter on agriculture in his memoirs with the words: 'Today's adult generation simply cannot imagine how things looked 50 or 60 years ago, either in Europe as a whole or in each individual community. Agriculture, industry, indeed all the economic activities and relations of the European nations, have experienced change on a scale unparalleled by anything seen in previous centuries for as far back as historical records extend.'[1] The passage is a subjective reflection of the profound and enduring experience of a historical process which, although already in motion before 1800, accelerated dramatically throughout Europe in the nineteenth century, and is usually described by the terms 'industrialization' and 'mechanization of everyday life'.

Since the second half of the eighteenth century, population density had been rising with demographic growth. All over Europe, people were pouring into the cities and the developing industrial regions. Urbanization was proceeding fastest in England, where more than half the population was already living in urban agglomerations by the middle of the nineteenth century. In Europe, an average 20 per cent of the population was living in towns, assuming that the border between town and country is drawn at communities with more than 5000 inhabitants. The most rapid increases in urban population during this period were taking place in Germany, Austria and Sweden (2 per cent per annum). The principal beneficiaries of this growth were the large metropolises such as London, Amsterdam and Berlin and the rapidly developing industrial towns. The population of the city of Dortmund, for example, rose by 1350 per cent between 1800 and 1875. In the same period the population of Berlin increased by 'just' 462 per cent, from 172,000 to 967,000. By 1910, 3.7 million people, representing 5.7 per cent of the population of the German Reich, were living in Greater Berlin. The population concentration was even denser in London, where no less than a fifth of the English population was domiciled at the beginning of the twentieth century.

Britain was the most heavily industrialized country of the nineteenth century. The highest rates of growth in industrial production, however, were in Germany and Sweden. Around 1830, Germany's share of world industrial production was just 3.5 per cent; by 1900 it had leapt to 13.2 per cent. Great Britain managed only to double its share during this period (from 9.5 to 18.5 per cent). Among the many technological innovations of the period, the construction of railways – which had been preceded by the invention of the steam-driven engine – was a particularly important factor in the rapid process of industrialization and urbanization. In 1840, the European railway network totalled roughly 3000 km. By 1880, this had risen to 170,000 km. Towards the end of the nineteenth century, Sweden possessed the densest railway network in proportion to population. Germany was slightly above, and Britain slightly below, the European average of 9 km per 10,000 inhabitants. The railways were used from the beginning to convey people as well as goods. In Germany alone, passenger rail traffic rose from 560 million to 6500 million passenger kilometres over a period of just thirty years (1850–80). People living in rural areas used the railway increasingly for shopping trips to neighbouring towns. Conversely, more and more city dwellers boarded the steam trains on Sundays and holidays for excursions to the countryside. The more regular and routine use of rail travel led to a 'new consciousness of space and distance'.[2]

As the nineteenth century drew to a close, the old horse-drawn trams were being replaced by electric trams in the inner-city areas of large metropolises such as London, Paris and Berlin. The switch from steam to electricity in transport technology was already apparent around the turn of the century, although it was not accompanied by any noticeable decrease in noise, dirt or noxious smells. The diesel- or petrol-driven motor vehicle first appears in traffic statistics in 1895. Three hundred automobiles were registered in France that year. Ten years later the number had risen to 21,500.

Human spatio-temporal consciousness was also altered by two other items of late nineteenth-century technology, namely the wireless tele-graph and the telephone. Roughly eight million telephone calls were made in Germany around 1883. By 1913, that number had increased 315-fold to 2.5 billion. In Europe and, above all, the United States local community action groups soon began to demonstrate against the disfigurement of the townscapes by rampant forests of telephone poles and thickets of wires. It was largely as a result of these rigorous campaigns that from the 1890s onwards – first in the USA and then in Europe – telephone lines were increasingly laid underground, where they were less conspicuous and obtrusive.

The increasing overstimulation of the senses

Industrialization, urbanization and the technological advances men-tioned above led to a change in perception which, as we shall see, affected primarily the sense of sight. But the other senses (hearing, smell, taste and touch) were also absorbed into the mechanization process to a greater or lesser extent. One of the early witnesses of this development was the Swiss man of letters Johann Jakob Bodmer (1698–1783), who spent the last years of his life in Zurich, living not far from the present university. On the side of his house that faced the city he kept the window shutters permanently closed, for the city was 'full of smoke, mud and din'.[3] A hundred years later most people, and not only in Zurich, were clearly still not accus-tomed to the ever-increasing noise and smell pollution, for public protests were becoming more and more frequent. Most of these complaints laid the blame on urbanization and the concentration of large numbers of people in small spaces. In 1899, for example, an article appeared in the Bern periodical *Der Neue Hausfreund* (The New Friend of the Family) under the title 'Über die Gefahren des Großstadtlebens' (On the Dangers of Living in Cities), which drew attention to the unhealthy consequences of urbanization: 'The tortured brain is occupied day and night; day and night it is an overheated machine operating under maximum steam pressure.'[4]

To stand any chance of success, these complaints needed to quote statistics, and in this context the then very recent science of occupational therapy was of particular relevance. In 1896, for instance, the Swiss doctor Théodore Vannod (1869–1938) had examined various school classes for signs of fatigue. His indicators for the deterioration of sense perception were skin sensitivity and sensitivity to pain.[5] The statistical records of the health insurance companies tended to support the claims of occupational therapists that the industrial process of production was proving to be increasingly damaging to the senses. According to the statistics of the Frankfurt compulsory medical insurance scheme for the year 1896, 6.7 per cent of male members fit for work suffered from eye complaints, and 1.8 per cent had impaired hearing. For insured women, the figures were only slightly lower, at 5.8 and 1.7 per cent, respectively. The role of these two senses as causes of disability in the period between 1891 and 1895 is also striking: 5 per cent of all insurance cases involved permanent damage to vision, and 0.4 per cent loss of hearing.[6]

In the light of these figures, it is hardly surprising that in 1888 the German Association of Public Hygiene passed a resolution calling for stronger measures for the protection of the senses of hearing and smell: 'The interests of public hygiene call for a legal framework for major municipalities, enabling them to exclude from certain districts the kind of manufacturing and industrial plants whose fumes, smoke or noise either pose a threat to the health of the inhabitants or detract from their residential convenience.'[7] Towards the end of the nineteenth century complaints were no longer confined to the ever more perceptible and visible effects of industrialization and urbanization on the senses of sight, hearing and smell. The hectic life of the large cities, unhealthy factory labour and above all the new transport and communication technologies were widely held to have a negative effect on sensory perception. People believed they could feel tension all around them, and they attributed the ostensible increase of nervous complaints (notably neurasthenia) to this phenomenon. In the essay entitled *'Cultural' Sexual Morality and Modern Tension* (1907) Sigmund Freud quotes at length from a work by the German pathologist and neurologist Wilhelm Erb (1840–1921), which had appeared in Heidelberg in 1893 under the title *Über die wachsende Nervosität unserer Zeit* (On the Increasing Nervousness of our Time). There Erb writes about 'the immense extension of communications' and the 'network of telegraphs and telephones' that had turned even holidays into nervous ordeals. Freud proceeds to quote the author's complaint that life in big cities had become ever more sophisticated and stressful: 'The exhausted nerves seek recuperation in increased stimulation and in highly-spiced pleasures, only to become more exhausted than before. Modern literature is predominantly concerned with the most questionable problems which stir up all the passions, and which encourage sensuality and a craving for pleasure, and contempt for every fundamental principle and ideal.'[8]

Shortly before the outbreak of the First World War, the German psychologist and politician Willy Hellpach (1877–1955) complained of similar symptoms of modern life in the city. His critique of civilization in a series of essays written at the beginning of the twentieth century is summarized in his book *Mensch und Volk der Großstadt* (Individual and People of the Big City, 2nd edn, 1952): 'The senses of the city have to operate with radically shortened comprehension and reaction times. They are forbidden to dwell on things, since they are subject to the functional law of haste.'[9] The well-worn topos of (healthy) country versus (sickly) city is indispensable to the argument: 'The senses have to make a much more conscious effort to open themselves up and are obliged to cope with a far more rapid succession of fleeting entities. This is not so much an intensification of our power of perception as its displacement. With his healthy senses, the countryman is alive to many things for which the city dweller no longer possesses an "organ".'[10]

In a detailed article on neurasthenia written at the turn of the century for a German standard medical work, the doctor and psychiatrist Theodor Ziehen (1862–1950) pointed out that the symptoms of this condition appeared somewhat more frequently in men than in women, and that they affected a strikingly large number of teachers. The author goes on to cite numerous examples of the highly variable sensory disorders characteristic of this 'modern' syndrome. Besides disordered and failing vision (sensitivity to light, narrowing of the visual field, misted vision, deterioration of visual acuity), he lists instances of more or less acute hearing impairment, such as extreme sensitivity to noise or reduction of aural acuity. Other sense organs were hardly affected, although occasional cases of 'cutaneous anaesthesia', or diminished skin sensitivity (sense of touch), had been observed.[11]

The argument that technological progress, or the Industrial Revolution, was responsible for this overburdening of the senses had already been advanced a few decades before the turn of the century, well before neurasthenia became the fashionable cultural malady of the *fin de siècle*. In the first volume of *Capital* (1867), Marx had argued that machine labour 'does away with the many-sided play of the muscles' and 'exhausts the nervous system to the uttermost'.[12] Apart from 'the new labour of watching the machine with his eyes and correcting its mistakes with his hands', the Industrial Revolution had left the workman 'the merely mechanical part of being the moving power'.[13] However, just a few decades later, American and German neurologists did not follow Marx in singling out 'machinery and heavy industry' as the principal causes of the increasing hypersensitivity of the senses. The main culprit in their eyes consisted of the new forms of transport and communication (railways and telegraphy). In 1892, the Jewish author and Zionist Max Nordau (1849–1923) summarized this critique of the technological factor by saying that civilized humanity had been taken unawares by its new sensations and advances. In other words, the senses still had to accustom themselves to new technological developments and changed conditions of living and working.

New technologies did not, however, automatically imply a threat to, or even a loss of, sense perception. The senses could also be greatly enhanced by them, witness the stethoscope, invented in 1819. From early times, people had dreamed of supplementing or even replacing individual sense organs with machines.[14] Consider, for instance, the stereoscope, invented at the beginning of the nineteenth century, with which it became possible to view objects three-dimensionally (as in the natural visual process) using a special configuration of lenses.

The rapidly advancing mechanization of the senses was reflected not least in nineteenth-century literature, for instance in the fantastic tales of the German writer E. T. A. Hoffmann (1776–1822). In Hoffmann's famous novella *The Sandman* (1817), a hypersensitive student named Nathaniel purchases a 'perspective glass' from Coppolo, a seller of weatherglasses. With it he is able to turn Olimpia, a female robot belonging to Spalanza, his physics professor, into a living being with alluring eyes. With the aid of the magic 'perspective', he as it were transfers his own eyes to the artefact, whose smouldering-eyed beauty then almost drives him insane.

The 'scopic regime'

No sense was more radically transformed by the onset of the Industrial Revolution than sight. While some early nineteenth-century thinkers continued to inveigh against 'the despotism of the eye' (Samuel Taylor Coleridge, 1772–1834), and called for a revaluation of hearing and touch, the 'scopic regime',[15] to use the now familiar term coined by the American cultural historian Martin Jay, was well on the way to becoming firmly established.

The growing dominance of sight in all areas of life is reflected in the way in which people perceived pollution. Contrary to what we might expect today, the smoke that began to belch from chimneys as the Industrial Revolution got under way was not at first experienced as smelly or pungent. The main complaint was rather that it obscured vision.[16] We find a further example of this privileging of sight in an article that appeared in a Württemberg newspaper in 1835, in which a journalist complains that the promenades of Stuttgart are littered with 'broken glass, old clothing, combs, weather-beaten wigs and dead dogs'. This deplorable state of affairs was 'as offensive to the eye as painful to the feet'.[17] He was apparently concerned less about the unpleasant smell of wayside rubbish than the unsightliness of these 'unofficial' dustbins. In those days, a walk in the countryside usually greeted the eye with positive and pleasant impressions. The growing enthusiasm for scaling towers, climbing mountains and taking trips in hot-air balloons was a sign of the definitive transformation during this period of *homo sapiens* into *homo videns* (Helmut Mayer).

From this time onwards, the sense of sight more or less assumed precedence over all the other senses, in theory as well as in practice. The layout of landscape gardens was one sign of this. In the late eighteenth and early nineteenth centuries, landscape gardeners began to devote more attention to the colour shades of flowers. Already popular at the time, roses began to be grown for the sake of their visual beauty, rather than their fragrance.[18]

The concept 'scopic regime' refers not least to a lack of ease with modernity that finds expression in the cultural criticism of the nineteenth century. One of the early representatives of this trend was the English writer and art theorist John Ruskin (1819–1900): 'The worst of me is that the Desire of my *Eyes* is so much more to me! Ever so much more than the desire of my mind.'[19] The author of a popular guide to correct behaviour wrote in similar terms: 'By saddling the eyes exclusively with the task of supplying the whole stock of intellectual knowledge, and by replacing memory and mental capacity with writing and print, we are treating the eyes in the way carters treat their nags.'[20] At the beginning of the twentieth century, the sociologist Georg Simmel (1858–1918) took up this theme of 'the enormous predominance of seeing over hearing', and made it the subject of his famous excursus on sensory perception: 'Before the development of omnibuses, railways and tramways in the nineteenth century, people were simply never in situations where they looked, or were forced to look, at each other without speaking for minutes or even hours on end. Modern transport is gradually consigning the major part of sensory relations between human individuals to the sense of sight, which will inevitably alter the basis of social feeling.'[21] One of Simmel's examples of such social change was the increasing isolation of people in large cities.

The 'sharpened' gaze

The 'scopic regime' was not established immediately. The transformation of looking occurred gradually, beginning in the pre-modern age and accelerating rapidly in the epoch of the Industrial Revolution with the arrival of new technologies that radically changed visual perception. The harbinger of this development was the enhancement of vision, which allowed the eye to venture into new, hitherto unknown, worlds. We are referring to the invention of the telescope and the microscope.

The telescope was invented at the beginning of the seventeenth century and created the conditions for the long-awaited departure into new realms of science. Historians remain divided on the question of whether the Dutch lens grinder Hans Lipperhey (c.1570–1619) was the sole inventor of the telescope. What is certain is that in 1608 Lipperhey applied for a patent for a telescope consisting of one convergent and one divergent lens. While the Dutch were still considering the potential military applications of his invention, Galileo Galilei (1564–1642), then living in Padua, was discovering its enormous importance for astronomy. With the aid of an imitation version, he discovered four of the moons of Jupiter. The first telescope with two convergent lenses was designed by Johannes Kepler and constructed by the Jesuit Christoph Scheiner (1575–1650).

An entry in the 1735 volume of *Zedler's Universal Lexicon* noted that the telescope had radically altered our image of the world: 'This is one of the most superb inventions of the last *saeculum*, for it opens the eyes of natural scientists to the form of things, transforming the sky into something quite different from what they had previously imagined it to be, and compelling nature to reveal things which would have otherwise remained forever hidden from our eyes.'[22] In the further course of the seventeenth and eighteenth centuries, the telescope became more than just a means of penetrating the firmament. It also saw action in the cause of colonization and the opening up of new territories for settlement (headword: Land surveying). In addition, it was used for all kinds of trivial purposes. Goethe was one culprit here. While supposedly watching an opera, he pointed one of the small telescopes that were the forerunners of today's binocular opera glasses at a woman who had caught his fancy in the audience, completely ignoring the singers on the stage.

As in the case of the telescope, the original authorship of the microscope is still a matter of debate. There is some evidence to suggest that the first to combine two lenses of extremely short focal length to form a magnifying glass was a certain Zacharias Jansen from Middelburg in Holland. The reputation of the microscope – according to the Italian art expert and natural scientist Francesco Algarotti (1712–1764), it could peer 'into the very heart of even the most hidden bodies'[23] – was largely established by the experiments of the Delft natural scientist Antoni van Leeuwenhoek (1632–1723). Van Leeuwenhoek made microscopes with magnifications of up to x270. His first microscopic experiments consisted of examinations of human and animal hairs and the surface structures of wood, grain and sand. He later explored the smallest life forms, dissected insects and studied their anatomies and nervous systems. He discovered water-dwelling infusoria and the spermatozoa of human and animal sperm and was also the first to observe the bundled fibres of the optic nerve.

Among the doctors who quickly realized the importance of the microscope were the Dutchman Reinier de Graaf (1641–1673), who described the follicles of the female ovary (known as Graafian follicles), and Pierre Borel (1620–1689), the personal physician of the French king. Borel not only conducted microscopic research but also published a book about the invention of the microscope (*De vero telescopii inventore*, The Hague, 1655).

Although the early microscopes were primitive, they introduced the observer to a hitherto unknown microscopic world. Each gaze, even at familiar objects, led to new discoveries, or as the 1746 volume of *Zedler's Universal Lexicon* puts it: 'The purpose of magnifying glasses is expressed in their observation of things invisible to the naked eye because of their smallness. These instruments are therefore an enormous contribution to the exact knowledge of nature.'[24] But it was not only natural science that profited from the invention. In the early eighteenth century microscopes actually became a kind of 'home entertainment', although they were so expensive that few people could afford to buy one. Those who did not own one could always enjoy the illustrations in the books of the Nuremberg councillor of justice Martin Frobenius Ledermüller (1719–1769), of which several editions survive. Yet, despite all the enthusiasm for the new possibilities it offered to the natural sciences, the new optical instrument was not without its critics. The Zurich scholar Johann Caspar Lavater (1741–1801) complained, for instance, that looking at things through a microscope caused people to lose their sense of the whole. Much more serious, on the other hand, were the reservations of those who thought that the microscope was a form of sensory delusion. Antoni van Leeuwenhoek's own contemporaries had accused him of having 'seen more with his imagination than with his glasses'.[25] It is evident from the detailed refutation contained in the 1746 volume of *Zedler's Universal Lexicon* that this criticism was still being heard in the middle of the eighteenth century: 'If we simply take exactly the same precautions against premature conclusions about the nature and con-stitutions of things as when looking at objects from a distance, we need have no fear of being misled by our senses in these cases.'[26] A few years later, this kind of criticism had been silenced. Henceforth, scientific research was no longer thinkable without the microscope, which underwent many technical improvements.

The 'disembodied' gaze

Another important milestone on the way to a new kind of seeing was the camera obscura. Its invention is generally attributed to Giovanni Battista della Porta (1543–1615). In the seventeenth century, this optical device became the symbol of Kepler's model of the visual process, which emphasized the importance of the retinal image in visual perception. But the camera obscura symbolized more than just the event of seeing as it was understood after the pioneering publications of Kepler, Descartes and Newton. As an optical instrument with numerous applications, it also represented a phenomenon in the history of vision that the American historian Jonathan Crary has called the 'disembodied gaze'. In order to understand this metaphor we need to know what the prototype of the camera obscura actually looked like. It consisted of a dark room which admitted rays of light through a tiny aperture. The observer positioned in the darkened room sees an inverted image of the objects of the outside world on the white surface of the wall opposite the aperture. Thus, the observer in the dark room represents the isolated, secluded and autonomous form of perception that we find reflected in the art of the seventeenth and eighteenth century (in Vermeer and Canaletto, for instance). Crary sees the camera obscura as 'a figure for both the observer who is nominally a free sovereign individual and a privatized subject confined in a quasi-domestic space, cut off from a public exterior world.'[27]

The laterna magica invented by the Dutch physicist Christian Huygens (1629–1695) quickly replaced the camera obscura as a fairground attraction. This was a very simple optical apparatus with the aid of which 'either by night, or in a darkened room, pictures painted on glass may be presented on a white wall, in their real size and in their natural colours.'[28] It consisted of a cardboard or tin box with a peephole and a projection device. By the middle of the eighteenth century, it could even be adapted for the projection of moving pictures.

The first German periodical specializing in projection, founded in 1877 by Dr Paul Eduard Liesegang (1837–1896), was named appropriately *Laterna magica*.

Strictly speaking, the optical instruments from which numerous eighteenth- and even nineteenth-century showmen made their living on the squares and streets of the cities were not magic lanterns, but 'show-boxes' or 'peep-shows' (Fr. *optiques*). The genuine magic lantern required projection onto a white wall, whereas the viewer had to stand right in front of the peep-show and peer laboriously through an aperture. The peep-show is thus related to the camera obscura, since it is based on the inversion of light effects. The original peep-show apparatuses were equipped with a mirror and a convex lens, so the eye of the viewer received a virtual image of the represented object. The popularity of these presentations of moving and still images at the end of the eighteenth century is demonstrated by a contemporary illustration bearing the following little jingle:

> There's the Italian calling by his peep-show box,
> heh! come and see something interesting,
> heh! come and see my marmot, come and see my raree-show
> a farthing won't make a hole in your pocket.[29]

In the nineteenth century the camera obscura-like peep-box even came to symbolize vision as such. In a book for children published in 1852, the English engraver and wood-cut illustrator Hablot Knight Browne (1815–1882) depicted the sense of sight in a vivid fairground scene. Two youths are gazing into a peep-box, while the showman stands by crying, 'Now then gents . . . open yr eyes – blow yr precious noses and don't breathe on the glasses.'[30]

The 'subjective' gaze

In the late 1820s, optical and sensory-physiological experiments with so-called retinal afterimages led to the development of a whole series of devices which exploited the familiar tendency of rapid sequences of sense impressions to merge into one. Thus at the beginning of the nineteenth century, the technology of vision was enlarged by a new variant, which the American cultural historian Jonathan Crary calls 'subjective seeing': 'The afterimage . . . and its successive modulations posed a theoretical and empirical demonstration of autonomous vision, of an optical experience that was produced by and within the subject.'[31]

One of the first apparatuses to exploit the illusionistic nature of afterimages was the so-called Thaumatrope (lit. magic turner), which was first introduced to the London public by a Dr John Paris in 1825. It consisted of a round disc on which there was a drawing of a bird and a cage. The rotation of the disc created the illusion that the bird was in the cage, the reason being that the image left on the retina by the first image briefly overlaid the second image. At the beginning of the 1830s, the Belgian Joseph Plateau (1801–1883) constructed his Phenakistoscope (lit. optical deception), which consisted of a single disc divided into eight or sixteen sections. Each of these sections contained a small slitted opening and a figure caught in a particular moment of motion. A mirror was fixed to the back of the disc. Having set the disc in motion, the viewer had to look through one of the slits. The 'persistence of the visual impression', as Plateau described it, created the illusion of figures in continuous movement. Another variant was the Zootrope (lit. wheel of life), invented by William G. Horner (1786–1837). It was sometimes called a 'magic drum' and consisted of a rotating slitted hollow cylinder. On the inside of the cylinder there was a strip of paper depicting the sequence of movements. Meanwhile in Vienna the physicist Simon Stampfer (1792–1864) was building his stroboscope, which was also called the 'wheel of life' and likewise based on the experiments with rotating cogwheels conducted by the distinguished physicist Michael Faraday (1791–1867). A particularly large version of this type of stroboscope could be seen in Frankfurt am Main in 1857. The cylinder was reputedly 18 feet in diameter (*c.*5.65 metres) and had more than thirty different show-boxes. By this point in time, therefore, a quite simple optical instrument, invented originally for research into subjective vision, had developed into an apparatus that was now used almost exclusively for the leisured amusement of the urban bourgeoisie.

In contrast to these optical devices, the stereoscope, which we have already mentioned in another context, did not create the illusion of movement. Together with photography, stereoscopy was the most common form of image production in the nineteenth century. The stereoscope also belongs in the context of research into subjective seeing in the 1820s and 1830s, and the revival of the debate on spatial perception that took place at the same time. It was invented by the Englishman Charles Wheatstone (1802–1875), who was particularly interested in human binocular vision. He discovered that the greater the angle of the optical axis during the act of seeing, the more realistic an object appeared. The effects of depth produced by the stereoscope, which exceeded anything that even gifted painters or graphic artists well versed in single-point perspective were capable of achieving in their media, fascinated and astonished even an experienced scientist and physiologist such as Hermann von Helmholtz (1821–1894). The inventor of the ophthalmoscope and discoverer of the close adjustment of the eye responded to his visual experience with great enthusiasm in 1850: 'These stereoscopic photographs are so true to nature and so lifelike in their portrayal of material things, that after viewing such a picture and recognizing in it some object like a house, for instance, we get the impression, when we actually do see the object, that we have already seen it before and are more or less familiar with it.'[32]

Like the Phenakistoscope and other optical devices not involving projection, the older stereoscopes required the viewer to stand close up to them and to keep to a fixed point of view. The spectator had to keep his gaze fixed on two mirrors positioned at right angles to each other in order to experience the spatially separate images mounted in slits on both sides as one unified image. He would then receive the impression (particularly vivid in the case of the advanced models which came onto the market in the 1860s) that he was looking at something right in front of him. Yet it was a pure illusion. More than any other optical instrument developed in those times, therefore, 'the stereoscope signals an eradication of "the point of view", around which, for several centuries, meanings had been assigned reciprocally to an observer and the object of his or her vision.'[33]

The ordinary public was naturally unconcerned with the subtleties of perception theory. It was simply fascinated by the simulation of a three-dimensionality that seemed close enough to touch. The demand for the instrument was correspondingly huge. Stereoscope mania reached a peak in the 1880s, by which time the number of image packages produced for these apparatuses ran into the millions.

The 'panoramic' view

Circular and semicircular panoramic images came into fashion at the end of the eighteenth century. They too presupposed the abandonment of a fixed angle of vision in that they enabled the viewer to alter his position and change the view presented to his gaze. In order to observe the entire picture, the spectator had to change his point of view, or at least to turn his head or move his eyes.[34] The invention of the 'panoramic' view is attributed to the Irish painter Robert Barker (*d.* 1806), who exhibited a panoramic image in London in 1789. Special buildings called 'panoramas' were soon erected to provide permanent accommodation for these large-format images, where they could be gazed at in wonderment for a small charge. One of the first such places was opened in 1794 in Leicester Square in London, where it attracted large crowds of visitors to a spectacular panoramic representation of the sea. A number of Barker's circular pictures were exhibited in Leipzig and Hamburg just a few years later.

The German tradition in this genre begins with the Leipzig theatre artist Johann Adam Breysig (1766–1831), who exhibited his first panorama in Berlin in 1800. Towards the end of the nineteenth century, the so-called Sedan-Panorama, commissioned by a joint-stock company for the railway station on the Alexanderplatz in Berlin, became a famous attraction. It was 39 metres in diameter and 18 metres high. The visitors stood on a revolving platform, the idea being to prevent the spectator from lingering for too long in one point of view. There was a restaurant on the ground floor, which together with the high admission charge was intended to help finance the enormous building costs (about one million Reichmarks). The selection of the panoramic subjects (depictions of battles, views of cities and landscapes, pictures of exotic animals) was usually decided by popular taste.

For millions of people, the panorama (along with the diorama which developed out of it) became 'a school for the gaze; an optical simulator, where an initially extreme, or unusually "sensational" sensory impression, could be experienced repeatedly and without risk, until it became a routine, everyday component of human seeing.'[35]

Among the disadvantages of both the panorama and its successor the diorama – which differed from its predecessor mainly in its use of sophisticated lighting effects (transparencies) – was the high cost, in time and money, of changing the pictures. In order to sustain public interest in such large-format images and to heighten the visual experiences they provided, Carl Ferdinand Langhans (1781–1869) developed the so-called Pleorama, which was presented to an astonished audience in Breslau in the year 1831. The *Breslauer Zeitung* of 11 June 1831 described its impact on the viewer:

> After many costly and laborious trials, this ingenious invention has now reached maturity. An unbroken series of pictures, stretching for several hundred yards, offers not only individual views of Naples, but actually moves the entire scene past us, so we experience it by embarking at Procida and travelling for several miles past some of the most famous landscapes in Europe, under glorious weather conditions. The mechanical devices responsible for the illusion of gliding past these shores (hence the name Pleorama) are so ingenious, and their effects so striking, that we actually feel we have been transported to a natural world unfamiliar to landlocked Europeans like ourselves.[36]

The Pleorama is one of the first intimations of an illusionistic art of mass effects that was to find its perfect form a few decades later with the invention of cinematography, whose contribution to the 'voyeurism' of twentieth-century humanity has been so immense.

The 'fixed' gaze

The idea of grasping the moment permanently, of recording the eye's fleeting images, was first expressed in a fantasy novel from the pen of the French doctor Tiphaigne de la Roche (1729–1774). A German translation of the book was published in 1761 under the title *Gyphantie, oder Die Erdbeschreibung*. The story describes how elemental spirits place objects which they wish to copy in front of a screen covered with a very thin and sticky substance. Once this varnish has hardened, the screen is removed to a dark place, whereupon a 'painting' appears on it, 'a painting that is all the more valuable for being more truthful than any art, and exempt from the ravages of time.'[37] The similarities to the daguerreotype process developed in France at the beginning of the 1830s by Josephe-Nicéphore Niepce (1765–1833) and Louis Jacques Mandé Daguerre (1787–1851) – exposure time, exposed coated film, darkroom – are striking.

A warning that was sounded in the *Leipziger Anzeiger* in 1839 gives some impression of the mixture of fascination and horror with which many contemporaries responded to the idea of seizing the world with the camera and capturing it on plates (later celluloid): 'As serious experiments conducted here in Germany have shown, the recording of fleeting reflexes is not only impossible, but the very idea borders on sacrilege. God created man in His own image, and no human machine may capture the image of God. God would need suddenly to have abandoned His own principles, were He to allow a Frenchman in Paris to bring an infernal invention like this into the world.'[38] However, photography was soon no longer the work of the devil but a medium that quickly became a tool of scientific investigation. Its primary purpose was to cater to the vanity (portrait photographs) and collectomania (photographic reminiscences of all kinds) of a mass middle-class public. As the French cultural sociologist Pierre Bourdieu has noted, photography, just a few years after its invention, was becoming an ever more popular 'means of dissolving the solid and compact reality of everyday perception into an infinity of fleeting profiles like dream images in order to capture absolutely unique moments of the reciprocal situation of things.'[39]

Today, we know just how easy it is to be tempted into accepting photographic reproduction as a substitute for reality. An early critique of the radical 'visualism' which prefers recorded reality to reality itself may be found in an essay by the American writer Oliver Wendell Holmes (1809–1894), which appeared in 1859. 'In fact, matter as a visible object is of no great use any longer, except as the mould on which form is shaped. Give us a few negatives of a thing worth seeing, taken from different points of view, and that is all we want of it. Pull it down or burn it up, if you please.'[40] Despite the millions of photographs taken of the Colosseum and Pantheon in Rome since Holmes's essay, no one so far has proposed demolishing these buildings on the grounds that we now have enough copies of them! However, museums are now increasingly dispensing with original works during exhibitions and making do with reproductions or facsimiles. One of the reasons given for this is that, in the 'age of mechanical reproduction' (Walter Benjamin), many visitors to exhibitions no longer experience the appeal of the real object or work of art with quite the intensity of former times.

The 'fixed' gaze of the camera's viewfinder and the supposedly completely faithful and detailed photographic reproduction of objects have brought about long-term changes in our visual apprehension of the world. What Friedrich Nietzsche noted as long ago as 1873 is probably far more true of the present: 'They [humans] are deeply immersed in illusions and dream images; their eyes merely glide over the surface of things and see "forms". Their senses nowhere lead to truth; on the contrary, they are content to receive stimuli and, as it were, to engage in a groping game on the back of things.'[41]

The 'breakneck' gaze

It was not only optical devices such as cameras and stereoscopes that were transforming the appearance of the world in the nineteenth century. The new transport technology was also creating entirely new visual experiences. The cultural historian Wolfgang Schivelbusch describes the view presented to the railway traveller as 'panoramic',[42] which is undoubtedly an accurate description of one aspect of the new form of seeing. For the history of sensory perception, however, another kind of visual experience was more decisive. Although it greatly irritated people at the time, no one takes very much notice of it today – unless of course they happen to be hurtling through the landscape at 150 miles an hour on a high-speed train for the first time. As one observer noted in 1843, the new sensation of high speed was already available to those who chose to travel by express mail coach: 'If you are travelling with the intention of gathering new impressions, you will certainly gain more by covering short distances slowly (e.g., on foot or horseback) than by embarking on a long journey at high speed, during which the fleetingness of the images is compounded by the feeling that you are receiving far too many of them.'[43]

Where the ordinary stagecoach, which was the traditional form of long-distance travel, usually offered only a restricted, curtained view of an outside world that slowly slipped by the traveller, the new and increasingly comfortable and luxurious railway coupés, with their large compartment windows, offered an almost unrestricted, albeit extraordinarily rapid view, of the countryside. In those days, people who had just made their first journey by rail frequently described the event as a novel and unfamiliar sensory experience. Take, for instance, the report by eighteen-year-old Niels Buch Breinholt from Lemvig in Jutland, who journeyed by train to Itzehoe in 1848:

> My first impression during this first railway journey was one of surprise that we were travelling so slowly, for having anticipated a lightning journey along the rails, it seemed that our speed was not significantly greater than what you could get from a fast horse on a good road. It gradually dawned on me that this was an illusion caused by the fact that my gaze had been fixed on distant objects. We were actually going so fast that a signal box standing close to the line flashed past me like a shadow, and I quickly withdrew my comparison with a journey by coach.[44]

In the age of rapid travel, we have grown more or less used to the occasional, though always somewhat astonishing, optical illusions we experience when glancing briefly out of the windows of train compartments, the side windows of cars or the little port-holes of aircraft.

The 'errant' gaze

We have also had to get used to another kind of gaze, which is often described in Anglo-American cultural studies as the 'mobilized gaze'.[45] This is the restless gaze of the *flâneur*, which was first described by the French poet Charles Baudelaire (1821–1867) in an essay on art entitled *The Painter of Modern Life* (1863). The perfect *flâneur* feels at home in the anonymity of the city. He is a born spectator, the universal onlooker who never feels that he is being looked at by others in return. It goes without saying that he is male, since it was unthinkable for a respectable nineteenth-century woman to wander about in public in this way.[46]

The glass-domed shopping arcades that sprang up in numerous European cities (notably in Paris) during the *fin de siècle* quickly turned into attractions for both serious shoppers and curious onlookers. As Walter Benjamin has suggested in his celebrated *Arcades Project* (begun in1935), the arcade was an ideal form of casual amusement, a place where one could allow one's gaze to wander freely and non-committally over the glittering goods and the streams of passers-by.

But there were also other places in the city on the Seine where one might show oneself without being seen, where one might, for a moment, fix one's eyes on another – in this case dead – person, before turning away from that brief satisfaction in order to pursue another. We are referring here to the voyeurism that propelled large numbers of people, including the typical *flâneur*, to the displays of corpses in the morgues.

According to Benjamin, the fleeting glances exchanged by men and women in the streets and brothels of a city like Paris were hardly any less morbid: 'With the rise of the great cities, prostitution acquires new mysteries. One of them is the labyrinthine character of the city itself. Prostitution seems to endow the labyrinth, whose image is etched on the body and soul of the *flâneur*, with a sort of coloured border.'[47] Here we are reminded of the revealing paintings of glittering Paris nightlife by Henri Marie de Toulouse-Lautrec (1864–1901) and the anonymous and voyeuristic milieu of prostitution. Baudelaire's *A une passante* (1861) also comes to mind, though in this poem, of course, the central event is not the *flâneur*'s brief eye contact with a girl of the streets but the fleeting capture of his gaze by a beautiful and erotically alluring woman who is swiftly swallowed up by the crowd.

The 'clinical' gaze

Also male, albeit of a quite different order, is the 'clinical gaze' that had been sharpened and applied to new fields of medical knowledge long before the actual rise of scientific medicine in the nineteenth century. The term is, of course, associated with the work of Michel Foucault (1926–1984) and refers to a form of medical scrutiny that began to gain acceptance in clinical practice and the study of medicine at the end of the eighteenth century. According to Foucault, the modern clinic is typified by 'a hearing and a speaking gaze'.[48] These two forms of perception subject the pathological symptoms of the body to a 'nominalist' and 'chemical' reduction. 'The clinical gaze', continues the French philosopher and scientific theorist, 'is not that of an intellectual eye that is able to perceive the unalterable purity of essences beneath phenomena. It is a gaze of the concrete sensibility, a gaze that travels from body to body, and whose trajectory is situated

—— 199 ——

in the space of sensible manifestations.'[49] This space is the modern hospital, with its institutionalized medical rounds, post-mortem examinations and expanding repertoire of modern visual diagnostic techniques (ophthalmoscopy, auriscopy, nasoscopy, endoscopy and, after 1896, X-ray photography). Along with the stethoscope, which called for finely tuned and sensitive hearing, the reflexive- or forehead mirror became the emblem of the modern doctor, who 'diagnoses illnesses using his visual sense'.[50]

This new way of looking at illness tended to sideline the patient, who had previously been the centre of attention, and it was not confined merely to the clinic or lecture theatre. In the late eighteenth century and particularly in the early nineteenth century, so-called medical topographies were increasingly important in medical practice. They served both as a medium for exchanging information and as an empirical basis for individual diagnosis and therapy. They also made exacting demands on their authors, whose eyes needed to be trained in several different ways, for, according to the Hanau officer of health, they undertook this important work not simply as general practitioners, but 'as natural scientists, physicists, chemists and arithmeticians'.[51]

The 'clouded' gaze

It was notably the doctors, with their practised 'clinical' gaze, who drew attention at an early date to the damaging effects of industrialization and technology on the senses in general and vision in particular. They were especially interested in the 'clouded' gaze, which was a collective name for a wide range of visual disorders which they attributed to the modern way of life and world of work. A dictionary of health published in 1842 complains of the phenomenon of failing vision: 'Which of the senses do the young people of the cities and the so-called better classes actually use in a proper manner? Not one of them. They accustom their eyes to short-sightedness and dull them with writing and artificial light.' The author is ready with advice: 'We must never simply abandon ourselves to sensory experience, for it is too manifold, confusing and distracting. We need to accustom ourselves from an early age to thinking and reflecting; to simplifying multiplicity and imposing order on diversity.'[52]

—— 200 ——

The nineteenth century undoubtedly made growing demands on the eyes of craftsmen, industrial workers and soldiers. Statistical research conducted by a German outpatients' clinic at the height of the industrial epoch shows that at that time short-sightedness increased by an average of 6 to 16 per cent when people entered the world of work. Those most affected were factory workers (17 per cent) and mechanics (20 per cent). One of the most hazardous professions of the time was typesetting, but there was a form of work which involved even greater risks. In some mills, 75 per cent of the carpet weavers were diagnosed as short-sighted.[53]

In German military circles, the visual acuity required of soldiers first became an issue at the time of the founding of the German Reich. One major in the medical corps made the pragmatic suggestion that a recruit's visual acuity should be considered adequate if he could recognize a non-commissioned officer's stripes when saluting him from a certain fixed distance. The specialist literature of the time argued about where to fix the norm and drew the boundary of average eyesight at anywhere between 20 and 50 per cent of perfect vision.[54] The procedures followed by other European countries during medical examinations for military service often varied considerably. At the beginning of the last third of the nineteenth century, the French army set short-sightedness at one-sixth of perfect vision. In the Danish army, on the other hand, it was one-eighth. A sample survey of recruits for the imperial German army at this time revealed that approximately 15 per cent of the young men had lower than normal visual acuity.

According to the records of the Reich insurance office, the frequency of severe eye injuries among the ordinary German population stood at 3.6 per cent around the end of the nineteenth century. However, as the high figure of 5.7 per cent suggests, industrial workers were much more at risk. As might be expected, metal workers were particularly exposed. It is again hardly astonishing that eye injuries to the gainfully employed were far more likely among men than among wage-earning women (ratio 6:1). Considered in terms of severity, the picture is as follows: one-quarter of all injuries involved the complete destruction of the eye, and half left the patient blind or barely able to see. The other injuries were relatively minor. Even in those days, occupational therapists were complaining about the indifference of workers to protective goggles.

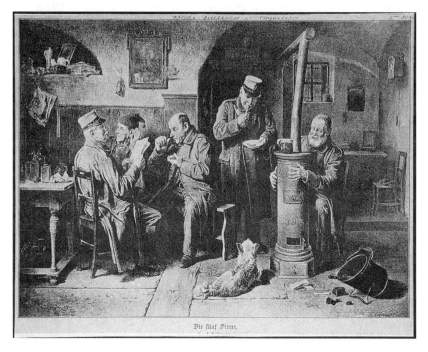

Figure 9.1   Soldier's quarters: allegory of the five senses; lithograph by
R. J. Friedländer (*c*.1850)

At roughly the time when the first detailed accident statistics were
being compiled in Germany, parapsychological groups were performing experiments with hypnosis in an attempt to prove that it was
possible 'to read without the use of the eyes',[55] although this was
undoubtedly more a bizarre coincidence than a desperate response to
the plight of the increasing numbers of those who had lost their sight
in battle or working in industry.

The advancing 'noise plague'

'Life in the past was silence. Noise came into being with the invention
of the machine in the nineteenth century',[56] declared the Italian futurist Luigi Russolo (1885–1947) in 1913. Next to eyesight, hearing

was undoubtedly the sense that suffered the negative side-effects of industrialization and urbanization most acutely. The 'noise plague' of the industrial age is a topic that has received a good deal of coverage in histories of the everyday life and mental attitudes of imperial Germany. One of the most frequently cited 'earwitnesses' of the age was Karl Lamprecht (1856–1915), who was also one of the most distinguished social and economic historians of the late nineteenth century. It was he who coined the no longer very common German term *Reizsamkeit* ('irritability') in order to describe the new phenomenon of increasing sensitivity to noise. Lamprecht made no secret of the fact that he was one of the afflicted: 'I suffer from the typical noises of the city and am particularly sensitive to their dissonance.'[57]

What were these 'typical noises of the city'? An article published in the *Deutsche Medizinische Wochenschrift* in 1912 lists four separate sources of noise: 1) industrial noise, 2) traffic noise, 3) noise in the private domain (blocks of flats, neighbourhoods) and 4) the noises which people made themselves, which they normally regarded as less disturbing.

Let us begin with the first category of factory noise. Increasing industrialization amplified the usual 'noisescape' with the din and hiss of steam engines, the nerve-racking clatter of mechanical looms, the monotonous whirring of automatic spinning machines and the hellish noise of riveting hammers and pneumatic drills. These noises were mostly muffled by factory walls, so the 'noise plague' affected mainly the workers employed in the plants behind them. Unfortunately, we have little information on how these radically new sensations were experienced by the people most affected by them. One of the few exceptions is the contemporary account of a metal worker, who, after more than forty years of service in the industry, found himself having to cope with the installation of the latest modern rollers in a plant that had relied hitherto on traditional methods of metal processing: 'I've worked for forty-two years without noise around me, so you can imagine how this sudden pounding and roaring affects an old man's nerves. I sweat all day long and have feelings of anxiety. I often cry like a little child and I can't sleep at night. I keep a light burning during the night which helps me to control my emotions.'[58] This earwitness goes on to say that he is not the only person to have this experience. Several of his workmates were similarly affected, and one had even committed suicide.

A medical investigation conducted towards the end of the nineteenth century found that miners, hammersmiths, boilermakers, rolling-mill workers, blacksmiths and metal workers had suffered considerable physical damage as a result of exposure to noise. A British study completed in 1886 reports that, after seventeen and a half years in the same job, the hearing ability of boilermakers was only 9.5 per cent of normal. The figure for postmen after an identical period was still 79 per cent. But there were also significant variations within the categories of noisy jobs. A handbook written by an ear specialist in 1892 noted that: 'While the incessant sounds and noises of the work and the working environment are the principal etiological factors in the damage to the organ of hearing suffered by boilermakers and related trades, the situation in other kinds of work is not quite so simple, for in those cases there is usually a combination of causes.'[59] Although the hazards of noise at the workplace had been fully examined by nineteenth-century statisticians, leaving little doubt as to the causal connections, it was not until 1929 that deafness from exposure to noise was finally recognized as an occupational disease.

The working women who suffered from the effects of permanent noise were employed mainly in the spinning- and weaving mills of the textile industry. But the category also included telephonists, which may strike us as somewhat surprising today. An explanation of this phenomenon is provided by an article that appeared in the *Zeitschrift für Ohrenheilkunde* (Journal of Ear Therapy) in 1890. Symptoms such as buzzing in the ears, headaches, dizziness and auditory hallucinations were traced to the discontinuous sound levels and piercing overtones that were a feature of the early telephones. It is evident from a French study of 1967, which describes the 'telephonist syndrome' (*névrose des téléphonistes*) in modern medical jargon, that this occupational disease (whose sufferers were largely women) did not disappear with the improvement of telephone technology. The cases discussed in this report involved 'serious psychic and physical asthenia with a crisis point in the evening after work, accompanied by loss of attention, concentration and memory; mood swings and instability, nervousness, irritability, anxiety attacks; and restlessness, noise sensitivity, hyperaffectivity with uncontrollable fits of crying and periods of depression.'[60] Thanks to the very latest telephone technology, the old-fashioned 'girl at the switchboard' has disappeared, but the operators (male and female) at the modern 'call centres' are now complaining of exactly the same symptoms.

The people of the nineteenth century undoubtedly found the increasing traffic noise worst of all, since it was impossible to avoid it, even on the way to work or during leisure hours. This modern cityscape of noise is described most impressively by the now forgotten German novelist Emmy von Dincklage (1825–1891) in a periodical article written in 1879:

> Future research will determine the exact percentage by which the lives of people with delicate nerves have been shortened by having to spend them in a busy part of a city. . . . How did we come to allow some appalling dog cart carrying a few empty milk cans to drown out the listening, conversation, thought, study, music and leisure of an entire street for a whole ten minutes? Why is it considered perfectly in order for them to assault our ear drums unnaturally, strain our nerves, provoke us into angry outbursts, turn healthy people morose, and make the sick even sicker? And the dog cart is by no means the only culprit, for it brings all sorts of other conveyances in its wake: clanging tramcars, creaking coal wagons, haulage vans and numerous other vehicles – all of which appear to have been constructed with the sole purpose of making the most excruciating din imaginable! And what are the consequences? The wildly excited airwaves rage and surge against the walls of houses, scattering in all directions in search of an exit like the waters of a canal, allowing no escape for anyone without a balloon to rise above them into quieter regions.[61]

It would be difficult to imagine a more vivid description of city traffic noise, and we are instantly reminded of Schopenhauer's impassioned protest in 1851 against 'the truly infernal cracking of whips in the echoing alleyways of the towns'.[62]

The growth of mass transportation during the last third of the nineteenth century produced a corresponding increase in the number of people who either felt disturbed by street noise or were convinced that it was damaging to their health. Complaints about the 'age of the bell', as the *Berliner Lokalanzeiger* aptly called it in its edition of 24 December 1909, did not simply die away. On the contrary: with the arrival of the new noise of automobile engines at the turn of the century, they simply grew louder and eventually led to the establishment of noise-abatement societies. In Germany, a citizen's action group inspired by American models was formed in 1908.

One of the co-founders of this association was the well-known German writer and publicist Theodor Lessing (1872–1933), who issued his own periodical.

Domestic noise was, and still is, considered a lesser evil, even though it too was extremely disruptive and draining on the nerves. Urbanization had led to increased population concentrations in the cities, where people were living closer and closer together. The noise pollution was particularly unbearable in areas containing large blocks of flats or, as in Berlin, tenement barracks. The idiosyncratic impressions of the young Franz Kafka (1883–1924) may be taken as entirely typical of the everyday experience of the urban middle and lower classes at the turn of the century: 'I sit in my room in the very headquarters of the uproar of the entire house. I hear all the doors close, because of their noise only the footsteps of those running between them are spared me, I hear even the slamming of the oven door in the kitchen.'[63] It is evident from the frequent disputes and court cases between residents, or between landlords and tenants, that by the end of the nineteenth century people were beginning to be bothered by the sound of carpet beating and the noise of children in courtyards and stairwells.

People were often not prepared to let matters rest at mere appeals for protection against noise. The anti-noise demonstrations were beginning to show results. More stringent building and trading regulations would help contain the growing industrial noise. Soundproofing measures were discussed at a fairly early juncture, though only rarely put into practice. One of the forerunners of Ohropax, a still popular personal sound excluder, was a product named Antiphon. Antiphon was an anchor-shaped metal instrument, at the end of which was a spherical ball that was inserted into the ear. The inventor was an army captain named M. Pleßner, who introduced the public to this 'Device for the Rendering Inaudible of Sounds and Noises' in 1885. Double windows and the asphalting of the main streets would help to contain traffic noise. It was already technically feasible to muffle the noise of trams, but since the project involved the costly modification of rails and points it was not carried out. In 1895, following a public complaint, the tram conductors of Hannover were ordered to stop their incessant bell-pulling, which had begun to get on people's nerves. It was also suggested to the railway companies that they might replace the shrill whistles of locomotives with bells. Better building regulations would help to muffle domestic noise, although before the First World War building acoustics was still a very new and undeveloped science.

Thus, the most effective weapon in the struggle against domestic noise usually consisted of the police courts, which had been expanding and acquiring more teeth in the last third of the nineteenth century, as more and more judgements were given in favour of noise-plagued plaintiffs. The legal foundations had been laid down by the Prussian higher administrative court. In the 1890s, this court ruled that ordinary citizens and persons 'whose resistance to loud noise . . . had been impaired by the disturbances of modern working life, particularly in heavily industrialized localities', would, where necessary, enjoy police protection against unwarranted and unhealthy noise.[64]

People who fled the infernal din of the city to seek peace in the countryside were often disappointed. The tolling bells of the many country churches were slowly coming to be regarded as disruptive by people who had come in search of recuperation and by the townies who travelled out from the cities – though rarely by the villagers themselves. For obvious reasons, the ringing of bells was usually experienced more intensely in the countryside than in the city. Alain Corbin describes the sounds typical of nineteenth-century French villages (and not only there) as follows:

> The countryside knew nothing then of 'the profane din' in which so many elements could be heard at once, and that constituted the background noise familiar to city dwellers. The auditory landscape, intercut with broad swathes of silence, here consisted of tollings and percussion that could be easily located. The hearing of sounds of metal against metal, wood on wood, or of human voices served to demarcate family or vicinity.[65]

This passage shows why the less intense, but nonetheless present, noise of rural areas was perceived in a way that, though different, was not necessarily less aggravating.

'City air stinks'

The French cultural historian Alain Corbin has given us more than just a fascinating account of the contrasting ways in which bells were perceived by townspeople and country dwellers in nineteenth-century

France. He is perhaps best known for his pioneering book on smell entitled *Le Miasme et la jonquille* (The Foul and the Fragrant, 1988). The central thesis of this book is that the period between the mid-eighteenth century and the end of the nineteenth century was a revolutionary era in the history of smell, during which human attitudes to odours were radically transformed. According to Corbin, the new form of sensory perception is reflected in the numerous attempts made during the period, first to describe smells, then to analyse and classify them socially, and finally to eradicate them, and not simply repress them or douse them with perfume. Corbin describes this process as a 'deodorization' of the environment that brought about permanent changes to the social life of cities.

In this context Corbin is not primarily interested in changes in house-building methods and transformations of traditional townscapes (e.g., as a result of extensive redevelopment) or the banishment of 'stinking' industrial plants to the outskirts of cities. His interest centres on the discourse of social hygiene which began long before the period of intensive industrialization. He is concerned with the changing attitude of the bourgeois elites to the lower strata of society, that is, to people who were supposedly responsible for spreading the 'stench of the poor'. Contemporary opinion saw the poor as a serious threat to hygiene, and one of the unfortunate consequences of this attitude, writes Corbin, was dissociation from the ordinary people, who smelled of death, decay and sin.

Even Corbin's critics concede the overall accuracy of his thesis, although they rightly complain that the restriction of his investigation to France and the early phases of the Industrial Revolution has produced distortions and occasional misinterpretations. So it is worth shifting our attention to the situation across the Rhine in Germany. Here, too, smell tolerance levels begin to fall towards the end of the eighteenth century. In 1796, for example, the doctor Carl Georg Theodor Kortum (1765–1847) spoke out against the unacceptable conditions in the town of Stolberg, near Aachen, which was a centre of early industrial metal processing: 'Small wonder . . . that notwithstanding the spaciousness of the valley, the thick, metallic and sulphurous smoke which pours from the oven chimneys eventually pervades the whole atmosphere and can be smelled everywhere.'[66]

But it was not just the stench caused by the rapidly expanding metal-working and chemical industries that Kortum and his colleagues perceived as exceptionally unpleasant and even classified as unhealthy. They also turned up their noses at the putrid smell of stagnant water, swamps, sewers and cemeteries. In the course of the nineteenth century, complaints were also raised about the stinking dunghills and cesspools of the countryside, but contemporary olfactory specialists constantly stressed the relative purity of country air. At the same time, however, the lowered smell tolerance levels of city people was increasingly evident: 'Excrement is the smallest but most disgusting and dangerous component of urban waste', wrote one observer at the beginning of the 1870s. 'The "soul of agriculture" may cause no offence in small farming towns, but it nauseates the more finely tuned senses of city dwellers. This is simply the hygienic instinct, although odourless is not of course synonymous with healthy, and bad smells are just one of the signs of danger.'[67]

Thus a smell was not just a smell. There were fine distinctions between smells, as Corbin shows in the case of France. Let us also attend to the words of a Berlin medical officer, who in 1878 published a book entitled *Gesundheitslehre für jedermann* (Hygiene for All):

There is no lack of 'scents' of all kinds out in the countryside, particularly in the manuring season, but they merely brush our nostrils superficially and pass away. Some enthusiasts even find them pleasant, for they represent the 'smell of the countryside'. In the city, on the other hand, smells seem to be condensed and concentrated in an oppressive mass, and are so intrusive that even the most patient of people let drop the euphemism 'foul smell' and complain of the stench. And their diagnosis is perfectly correct: city air stinks![68]

In the Middle Ages, the phrase 'town air makes you free' was an allusion to the privileged legal position of the towns. In the industrial age, however, the image of the city was shaped less by the social and professional opportunities it continued to offer than by the foul air of its huge conurbations.

As numerous historical studies of the development of environmental consciousness and social hygiene in Germany and neighbouring European countries have shown, the nose maintained its position as 'a sensitive instrument in the struggle against the threat of air pollution'[69] until the mid-nineteenth century. In 1857, when a group of farmers from Werther (Westphalia) protested against the expansion of the factory of a firm that extracted mineral oil and paraffin from bituminous slate, they received the following rejoinder from the owners: 'The protestors have been incited by agitators, for they are all farmers in daily contact with ammonia-based fertilizers. Their sense of smell is so underdeveloped and undiscriminating that under normal circumstances they would think that oil was perfume.'[70]

It was not only laymen who relied on their olfactory organ to track down smells. In 1866, a Zurich district health officer conducted old-style 'scent-samplings' in a hundred households: 'I hereby confirm that I performed an impartial assessment of the situations I examined there. Lavatorial gases are a 'conditio qua non' of our water closets and our olfactory organs should not make exaggerated demands.'[71] But as early as the 1850s, there had been a number of promising 'on-site' attempts to measure and determine the quality of the air of latrines using modern scientific methods.

If Corbin is basically right in assuming that olfactory perception had become manifestly more discriminating among the urban upper and middle classes since the end of the eighteenth century, then we need to ask what kind of 'deodorizing' measures were either contemplated or put into effect at the time. One rather curious method was reported in one of the 1864 issues of the *Monatsblatt für medizinische Statistik und öffentliche Gesundheitspflege* (Monthly Bulletin of Medical Statistics and Public Hygiene). After what appears to have been a general collection of rubbish, during which all the smelly refuse had been swept to the edge of the gutters, the mayor of an unnamed town in Saxony was forced to admit that the operation had resulted in the creation of 'an enormously disgusting smell'. This would not, in itself, have moved him to take further action, had he not received the unexpected news that the king was about to visit the town. In this state of emergency, and given the need for rapid action, the 'brilliant' idea of one of the town councillors seemed to offer a solution. It was no sooner said than done: 'The prisoners and vagrants were released from the jail and the town-hall cellars and told to line up in front of the evil-smelling places and breathe in the smell, rhythmically opening and closing their nostrils as ordered.'[72] This story may be too good to be true, but it does have the merit of underlining the importance of the organ of smell in those days as a weapon in the struggle against air pollution. The sense of smell retained its time-honoured function throughout the nineteenth century. The stink informed the citizens and the city fathers, as well as distinguished medical experts such as the Munich professor of hygiene Max von Pettenkofer (1818–1901), that the filth of the streets, the foul-smelling sewage, the contaminated rivers and the polluted air harboured dangerous miasmata and the germs of disease.

When the stench of the rapidly growing towns became even worse and people had literally 'had it up to their noses', the roads were torn up everywhere, and sewage pipes were laid to carry the refuse into the rivers, with the result that, although inner cities became less smelly in the nineteenth century, people in the surrounding areas began to complain of stinking rivers. By 1907, forty German cities already had discharge tunnels. Scientific reports based on water samples and chemical analysis played a large part in the expensive extension and improvement of municipal water supply and sewage systems in the second half of the nineteenth century.

From the end of the eighteenth century onwards, as the modern city gradually got rid of its smells and the fledgling health and hygiene movement – with the enthusiastic support of the soap and perfume industry – began to shift the site of the struggle to body odour, the vocabulary of smells began to shrink. Today, only a quarter of the words that have been used to describe the various sensations of smell since the New High German period are still current in modern German. Of the sixty-two relevant root words established by linguistic historians for Old and Middle High German, only the following could still be found in early nineteenth-century dictionaries: *aromatisch* (aromatic), *bitter* (bitter), *Bracke* (brackish water), *Brodem* (visible vapour), *Duft* (scent), *dumpf* (musty), *eifer* (pungent, sharp), *faul* (foul, rotten), *garstig* (nasty, horrible), *hantig* (Upper German for bitter), *herb* (sharp, bitter), *köhren* (to sample with the senses), *kosten* (to taste by smelling), *lecken* (to lick), *moderig* (mouldy, musty), *muffen* (to sniff out), *riechen* (to smell), *schmecken* (S. Ger., Aus., Sw.: to smell), *schmirgeln* (to smell like rancid fat), *stinken* (to stink), *Ulm* (the smell of rotting wood), *wittern* (to sniff the air, sense or scent) and *Würze* (aroma).[73] Although a few new words have been added over the years – *brenzlig* (smell of burning), for example, or *milde* (mild), both of which meant something different in Middle High German – very few of the terms mentioned here are still in use today.

Aberrations of the sense of taste

According to the German sociologist Eva Barlösius, the period since the nineteenth century is marked by a 'synthesis of taste formation and pleasurable perception' which has contributed to the 'cultivation of the senses' and their 'liberation from centuries of denigration'.[74] The thesis sounds plausible. Nevertheless, if we discount the few economic-, cultural- and nutrition-historical studies of the much-cited changeover to sweet taste, it has to be said that we still lack a historically grounded cultural psychology of changing taste. Historians have for the most part ignored the question of the extent to which industrialization and the rise of the nineteenth-century food industry have also altered other tastes (sour, bitter, salty). So here we are able to present only a few facets of the exciting story of changes of taste over this period.

The article entitled 'Sense of taste' in the *Encyclopädie der medicinischen Wissenschaften* (Encyclopedia of Medical Sciences, 1831) begins with a treatment of the four universal forms of taste (sour, bitter, salty, sweet), before going on to consider the so-called varieties in greater detail. It includes a critical discussion of the theories of the French physiologist Marie-François-Xavier Bichat (1771–1802). The latter had claimed that, 'in so far as it reserves the right to the final word on taste, habit causes this sense to deteriorate.'[75] The author of the article disputes this, agreeing only that the 'abuse of strong alcoholic drinks, strongly stimulating food and spices' may lead to a dulling of the sense of taste. His words provide a clue to the factors responsible for the mutation of taste in the nineteenth century: the increasing consumption of alcohol and the addition of new, semi-luxury items (e.g., coffee) to the daily menu.

Let us begin with the sharp-tasting alcoholic spirits that are supposedly capable of causing a permanent loss of taste. The contemporaries of Goethe were already aware that, with regard to alcohol, the problem was not so much the rising consumption of wine and beer as it was the rapid rise in the consumption of spirits after the eighteenth century. In 1796, the author of a medical topography of the city of Berlin declared that spirits were 'the preferred drink of the common man', and that they 'are now almost as much of a daily necessity as bread.'[76] According to reliable estimates, the consumption of spirits quintupled in the first three decades of the nineteenth century, owing not least to the flooding of the market with cheap potato schnapps in the 1820s. In some parts of mid-nineteenth-century Germany and Austria-Hungary, the annual per capita consumption of schnapps was just over 10 litres. One hundred years later, the per capita consumption of schnapps in the German Federal Republic was a mere 1.1 litres.

However, the much-debated nineteenth-century 'alcohol problem' will not concern us here, since we are interested in this conspicuous form of popular consumption primarily as the manifestation of a change of taste. It is plain that we are dealing here with a reaction to the extreme monotony of the nineteenth century diet, which consisted largely of bread and potatoes, with very little meat. As the physiologist Max Gruber (1853–1927) pointed out in 1888, a strong drink such as schnapps was a relatively cheap and effective way of breaking the gustatory monotony: 'Anyone who tries eating 1000 grams of bread or 2000 grams or more of potatoes day after day will soon be persuaded of the joys of replacing a tenth of this bulk with a strong and sharp-tasting liquid.'[77] So it was not spirits that dulled the sense of taste, but the other way round: large sections of the working population resorted to this little luxury because of the monotonous fare to which they were condemned by their low wages; it provided a change of taste and stimulated the taste buds.

Another very bitter, albeit non-alcoholic, drink that had been consumed in large quantities by the less well-off since the eighteenth century was chicory coffee. This popular substitute for real coffee was made from bitter-tasting chicory root (Cichorium intybus), with added sugar beet, fat and alkali carbonates. It was also known as Prussian coffee. In 1862, 80,000 metric tonnes of powdered chicory coffee were produced in Prussia alone. The economic historian Hans Jürgen Teuteberg assumes that its cheapness was not the only factor in the increasing consumption of the drink. In his opinion, we really need to establish the extent to which 'the bitter taste of real coffee which, until the end of the nineteenth century, was only rarely sugared and taken without milk or cream because of the expense, actually furthered the remarkably long career of ersatz coffee.'[78] For the present, however, we are still awaiting a mental- and cultural-historical study of ersatz coffee consumption that takes account of this factor.

Considering the importance of salt before the development of modern food-preservation technology, it is reasonable to assume that people were accustomed to eating salty foods such as salt meat and pickled vegetables until well into the nineteenth century. How far this has brought about a permanent impairment of taste, or rather an enduring predilection for all manner of salted foods, remains a matter of speculation. In any event, it is noticeable that the average per capita consumption of table salt in Germany has not gone up since the last third of the nineteenth century. Around 1896, it stood at 7.78 kilograms per year, the same as in 1871, the year of the founding of the new German Reich. This is just a little more than the 7.75 kilograms per year which *Meyers Konversationslexikon* of 1878 lists as the body's normal requirement.

And what about the taste for sour food? Here, too, a change of taste seems to have set in by the nineteenth century at the latest. As the folklorist Günter Wiegelmann has shown in his study of spiced bread, the taste for sour and bitter-spiced foods (bread, cheeses and sausages) typical of large areas of Central Europe until well into the early modern period was no longer encountered in all of these regions in the nineteenth century. The late eighteenth century saw the development of a low-spice zone that covered the Rhineland, Saxony and Mecklenburg. In these areas, unspiced bread (i.e., bread without added caraway, fennel and aniseed) began to gain ground. It is thought that the early arrival of coffee-drinking in these areas must have produced a change of taste, for since the nineteenth century people there had been accustomed to eating sweet items such as cakes, biscuits and tarts as an accompaniment to unsweetened coffee on festive and ceremonial occasions, or when paying social calls. On ordinary weekdays, they ate bread spread with sweet marmalade or sugar-beet syrup. For this reason, more and more people had begun to prefer bread 'with a neutral taste'. Wiegelmann therefore interprets the disappearance of the former variety of spices as the sign of a 'modernization' of gastronomic culture and taste.[79]

The change of preference to sweet-tasting food that may be observed among all classes of society from the early nineteenth century onwards has been thoroughly charted. As early as 1805, the student of public affairs and technical historian Johann Beckmann (1739–1811) remarked that: 'sweet things were so popular in former times that people tended to judge the quality and taste of a meal according to its degree of sweetness', and went on to add: 'This is a view still held by the larger part of the poorer classes of our country who cannot afford to keep up with the latest culinary fashions of the rich.'[80] Sugar consumption had been rising steeply in all sectors of the population since the mid-nineteenth century. In the German Reich, the consumption rate stood at about 1 kg per inhabitant around the year 1800, rising to 2.7 kg in 1850, and touching 12.63 kg by 1900. Sugar consumption had thus increased twelvefold over a period of just one hundred years.

'The taste for sweetness', writes Wiegelmann, 'began to encroach on all the various mealtimes, beginning with the food served with coffee during social visits and then proceeding to ordinary afternoon coffee (working days included), before advancing finally on breakfast and morning coffee.'[81] Popular meals consisting of a simple bowl of soup were also affected by the trend. Sugar is featured as an ingredient of just 15 per cent of the soup recipes in one of the most renowned cookery books of the sixteenth century. In the middle-class cookery books of the first half of the nineteenth century, on the other hand, about 49 per cent of the soup recipes are for sweet soups. Chocolate products of all kinds were becoming more and more popular at this time, with sweet milk chocolate replacing soft bitter chocolate. The extent to which sweet tastes were coming to dominate all the others is demonstrated by the large-scale advertising of drinking chocolate and cocoa, both of which were drinks that had been upper-class status symbols under the *ancien régime*. A notable feature of the advertising slogans for these products was their tendency to place tastiness or 'palatableness' almost on a level with nutritional value.[82]

We should also not neglect to mention the changes of taste connected with the meteoric rise of the nutrition and semi-luxury food industry.[83] After the invention of the milk centrifuge in 1877 and the introduction of pasteurization (preservation of milk by heat processing) in the 1880s, people began to complain that milk no longer tasted of 'cow'. This did not, however, prevent them from perceiving the economic and hygienic advantages of the new processes. Other food products, such as bread, sausages and cheese, only began to change and lose something of their traditional aroma in the course of the twentieth century. Such losses were offset, or at least hidden, by the addition of taste concentrates.

The last third of the nineteenth century also saw the beginning of a trend away from traditional, top-fermented types of beer towards bottom-fermenting brewing methods, which yielded a different, rather bitter taste. Finally, we must note the triumphal entry of meat extract, which began in the 1860s and was clearly to the taste of large sections of the population. As early as the end of the nineteenth century, advertisers were claiming that this most successful of all the products of the modern food industry would 'enhance the flavour' of soups, sauces, vegetables and meat. As one German nutritionist noted soberly shortly before the First World War: 'Industry has managed to simplify not only the consumer's sense of taste but also the domestic use of these products for the seasoning of dishes and the preparation of consommés.'[84]

The deterioration of tactility

The transformation of the sense of touch in the industrial age is still uncharted territory. There is no historical research on the subject, so we are compelled to rely on guesswork and a few pointers in the available sources. A clue is provided by an article entitled 'The sense of touch' in the *Encyclopädie der medicinischen Wissenschaften* mentioned above. This states that the sense of touch 'is crude and imperfect among people engaged in the kind of heavy manual labour that turns the skin of the hands horny.'[85] The question is how far this applies to the growing number of industrial workers. Karl Marx, as we have seen, noted that the lathe had largely replaced the human hand in the production of tools and machines. Nevertheless, machines could not replace much heavy and hazardous manual work, so that calloused hands undoubtedly continued to be a characteristic physical feature of the industrial and manual worker as the nineteenth century wore on. In this context, we might note the observations of the historian Michael Giesecke. In an essay on the history of printing, he wonders whether, in addition to reinforcing our 'tactile sensoria', the use of tools might have led to a shifting of the 'sensorial boundaries of our hands'.[86]

But touch is not simply localized in the hand. Did the long-term changes in the world of life and work (technologization, industrialization) also lead to a deadening of the tactile sense in other sensitive areas of the body? The medical literature of this period offers a preliminary purchase on the question. The statistics for skin diseases which are available for some countries from the nineteenth century onwards, report no abnormal increases in loss of dermatological sensitivity that might indicate a rise or reduction of normal thresholds of tactility. According to a statistical report by the American Dermatological Association, there were only fifty-six cases of anaesthesia (total loss of sensation) in the USA in the period between 1878 and 1911. Ninety of the cases reported were diagnosed as hyperaesthesia (acute skin sensitivity). These two conditions represent a bare 0.09 per cent and 0.014 per cent, respectively, of all 'skin diseases' reported in the period![87]

In a noteworthy study published in 1896, the Swiss educational hygienist Théodore Vannod demonstrated that the increasing demands of a changing work- and lifestyle could lead to the temporary and even permanent deterioration of their 'levels of receptivity' (Wilhelm Wundt). Vannod's indicators for mental and physical overexertion among his experimentees were the sensitivity of their skins to tactile stimulation and their sensitivity to pain. The results were unambiguous. For Vannod there was only one possible conclusion: afternoon lessons in Swiss schools had to be abolished. One wonders what this Swiss investigator of 'overburdening' would have recommended, had his physiological experiments included the vast army of employees and factory workers who knew neither the eight-hour day nor the five-day week.

— 10 —
Experimental Physiology and the Separation of the Senses

> Observation and experiment may grasp and represent each sense, both in its independent existence and in its particular way of responding to the external world.
>
> Johannes Evangelista Purkyně, *Towards a Subjective Understanding of Vision* (1819)

The 'law of specific sensory energy'

If one looks today at the huge number of scientific publications on the subject of the senses, the question of disciplinary jurisdiction appears to be resolved: the senses are no longer so much a matter of philosophical enquiry, but in the first instance a branch of physiological research. However, this is not the subject of the ensuing chapter.

The beginnings of sensory physiology reach back far into the eighteenth century, but its real founder is considered to be Johannes Müller (1801–1858). 'The philosophy of the senses has been derived by Müller entirely from nature',[1] wrote Rudolf Virchow (1821–1902), who was probably the most famous German doctor of the second half of the nineteenth century. By finding a new, scientifically verifiable basis for the individuation of the outer senses, Müller, who taught physiology in Bonn before moving to Berlin, transformed the five senses into a rapidly propagating number of sensorial modalities that could be investigated experimentally, and without reference to their social or natural-philosophical context.

Published in 1826, Müller's pioneering work on the comparative physiology of the visual sense formulated the 'law of specific sensory energy', which was still being discussed by scientists in the twentieth century, albeit in a modified form. It is based on the assumption that each kind of nerve (optical, cochlear, olfactory, etc.) possesses its own inherent specific energy which is incapable of further physical definition. Müller cites the example of the sense of sight. Regardless of the kind of stimulus (electrical, chemical or mechanical) applied to the optical nerve, the latter will invariably produce sensations of light, darkness or colour. According to this theory, it is not the stimulus that is sensed, only 'that which is perceptible' to the particular sense concerned.

In *Elements of Physiology* (2 vols., 1834–40), which was long considered to be the standard work on this new fundamental medical subject, Müller expanded his sensory-physiological theory and summarized it in the form of ten theses. The eighth of these states, for example, that:

It is true that the sensory nerves initially perceive only their own situations, or that the sensorium responds to the conditions of the sensory nerves. However, these sensory nerves share, as bodies, the characteristics of other bodies, since they are extended in space and susceptible to communicated impulses and chemical modification by heat or electricity; so that when they are affected by external causes they will inform the sensorium of qualities and changes in the external world, in addition to registering changes in their own state. Such changes will vary according to characteristics and sensory energies specific to the particular sense concerned.[2]

In other words, each sensation depends on a particular state of the nerves. It is not the qualities of the objects operating on the senses from outside that are conducted to the sensory centre, but the various sensory energies. Precisely what these specific qualities of the senses are is a question that Müller leaves open. It is, for instance, unclear whether the various sensory energies are localized in parts of the brain or in the spinal cord (seventh thesis).

In order to understand the historical-scientific status of the 'law of specific sensory energies', and to explain its enormous influence on later nineteenth-century research, we must bear in mind that when Müller formulated his theses it was not known that nerve fibres are merely extensions of nerve cells, and that the latter are themselves excited by short electrical pulses. Instead, the human nervous system was thought to be a tissue of fibres which transmitted the stimuli from the external sense organs to the brain. The rapid acceptance of the theory of specific sensory perception was owing not least to the fact that it accorded with modern technological understanding, and also opened the way to arguments by analogy. In one of the later editions of his *On the Sensations of Tone* (1863), Hermann von Helmholtz writes:

> Nerves have been often and not unsuitably compared to telegraph wires. Such a wire conducts one kind of electric current and no other; it may be stronger, it may be weaker, it may move in either direction; it has no other qualitative differences. Nevertheless, according to the different kinds of apparatus with which we provide its terminations, we can send telegraphic dispatches, ring bells, explode mines, decompose water, move magnets, magnetize iron, develop light, and so on. *So with the nerves.*[3]

Recent histories of science have attempted to establish parallels between Müller's and Helmholtz's rigid separation of the individual senses and Karl Marx's differentiation of the senses and assertion of their autonomy. These studies refer to a passage in the *Economic and Philosophical Manuscripts* of 1844 where Marx states that: 'An object appears differently to the *eye* than to the *ear*, and the object of the eye *is* different from the object of the ear.'[4] But for Marx as a philosopher, the problem was not the scientifically explicable separation and specialization of the senses, but the alienation of the senses within the property relations of capitalist society.

Müller's theory of specific sensory energy was expanded and modified by Hermann von Helmholtz – probably the most important German physiologist of the second half of the nineteenth century – on the basis of his own sensory physiological research, which was concerned largely with the sense of hearing. Helmholtz assumed, for instance, that the perception of sound at any level corresponded to the excitation of a particular fibre of the cochlear nerve. In the case of colour perception, on the other hand, only three nerve fibres needed to be distinguished, which transmitted the perception of blue, yellow and red respectively. He further distinguished between the qualities already mentioned (the three basic colours, high and low tones) and the so-called modalities (e.g., sensations of light and sound), in which there were, according to him, no transitions. New sensorial qualities arose only as a result of mixing the basic qualities.

In 1893, the psychologist of perception Oswald Külpe (1862–1915) added up the sense perceptions as they were then known and came up with 694 different sensations of brightness and 150 colour shades for the sense of sight, 11,063 tones for hearing, three or four qualities of taste and touch, and an indefinite number of smells. At almost the same time, his English colleague Edward Titchener (1867–1927) arrived at 32,820 colours and 11,600 sounds, which were allegedly distinguishable on the basis of existing studies of optics and acoustics and with the assistance of the sense organs concerned.[5]

The physiologist Ewald Hering (1834–1918), who succeeded Johannes Evangelista Purkyně at the University of Prague, attempted to relate Helmholtz's theory of perception to certain processes taking place in the brain. He thought that all phenomena of sensation, perception and cognition could be explained by studying the physiology of the brain. According to Hering, the brain cells were excited by stimuli from the sensory nerve fibres, 'and depending on the capacity of a brain cell easily and frequently to receive the stimuli arriving from one sense organ or the other, or from this or that particular sensory nerve fibre, it will develop a specialization for the specific qualities of precisely those kinds of stimuli.'[6] Thus, sensory experience implied the specialization and individualization of the activities of particular parts of the human brain. The 'sensory energies' developed in the course of this process were, in Hering's opinion, nothing less than the 'organic expression of our individual memory'. He was, thus, concerned primarily with the interactions of cerebral functions and perceptions. With these experiments, Hering paved the way for twentieth-century brain research, which uses both physiological and psychological methods to explore the cerebral mechanisms of perception and cognition.

The discovery of new senses

Johannes Müller's physiology of the senses called for a separation of physical phenomena from the phenomena of perception, which led to a shift of attention from the object of perception to the particular form in which it was perceived. As the sociologist of knowledge Dieter Hoffmann-Axthelm has stressed, 'this meant that from now on the line dividing the outer from the inner perception of objects and feelings was a matter of indifference; for regardless of where the stimuli originated, everything was produced by inner sensation.'[7] So the way was now clear for the discovery of new senses. One sense in particular, the so-called muscular sense, had failed to fit into the earlier scheme, and this could now be defined.

At the beginning of the nineteenth century, a number of physiologists had already tried independently to prove the existence of a muscular sensation. Following the sensory-physiological theories of Müller and Helmholtz, later physiologists attempted to provide experimental verification of the existence of feelings and perceptions specific to this sense. They believed, for instance, that the sensation of active or passive movement and the sense of position, weight and resistance were coupled to the muscular sense. It was, on the other hand, rather more difficult to determine which perceptions we owe to this sense. The example most frequently cited is our idea of the magnitude of a weight or load supplied by the various tensings of a muscle. Ernst Heinrich Weber (1795–1878) was the first to undertake a more precise description of the muscular sense. His experiments showed that this sense even enabled humans to distinguish between barely perceptible degrees of heaviness. Weber's method of testing the muscular sense was to wrap weights in a cloth, which then had to be lifted up by grasping the knotted ends with the hands. The idea was to prevent the sense of touch or, rather, pressure from influencing the perception.

Despite these extremely elaborate investigations and measurements, many nineteenth-century physiologists denied the existence of this sense. The Graz physiologist Alexander Rollet (1834–1903) summarized their arguments as follows:

> The actions of this muscular sense are entirely analogous to those produced by the skin's sense of pressure or space, or by the retina of the eye. This is why the very existence of a muscular sense, or at least the dependence on the muscular sense of some of the perceptions mentioned earlier, has been denied by various scientists, who have ascribed some or all of these perceptions either to the domain of the skin's sense of touch, or to the sense of sight.[8]

Those who accepted the theory of a separate muscular sense, however, pointed to the presence of sensitive nerve fibres within the muscles (e.g., Ernst Heinrich Weber and Charles Bell) or to sense impressions peculiar to the muscular sense (Wilhelm Wundt).

New methods of physiological measurement

In a remark that was entirely in keeping with the ideas of his celeb-rated colleague Johannes Müller, the physiologist Friedrich Tiedemann (1781–1861) noted in 1830 that: 'When taking an empirical approach to physiology, we first try to grasp the relations of living bodies and their characteristics to our senses, and to investigate their appearance and practical manifestations by means of those senses. . . . We per-form our observations and experiments either by means of the naked senses or with the aid of various instruments.'[9] In investigations of the visual sense, for example, the ophthalmoscope is used to look into the depths of the eye, the ophthalmometer to measure the curvature of the cornea and the spectrophotometer to determine the intensity of monochromatic light. All these instruments were invented by Hermann von Helmholtz in the mid-nineteenth century to assist his experiments in physiological optics and colour perception.

Other investigational and metrological methods were developed or refined in the course of the nineteenth century. In 1835, the Bremen doctor and biologist Gottfried Reinhold Treviranus (1776–1837) published the results of his microscopic investigations of the retina. They marked the beginning of a new field of research known to the history of science and medicine as 'microphysiology'.[10] His well-known and much-cited tuning fork experiment of 1834 gave Ernst Heinrich Weber the idea that sounds that are reproduced in the inner ear via the bones of the skull are received by the cochlea, while sound waves are carried by air to the vestibulum or the fleshy part of the bony labyrinth of the inner ear. This reflection gave birth to a test that is still used today in the examination of hearing disorders. Ewald Hering developed a so-called aesthesiometer for the measurement of the sense of touch. It consisted of twelve cylindrical rods, of which only one was smooth, while the rest had varying degrees of roughness (ran-ging from 0.11 micrometers to 1.0 micrometers). The experimental subject was required to indicate which of the rods still felt rough to the touch. The Dutchman Hendrik Zwaardemaker (1857–1930) invented the olfactometer, which calibrated thresholds of sensitivity to various odorous substances. This simple device consists of two tubes of different lengths which can be pushed over each other. Pushing the outer tube forwards exposes more of the surface of the other tube, which is coated with a scent. Using this method, it is easy to ascertain the acuteness of a person's sense of smell. In the physiological study of taste, the quality-priority saporimeter was joined at a relatively early stage by the quantity-priority gustometer.

A concept introduced into sensory physiology by the still well-known psycho-physicist Gustav Fechner (1801–1887) acquired importance in the context of the new measuring techniques of those times. By 'stimulation threshold' Fechner meant the degree of intensity required for a stimulus to produce a sensation that was still just about perceptible. The equation named after him states that the strength of a sensation increases in proportion to the logarithm of the strength of the stimulus. Fechner had discovered that the intensity of light perception was not directly proportional to the intensification of the physical stimulus. The 'difference threshold' was Fechner's term for the smallest difference of stimulus that is still capable of rendering perceptible a difference in the intensity of a sensation. Fechner's equation soon entered the textbooks. 'To determine the value of this difference threshold experimentally', states an introduction to psycho-physics published in 1878, 'we can first use the so-called method of the just-noticeable difference, whose use and verification procedures do not appear to require any further assistance from mathematics.'[11] On the basis of Fechner's discovery, it was thought that sensory perception consisted of a succession of magnitudes of varying intensity which could now be measured quantitatively, as a result of which human sensation would become to a large extent calculable.

The physiology of the sense of vision

Many of the revolutionary nineteenth-century discoveries in the field of sensory physiology derived from experimental investigations into the sense of sight. The theory of vision developed by Johannes Müller and extended by Hermann von Helmholtz deserves special mention in this context, for it was largely owing to this theory that the sense of sight ceased to be regarded as a privileged form of knowledge and became a quite normal object of experimental scientific enquiry.

As already indicated, the basic outlines of this new approach are already present in the work of Johannes Müller. He was the first proponent of the pioneering view that it could be shown experimentally that, 'when we see, we are experiencing the state of the retina and nothing more than this, and that the retina is, so to speak, the visual field itself; dark when at rest and light when excited.'[12] Müller believed it was possible to explain the then still unexplored collaboration of mind, brain and retina by assuming that 'the mind continues to have an effect on the nerve endings to the extent that the sensory nerves are merely processes of the sensorium.'[13] This later earned him the accusation of 'nativism' from Helmholtz, by which he meant that Müller subscribed to the view that certain ways of thinking, acting and feeling were innate. In contrast to Müller, and drawing on the ophthalmological research of his own time, Helmholtz insisted that the relations of corresponding positions of the retina observed by Müller were not given in nature, but had to be learned, and were therefore subject to alteration and change.

The centrepiece of this emphatically empirical theory of vision was the doctrine of the semiotic character of sense perception which Helmholtz formulated in his *Handbook of Physiological Optics*: 'Our ideas of objects can only be symbols; naturally given signs for the things we learn to use in order to regulate our actions and movements. If we have learned to read these symbols correctly, we will be in a position to organize our actions with their help, so that they accord with our wishes; in other words, any new sensory experiences will occur as expected.'[14] This semiotic theory of perception was the subject of heated controversy in Helmholtz's own lifetime, although in the further course of the nineteenth century it proved to be particularly fruitful in the science of the physiology of seeing.

Helmholtz was also the co-founder of the so-called trichromatic theory of vision. His first publication dealing with colour perception appeared in 1852. Here he returned to the concept of Thomas Young (1773–1829) of the three basic colours of the spectrum – red, green and violet – and expanded it into a trichromatic theory of colour. The theory states that, according to the way they are mixed, the three basic colours mentioned are sufficient to produce every shade of colour in the spectrum. Investigations of congenital colour-blindness and so-called dichromatism (two-colour vision) seemed to confirm this trichromatic theory. Ewald Hering, on the other hand, held to his own 'Opposite Colour Theory', which states that colour perception falls into three contrastingly structured pairs of colours (red/green, yellow/blue, white/black). Both these colour theories were hotly debated until well into the twentieth century.[15] 'In historical retrospect', wrote the Berlin neurophysiologist Otto-Joachim Grüsser (*d.* 1995), 'it is satisfying to note that each of these two great adversaries of the second half of the nineteenth century has turned out to be correct in one of the branches of the physiology of colour perception.'[16] Today, we know that the distinction of colours also involves cerebral mechanisms which did not become a topic of intensive neurophysiological research until the last three decades of the twentieth century.

The physiology of the sense of hearing

There were occasional physiological experiments with the organ of hearing in the eighteenth century, but the real breakthroughs of experimental research occurred in the first half of the nineteenth century. One of the initiators of the modern physiological approach was François Magendie (1783–1855), a professor at the Collège de France in Paris. Magendie's experiments showed that the skin of the external auditory meatus was particularly sensitive. He also noted that high-pitched sounds were painful to the ear, and described the regression of hearing in old age as an effect of 'the deteriorating sensitivity of the cochlear nerve.

Among Magendie's notable German contemporaries was the doctor and poet Justinus Kerner. Under the supervision of his Tübingen teacher, Johann Heinrich Ferdinand von Autenrieth (1772–1835), himself the author of a well-known textbook on human physiology (1802), Kerner had written a much discussed medical dissertation on animal hearing. His fellow student Karl August Varnhagen von Ense (1785–1858) described his animal and sensory-physiological experiments as follows: 'He has chosen the sense of hearing as his dissertation subject, which has involved him in some quite new experiments with animals. . . . The experiments are clever and imaginative and he does his best to avoid cruelty to the animals.'[17] In the light of the modern debate on the necessity of animal experiments, many of Kerner's vivisections (e.g., the removal of a cat's outer ear) may now strike us as highly questionable. Yet it must be conceded that they are not without a certain originality. The same applies to the experiments with which Kerner discovered that animals respond to both pitch and tone colour and that their directional hearing varies from species to species.

The physiology of the organ of hearing is also indebted to Johannes Müller for numerous fresh discoveries. His investigations of sound conduction in the tympanic cavity were a major advance. Among his other achievements was his discovery, when experimenting on himself, that the hearing is muffled if the eardrum is subjected to extreme pressure by either rarefying or compressing the air in the tympanic cavity.

Ernst Heinrich Weber's work on the functioning of the inner ear represents further progress. Weber did not experiment with animals, but based his theory on the physics of acoustics. 'Weber's test' became famous. Here, the experimental subject blocks his ears by clamping his hands firmly against them. This makes his voice sound much louder to himself than when his ears are open. If only one ear is closed, the voice sounds much louder through that ear than through the ear left open. The same effect is produced by the tuning fork experiment already mentioned in another context. Weber was actually convinced from an early stage that the tuning fork would play an important role in the diagnosis of auditory deficiencies.

The first half of the nineteenth century witnessed the first attempts to measure hardness of hearing precisely. Various kinds of measuring devices were developed, with the pocket watch eventually emerging as the standard audiometer. Best known was the method used by the now completely forgotten Viennese doctor Franciscus Polansky. It consisted of a rod-shaped device with a sliding watch attached to it. The rod bore a mark representing the distance at which a person of normal hearing would hear the ticking of the watch, with both ears closed and the end of the rod held between his teeth. Any deviation from this standard was then the measure of the degree of diminished hearing. According to the celebrated Viennese ear specialist Adam Politzer (1835–1920), the author of a history of otology, 'one might also ascertain the acuteness of a patient's hearing by speaking sentences out loud.'[18] Politzer was also the inventor of an audiometer named after him, which is still in use today. With this apparatus, a rhythmical tone is produced by striking a steel cylinder, the distance at which the standard tone is still audible serving as the yardstick of aural acuity. From the 1850s onwards, the auriscope was used to examine the acoustic meatus and eardrum. The initial light source was daylight, but artificial light (gas lamps and electric light) was used more and more towards the end of the nineteenth century.

Hermann von Helmholtz's pioneering research was not confined to the field of the physiological. His book *On the Sensations of Tone as a Physiological Basis for a Theory of Music* (1863), which took him seven years to write, became a standard text of modern acoustics. Its starting point was the experimental research on the speed of nervous impulses which he had begun in Königsberg. He demonstrated that this speed was a variable quantity which was determined by physical conditions (e.g., temperature). The experiments in physics that he completed in Heidelberg led to the modification of the hitherto unchallenged acoustic law of the physicist Georg Simon Ohm (1789–1854), which stated that the human ear could receive only simple harmonic vibrations. Helmholtz showed that almost all the tones produced by musical instruments were composite in character, and that the precise combination of the overtones was the decisive factor in tone colour. The presence of overtones that could not be immediately heard had not been suspected up to that point. Helmholtz also discovered that the floating rhythms created by the mutual interference of notes with the same oscillation periods were an essential element of musical sound effects. In addition, his researches led him to the formulation of a resonance theory of hearing, which was to remain more or less unchanged for decades, and he proved by experiment that the overtones of vowels change according to the position of the oral cavity.

The works of the physicist Ernst Mach (1838–1916) occupy a special place among the numerous studies of the physiology of hearing that appeared in the second half of the nineteenth century. Mach discovered, among other things, that the semicircular canals next to the cochlea were a sense organ for the perception of rotary motion. Even before Helmholtz, Adam Politzer had discovered (in 1861) the vibrations of the auditory ossicles during the transmission of sound. According to his own graphic account, he did this by 'exposing the hammer-incus joints of fresh human hearing organs and sticking glass threads to the hammerhead, whose vibrations were then recorded onto a piece of paper covered with a layer of soot.'[19] We should also mention the investigations into the rapid exhaustion of the ear (e.g., by continuous high-pitched whistling sounds) and the studies of so-called after-sensations, which Fechner describes as the 'souvenirs' of sound impressions which have already died away. Finally, there were the animal experiments conducted by some of Helmholtz's pupils on the damage to hearing caused by long and continuous exposure to loud noise, which were of enormous practical significance in the then still very new discipline of occupational medicine.

The physiology of the sense of smell

Compared to the work completed on the senses of sight and hearing, the physiologists of the eighteenth and nineteenth centuries were only marginally concerned with smell. The schematic division of smells into seven different types (aromatic, scented, ambrosial, garlic-like, stinking, repulsive and disgusting) by the Swedish doctor and botanist Karl von Linné (1707–1781) was still being discussed seriously in the nineteenth century. The first comprehensive work on the sense of smell emerged from the pen of the Paris anatomist Hippolyte Cloquet (1784–1840) in 1821. A German translation appeared three years later under the somewhat elaborate title *Ophresiologie, oder Lehre von den Gerüchen, von dem Geruchsinn und den Geruchsorganen und deren Krankheiten* (Ophresiology, or The Theory of Smells: On the Sense of Smell and the Organs of Smell and their Diseases). From an anatomical and physiological basis, Cloquet devotes more than 500 pages to the 'nature' and classification of smells, as well as the olfactory nerves and the 'conditions of smelling'. Concerning the seat of the sense of smell, for instance, he writes: 'Henceforward, we are no longer dealing with guesswork. We may state as a general principle that in humans and most of the animal vertebrates the nostrils and mucous membranes are assuredly the parts where the sense of smell has its seat, and that they perform the work necessary for the exercise of this particular sensory power.'[20]

Just how little was known about the physiology of the sense of smell in those days is clear from Cloquet's extremely vague remark about the olfactory nerves: 'The nerves of the mucous membrane are manifestly of two kinds; some serve the purpose of smelling, and these are the branches of the olfactory nerves, or the first pair, while others perform the task of preserving the life of the smell in the skin.'[21] The separation of the olfactory mucosa (*regio olfactoria*) from the ordinary nasal mucous membrane that is touched on here was not examined experimentally until the 1850s, when several studies appeared.[22] Among them was an essay whose title, 'Untersuchung des Retinazapfens und des Riechhautepithels bei einem Hingerichteten' (Investigation of the Retinal Ganglion and Olfactory Epithelium of an Executed Male), blandly reveals the use of experimental materials which would nowadays be regarded as ethically questionable in the highest degree.

The connection between the fibres of the *nervus olfactorius* and the sensory cells of the mucous epithelium remained a contentious issue for a long period of time, and was only clarified histologically at a much later date. The tiny sensory hairs of the olfactory cells – whose structure is now fully known, following examination by modern electron microscopes – were discovered and described by Max Schultze (1825–1874) in 1856.

Thus, the physiology of the sense of smell made little progress until well into the second half of the nineteenth century. Nevertheless, the number of pages devoted to the subject of smell in the physiological textbooks began to increase. Where it had been dismissed in eleven pages in Rudolf Wagner's *Handwörterbuch der Physiologie* (Concise Dictionary of Physiology) of 1844, it managed to get sixty-two pages in the physiological lexicon published by Ludimar Hermann (1838–1914) in 1880. The smell receptors in the nasal mucous membrane were first described by Max Schultze in 1863. In 1886, Emil Aronsohn (1863–?) published his experimental investigations into olfactory physiology, in which he dealt with the habituating effects of smelling. It was not until Hendrik Zwaardemaker's invention of the olfacto-meter in 1884 that research in the field received another boost. Using Zwaardemaker's smell gauge, it was at last possible to measure keenness of smell. His new method enabled Fechner's law of the proportional increase of sensitivity thresholds to be applied to the sense of smell.

The use of rhinoscopy for the diagnostic examination of the nostrils begins with Joseph Czermak (1825–1872). Czermak introduced the new procedure in an article in the prestigious *Wiener Medizinische*

Wochenschrift (Vienna Medical Weekly) in 1858. The instrument consisted of a double tube, which could hold the tongue flat at the same time. After the 1860s, doctors also increasingly used funnel-shaped mirrors to examine the nasopharynx.

In the second third of the nineteenth century, so-called mental chronometry found a role in the discipline of physiological psychology established by Wilhelm Wundt (1832–1920). The biologist Gustav Jäger (1832–1917) – or 'Soul Sniffer', as he was known to his detractors – believed that its methods should also be used to investigate the sense of smell. With the aid of a Hipper chronoscope, or chronometer, Jäger examined a host of scents for their effects on the nervous apparatus. Jäger's neuroanalysis, as he called it, proceeded as follows: 'I took two successive measurements before and after the inhalation of a scent, and then took the averages and compared them. If the second figure was lower than the first, it proved that my nervous excitability had risen as a result of the inhalation; if the second average value was greater, it meant that my excitability had decreased.'[23] Once he had made enough of these measurements on himself and his voluntary guinea pigs, it seemed clear beyond reasonable doubt 'that the fleeting substances that affect the nose pleasantly produce an acceleration of time, or in other words an increase of excitement. The unpleasant ones, on the other hand, have a retarding or depressing effect on the sensibilities.'[24]

Although highly controversial in the scientific world of the second third of the nineteenth century, Jäger's theory of smell became extremely familiar to the world at large, for it provided the basis of a hygienics oriented on the deodorization of the body. His popularity made Jäger even more suspicious in the eyes of his opponents. His scientific presentation of his neuroanalysis to the fifty-sixth Congress of German Scientists and Physicians at Baden-Baden ended in uproar when he began to wind up his lecture with a description of the so-called defecation experiment. Jäger's words and the heckling from the audience were recorded in the proceedings. Just as Jäger was turning to his neuroanalytical scent graph and explaining that the 'two first averages [were taken] before the act of defecation, the other three averages post actum defecationis . . . and the last after the exhalation of this smell into the fresh air',[25] he was simply shouted down with cries of 'Stop, stop!' Although this scandal undoubtedly damaged his scientific reputation, it clearly failed to depress sales of his highly successful 'perspiration-promoting' woollen clothing (the 'Jäger uniform'), which numbered the Württemberg industrial magnate Robert Bosch (1861–1942) among its patrons.

The physiology of the sense of taste

In the physiological manuals of the late eighteenth and early nineteenth centuries, the sense of taste was treated more or less as perfunctorily as the sense of smell. We have seen that Aristotle distinguished between seven qualities of taste (sweet, sour, salty, bitter, sharp, tangy and astringent). In the year 1751, Karl von Linné and Albrecht von Haller (1708–77) located eleven and twelve different kinds of taste, respectively. In the first half of the nineteenth century, however, this number is sometimes radically reduced. The more experimentally minded physiologists initially acknowledged just two tastes: sweet and bitter. On the basis of his own research, the Innsbruck physiologist Maximilian von Vintschgau (1832–1902), who wrote the entry on smell in Hermann's *Handbuch der Physiologie* (Manual of Physiology, 1880), came to the conclusion – still valid until quite recently – that there were just four basic taste sensations, that is, sweet, salty, bitter and sour. More than two decades were to elapse before this quadripartite division was generally accepted. It was not until very recently that biochemists were able to demonstrate the existence of a fifth variant of taste: umami.

In those days, the sense of taste was generally tested using syrup, quinine, a concentrated solution of common salt, and extremely diluted hydrochloric acid or acetic acid. An early standard work on the physiology of taste published in 1825 by Wilhelm Horn (1803–1871) allows us a glimpse of the already very systematic procedures followed by early nineteenth-century scientists:

> I took the liquid substances or crystals on a brush and, after rising in the morning, washing out my oral cavity and drinking a glass of water, I applied it to several of my lingual papillae in front of a mirror. I was possibly able to do this more easily than some because I have a number of papillis fungiformibus on the middle of my tongue, which are quite separate from the others. I then coated my soft palate and the other areas of my oral cavity and wrote down the title of the experiment.

Before applying the substance to another type of papillae I naturally washed my mouth with water. . . . I repeated the experiments with impartial friends and we obtained the same results.[26]

Qualitative testing was normally considered sufficient, but quantitative methods of measuring taste (gustometry) were also introduced later.

The Berlin physiologist Johannes Müller, whom we have often had occasion to mention before, was interested mainly in the taste nerves and knew of Horn's experimental demonstration of the differential sensitivities of the papillae. Like Albrecht von Haller and Charles Bell (1774–1842) before him, he concluded that these leaf-shaped little warts on the tongue were in fact organs of taste. It was not until 1867 that the taste buds were discovered independently by Gustav Schwalbe (1844–1916), a pupil of Max Schultze, and the Swede Otto Christian Lovén (1835–1904), but their exact number remained a matter of speculation for quite some time. Only in 1906 was the anatomist Friedrich Heiderich (1878–?) able to show that one papilla contained a maximum of 508 and a minimum of thirty-three taste buds. In 1892, the physiologist Lewis E. Shore demonstrated that the tongue's sensitivity to taste not only was greater in some areas than others but also varied according to the quality of the sensation.

The physiology of the sense of touch

The first physiologist to undertake a systematic experimental investigation of the sense of touch was Ernst Heinrich Weber, whom we have already encountered in an earlier context. His interest in the subject was purely pragmatic: 'The exact investigation of the sense of touch and the common sensibility of the skin and muscles is of particular interest, for no other sense organ offers so many opportunities for experiment and measurement without risk to ourselves.'[27] Weber was aware from the outset of the difficulties of experimental work in this field, realizing at an early stage that 'pure sensation tells us nothing about where the nerves that produce the sensations are being stimulated' and that 'all sensations are originally only conditions that stimulate our consciousness. Although such stimuli may vary in quality and degree, they do not make us immediately conscious of spatial relations.'[28]

Knowledge of the fine structure of the skin was sketchy at the time that Weber began his experiments. Although the vital importance for the perception of vibrations of the large, lamellae-like corpuscles at the end of the nerve fibres of the subcutis (Pacinian corpuscles) was already recognized, their function as receptors was still a matter of debate. So it was not surprising that Weber should continue to assume that the skin's senses of heat and pressure were one and the same thing. It was not until the 1880s that Magnus Gustaf Blix (1849–1904) in Sweden and Alfred Goldscheider (1858–1935) in Germany demonstrated that the skin contained both temperature and pressure points by subjecting tiny areas of skin to electrical stimulation.

'Sensorial circles' was Weber's term for highly sensitive areas of the skin. He thought that their anatomical substratum was the skin nerves and assigned a particular nerve to one or more of the circles. He also noted that, when he applied the points of a pair of compasses to the skin, the pricks could not be experienced as two distinct sensations beyond a certain distance. This marked the discovery of a phenomenon described towards the end of the nineteenth century as the 'simultaneous space threshold' by Max von Frey (1852–1932), who was a pupil of the celebrated Leipzig experimental physiologist Carl Ludwig (1816–1894). As late as the 1960s, physiologists were still using Weber's compass to measure the sensitivity of various areas of the hand.

We have already mentioned Weber's pioneering exploration of the sense of pressure which led to the law of just-noticeable differences named after him (Weber's law). As we have seen, Weber rejected the idea of a specific epidermal temperature sensor, but this did not deter him from looking for areas of the skin that were more sensitive than others to heat and cold. The role of the so-called pain sense, which can also be localized on the skin, was relatively minor, for he lumped pain together with the 'common sense', about which it was impossible to obtain scientifically exact information.

Weber's achievements in the physiology of skin sensation have been acknowledged by many medical and scientific historians.[29] His famous treatise *Tastsinn und Gemeingefühl* (Sense of Touch and Common Sense, 1846) not only included important research results in the field of the physiology of the skin but also gave a boost to sensory physiology in general. Terms still in use today in physiological research, such as 'threshold of stimulation', 'temperature sense' or 'simultaneous spatial threshold', were either first coined by Weber or named after his experiments.

Towards the end of the nineteenth century many of the questions which had either been left open or simply not considered in Weber's theories of the skin senses were finally answered by the Würzburg physiologist Max von Frey, whom we have already mentioned. In 1894, he proved the existence of pain points. In so doing, he added a fourth sense to the senses of pressure, warmth and coldness. A year later, he discovered that each of these four forms of sensation or modalities possessed its own organ. The so-called Krause-Endkolben (Krause's corpuscles), for example, were responsible for the sensation of coldness. These form a sensitive receptor, consisting of a round or oval body with built-in nerve threads, which is situated in the epidermis.

For his experiments Frey constructed a simple device that enabled him to apply tiny stimuli to the skin. It consisted of a series of brushes of different degrees of stiffness which were fixed with sealing wax to a movable rod. This instrument, known universally in physiological research as the 'Frey brush', is used to locate pain points and to determine their threshold values. The experiments performed on prisoners of both sexes without their consent by Cesare Lombroso (1836–1909) in the 1880s show how such pain-measuring instruments could also be used for inhumane and scientifically dubious investigations. 'The criminal's predilection for a painful and risky operation such as tattooing', wrote Lombroso, 'led me to conclude that, like many lunatics, criminals are less sensitive to physical pain than normal people.'[30] This Italian psychiatrist and criminologist attempted to substantiate this ideologically loaded theory of the inferior physical sensitivities of professional criminals by means of a whole series of physiological experiments. To test the reflex responses of his human guinea pigs, he stuck needles into them and treated them with electric shocks, and must certainly have left them with more than merely unpleasant sensory impressions.

To summarize: the experimental sensory physiology of the nineteenth century is characterized by the definition of the senses according to sensory modalities. In contrast to earlier times, it is now no longer the individual senses that are enumerated and classified, but sensory perceptions of all kinds. The reinterpretation of the sense of touch as a skin sensation consisting of a number of discrete aspects (pressure, heat, cold and pain) may be regarded as typical. The methods and instruments developed by leading nineteenth-century sensory physiologists produced results that are still valid today, although they are hardly compatible with traditional ideas of the five senses and have fostered the separation of the senses.

Part IV

The 'Rediscovery' of the Senses in the Twentieth Century

— 11 —

Touching – or The New Pleasure in the Body

The hand will replace all other instruments, and by allying itself to the intellect will secure the latter's universal domination. . . . It is impossible to say what will happen when the hand is raised from the gutter to the ranks of the high nobility.

Gerhard Hauptmann, *The Island of the Great Mother* (1924)

A 'haptic age'?

According to an article in the *Stuttgarter Nachrichten* of 18 October 1999, we have now entered a 'haptic age', and the writer was not just referring to a new trend in underwear. The piece also noted other signs of the changing times: for instance, the stress on tenderness in sexual therapy, as well as the increasing demand for healers with 'magic hands' (animal magnetopaths, masseurs and chiropractors) and the supposedly growing number of adults in need of 'loving sex' – to whom the advertisers have been more than happy to respond ('tender as a cuddle', 'soft as a caress'). Two years before this, the German weekly newspaper *Die Zeit* (11 April 1997) published a 'Manifesto for the Emancipation of the Sense of Touch', which appeared to reflect a 'new pleasure in touching'. So was the twentieth century perhaps signing off with a new variant of Descartes' famous *cogito*: 'I fondle, therefore I am'? Historians, whose task it is to take stock of a variety of different sources, will obviously find this question more difficult to answer than journalists, with their penchant for catchphrases and oversimplifications.

The historian of philosophy, for instance, will note conflicting tendencies. In the first half of the twentieth century some thinkers were maintaining that the sense of touch was losing its significance in sensory knowledge, while others were insisting on the epistemological priority of haptic experience. Hermann Friedmann (1873–1957), an adherent of the then up-and-coming *Gestalt* theory of the psychology of perception, declared in 1930 that the objects of tactile experience were eking out 'a brief and wretched existence in a stunted tactile memory and the aesthetically impoverished realm of tactile fantasy'.[1] The Hungarian psychologist Geza Révész (1878–1955) took an opposite view. In the early 1940s, he stressed that knowledge acquired by means of the sense of touch was more convincing and persuasive.[2] Moving forward to the philosophy of the present, we encounter Jean Baudrillard's theory that the hand is 'no longer the prehensile organ that focuses effort: rather, nothing more than the abstract *sign* of manipulability, to which buttons, handles, and so on are all the better suited.'[3] The invention of 'touch screens', interactive monitors which dispense with the keyboard and mouse, making computers easier to use than ever, would appear to bear out Baudrillard's theory that the increase of tactile experience in the media age has not necessarily produced an enrichment of sensory perception.

The cultural historian will note that, while the gesture of the handshake remains the most frequent form of public tactile contact in the Western cultural region, other forms of interpersonal physical contact have atrophied in post-modern industrial society, and are now largely accidental. The chances of casual tactile encounter may well increase during journeys by overcrowded public transport, or in the jostle of department stores and pedestrian zones, but such random brushings lack a positive charge and are normally accompanied by more or less effusive apologies.

In the face of the increasing lack of affectionate and intimate bodily contact in the twentieth century, the American futurologist John Naisbitt called for a new form of social behaviour, for which he coined the term 'high touch'.[4] It addresses the growing need for a kind of closeness and togetherness that might compensate for the negative aspects of high-tech society. He sees the rapid growth of self-help groups and the world-wide boom in new systems of learning and therapy as early signs of a development in this direction. On the other hand, the late 1960s witnessed the beginning of a remarkable rediscovery of the sense of touch. For it was around this time that a generation which had grown up with television began to discover that, in addition to the ever more dominant sense of sight, there was also a sense of touch. Besides the sit-in, the flower-power generation and the hippie movement also invented the 'touch-in', at which people who had never met before would kiss and embrace and seek to offer each other tenderness. The rise of the commune movement and the practice of group hashish smoking, during which 'joints' passed from hand to hand, were part of the same scene.

At almost the same time, towards the end of the 1960s, the American media theorist Marshall McLuhan took many critics of the television age by surprise with his thesis that, contrary to what its name appeared to suggest, television was a tactile rather than a visual medium, since the cathode rays which produced television images actually 'stroked' the retina of the eye. Hence the title of his famous book *The Medium is the Massage* (1967). According to the media expert Derrick de Kerckhove, McLuhan's proposition may also be taken to mean that 'television is a multi-sensory experience that indirectly supports and underlines the importance of the sense of touch in other areas of competence.'[5] On the other hand, McLuhan's dictum may simply mean that the TV massage is a subtle form of brainwashing. Today, in the multimedia age, it has acquired new associations: our continuous zapping between dozens of channels provides plenty of exercise for the sense of touch.

The growing interest in body therapy

The rediscovery or revaluation of the sense of touch in the twentieth century is attested by the recent upsurge of interest in body therapies. The therapeutic touching of one's own or another's body has become a major industry. The health market now offers a bewilderingly vast array of products, ranging from functional body methods (sensory awareness training, the Alexander technique, and all sorts of massaging procedures, e.g., the Rolfing method) to conflict-oriented physical treatments (feeling therapies).

One trustworthy indicator of the trend is the flood of new publications on massage that has been swamping the German book market for more than three decades. The number of publications on the subject fluctuated between eight and eighteen per decade in the 1950s and 1960s, but rose steeply thereafter. Fifty titles appeared in the 1970s, more than twice that again (116) in the 1980s, and a record 198 in the 1990s. Particularly noticeable is the boom in books dealing with Far Eastern massage techniques that was such a feature of the 1990s. It is not only the German actress Marie-Luise Marjan – better known as Mother Beimer in the TV series *Lindenstraße* (Lime Street) – who goes into raptures about ayurvedic massages with sesame oil and feels she is 'floating on clouds' after her treatment session. Other celebrities too swear by the *Panchakarma* purification course, with its well-being inducing, whole-body synchronized massages, special herbal enemas, steam baths, customized diets, yoga and meditation. The bandleader Paul Kuhn recently told the press that he felt 'fit as a fiddle' and at last rid of his sinus trouble after one of these cures.

Two hundred years earlier, a companion of the explorer and circum-navigator James Cook had a similar experience in Tahiti. This is what he had to say after he and his fellow Europeans had enjoyed an unfamiliar kind of massage treatment on the paradisal island:

We were invited to sit on an elaborately woven mat which had been laid over the dry grass in one corner of the hut. The daughter of our host, who clearly excelled the other beauties of Tahiti in point of regularity of limb, skin colour and facial features, smiled at us in a friendly manner and joined her companions in obliging us. To relieve us of our fatigue, she stroked our arms and legs and gently kneaded our muscles with her hands. The sensation was extremely gratifying. I will not attempt to judge whether these manipulations encouraged the circulation of the blood in the finer vessels or were able to restore the elasticity of the tired and slackened muscles; suffice it to say that they restored our energies and banished our fatigue.[6]

Today, of course, when most modern European countries offer an enormous range of oriental therapies, we do not necessarily need to fly off to Tahiti or the Far East to enjoy the regenerative effects of exotic massage.

Psycho-physical body treatments have also grown in popularity throughout the Western world over the past thirty years. Their adop-tion in the USA was accompanied by the publication of popular scientific works describing the skin's sensitivity and promoting the rediscovery of the sense of touch. Jane Howard's *Touch Me!* (1971) is a typical example of the genre. At roughly the same time, the Esalen Center in California developed a new ('gentle') massage technique which involved the exaggeratedly slow stroking of the body. The bioenergetic therapy developed by Frederick Matthias Alexander (*b.* 1910) under the influence of Wilhelm Reich (1897–1957), which includes an exercise called 'grounding', or learning how to feel bonded to the earth, should also be mentioned in this context.

Finally, there is the method whose very name proclaims the re-valuation of the sense of touch: 'feeling therapy'. It was developed in Los Angeles by the physical therapists Werner Karle and Alan Switzer. Its aim is not only 'to alter the patient's bodily structure, but also to reorientate it in a way that opens it up to the influx of feeling, enabling it to live a more flexible life.'[7] The following passage from one of the treatment records shows how it works in practice:[8]

> THERAPIST: . . . Don't think. Just feel with your hands. What do you feel?
> PATIENT: (weeping): I feel soft skin and warm . . . so good . . . (sobbing)
> THERAPIST: Don't go away.
> PATIENT: Yes . . . I'm going away . . .
> THERAPIST: No. Stay. Just describe what you are feeling now; that's all you have to do.

Such exercises in feeling and touching are intended to reactivate the more basic feelings, smooth away blockages in the body's perception and restore that lost 'interactional reality of feeling' which we per-haps once inhabited in childhood.

Physiotherapy too has received a new impetus. The classical manual massage has enjoyed a renaissance, and not just because it happens to be covered by medical insurance (in Germany at least). How different things were in the last third of the nineteenth century. In those days, the eminent surgeon Theodor Billroth (1826–1894) felt that he had to play his part in securing the official medical recognition of this physiotherapeutic treatment. In 1875, he launched a plea in the respected *Wiener Medizinische Wochenschrift* (Vienna Medical Weekly): 'I can only agree with my colleagues von Langenbeck and Esmarch that in appropriate cases massage undoubtedly merits more attention than it has received in German-speaking countries over the last few decades.'[9] But the medical community remained split by the issue for some considerable time. In the jubilee edition of *Das neue Naturheilverfahren* (New Natural Healing, 1902), of which a million copies had already been sold, the manufacturer and 'naturopath'

Friedrich Eduard Bilz (1842–1922) complained that: 'Even after science had, so to speak, rediscovered massage, and French, Dutch, Swedish and Scandinavian doctors had begun to practise it with great success, German Aesculapians, in common with the lay world at large, remained cool and diffident.'[10]

It also took some time for this particular branch of therapy to gain professional status. In Switzerland, the first diploma courses for prospective masseurs were established in 1917. Two women and seven men subscribed. A Swiss professional association of state-licensed masseurs and masseuses was founded two years later. In Switzerland, and later in Germany, the main reason for this incorporation was to create a clear distinction between physiotherapy and the world's oldest profession, prostitution. As the Swiss medical historian Sabine Ruth Welti has noted, 'The principal beneficiaries of the professional organization were the masseuses, who valued its support in their struggle against the dubious massage advertisements published in the newspapers.'[11] Similar professional bodies had already been established in other countries before the end of the nineteenth century (the Netherlands, 1889; England, 1894).

The use of massage in gynaecology was long regarded as particularly problematic. A technique of massaging the lower abdomen invented by a former major in the Swedish army named Thure Brandt (1819–1895) was clearly very popular among female patients, but the medical profession did not abandon its strong moral and ethical reservations towards it until the twentieth century. One medical writer suggested a modification of the method, whereby the female patient did not have to undress completely and her entire body was shrouded in a 'massage blanket'. He reasoned as follows: 'The adoption of this method removes anything embarrassing, distasteful or indecent from the situation. Observe the difference between this and Thure Brandt. According to his method, the patient must surrender to two masseurs at once, who subject her to manipulations that are disrespectful in the highest degree, and deeply offensive to a woman's sense of honour, however indispensable they may be to the treatment.'[12] Furthermore, it was essential that a woman who freely consented to submit herself to such 'shameless' therapy required protection against herself: 'A sensual woman who discovers that this form of massage may be accompanied by sexual arousal will tend to make a virtue of necessity.'[13]

A few decades later, the psychiatrist Wilhelm Reich was to bear the full brunt of the suspicion that medically therapeutic bodily contact was an open invitation to the therapist to indulge in sexual acts with the patient. An attempt was made to brand Reich as a criminal deviant because he had allegedly used his therapy sessions for the purpose of getting his male and female patients to masturbate.

The same moral objections were voiced at the beginning of the twentieth century, when doctors and psychiatrists began to prescribe electric vibration massage as a treatment for female patients diagnosed as hysterical or neurasthenic. As soon as new, user-friendly and inexpensive self-treatment apparatuses began to appear on the market (at first in the USA), male and female patients were no longer dependent on the goodwill of doctors. They could try out the effects of a soft vibrator massage in their own homes. In 1906, an American women's magazine extolled the advantages of electrotherapeutic techniques as follows:

> Why has electrical massage taken the place of the manual, or Swedish method? Simply because it can be applied more rapidly, uniformly and *deeply* than by hand, and for as long a period as may be desired. The professional masseur can not only not reach as deeply as can mechanical vibration, but is manifestly not able to prolong his treatment for a sufficient length of time to accomplish the results attained by modern vibratory machinery, which never tires. The number and strength of the movements that can be applied by hand are extremely limited; the perfectly adjusted American Vibrator runs *indefinitely* and is susceptible of a variety and rapidity of movements utterly impossible of human attainment.[14]

The White Cross Electric Vibrator, which was advertised as bringing Swedish massage directly into the home, was another device that sold extremely well in the years before the Second World War.

Germany was rather behind the times with regard to vibrators. A popular manual of natural healing published in 1907 informs us that: 'Unfortunately, most of the vibration machines on the market are so expensive that only doctors and heads of institutes can afford to buy them. The single exception is the hand-operated "Venivici" vibrator, whose undoubted merits have ensured wide distribution.'[15] A glance at the illustration of the extremely clumsy-looking contraption that accompanies this text is enough, however, to make us wonder how a mechanical vibrator like this could ever capture the popular imagination, although its Latin name is clearly intended to announce its impending conquest of the health market.

In the USA, advertisements for electric massage machines disappeared from women's magazines and domestic-appliance catalogues a few years before the Second World War. When the vibrator re-emerged during the sexual revolution of the 1960s, it was no longer camouflaged as a health-care product, but openly marketed as a sex toy for men and women alike. This was not simply a matter of changing the old labels, for the action marked a radical refunctioning of a device that began its life as a strictly medical, therapeutic apparatus.

The discovery of erogenous zones

So far we have been speaking of the 'instrumental forms' (Jens Loenhoff) of tactile experience and behaviour. In addition to the manipulations of masseurs and masseuses just mentioned, these include the professionally contingent and socially legitimated touchings of hairdressers, doctors, and the sales staff of fashion shops. Yet it is above all the more exclusively intimate forms of touching that took on greater significance in the twentieth century. Here too, we need to distinguish between different degrees and stages, as the German Romantic poet Novalis was already well aware: 'The gaze – (speech) – the touching of hands – the kiss – the touching of breasts – the grasp of the private parts – the act of embrace – these are the rungs of the ladder – down which the soul descends – opposite to this stands another ladder – up which the body ascends – to the instant of embrace.'[16] These forms of touching take place in public only up to a certain point, even in a socially more permissive climate such as that of the late twentieth century. An empirical survey like the one conducted at a British seaside resort in 1939 would have been quite unimaginable a hundred years earlier.[17] On this occasion, a diligent and impeccably scientific observer counted 252 couples on the promenade between 11.30 a.m. and midnight. Of these, 120 embraced while seated, forty-two held each other affectionately in a standing position, forty-six lay cuddling on the sand, twenty-five kissed where they sat, three kissed each other as they walked, nine embraced in various kinds of conveyances, and seven women or, rather, young girls were observed sitting on the knees of men, which was apparently regarded as particularly indecent. There is of course nothing new about the exchange of tactile endearments between couples. But in the twentieth century these intimacies not only became more publicly conspicuous, but the whole manner in which they were perceived changed in response to the new psychoanalytic and sexological emphasis of the role of the 'erogenous zones' and the sense of touch in the sexual gratification of the man, and particularly of the woman.

In his book on the education of the senses in the bourgeois era, the American cultural historian Peter Gay draws attention to the key role of Sigmund Freud in the rediscovery of female sensuality. In the famous *Three Essays on Sexual Theory* of 1904–5, the founder of psychoanalysis claims that 'satisfaction arises first and foremost from the appropriate stimulation of what we have described as erotogenic zones.'[18] In other writings he notes the significance of 'tactile sensations', 'touching as a source of pleasure' and 'erotic touching'. The taboo on touching is 'one of the oldest and most fundamental commands of obsessional neurosis'. 'Eros', says Freud, 'desires contact because it strives to make the ego and the loved object one.' His sexual theoretical writings also consider the common equation of tactile stimuli with the sexual act and sexual desire: 'To "touch" a woman has become a euphemism for using her as a sexual object. Not to "touch" one's genitals is the phrase employed for the prohibition of auto-erotic gratification.'

Despite what the older tradition of Freudian research would have us believe, the discovery of the role of the sense of touch in human sexuality was not just the work of Freud. In this context, the German psychiatrist Albert Moll (1862–1939) merits particular attention. Moll's famous *Libido sexualis* (1897), which describes the decline of sexual stimuli in the course of human history (following the introduction of clothes, perfumes and standards of cleanliness, etc.), confirmed Freud's view that in the course of human evolution there had been a 'shutdown of formerly erogenous zones', which was connected to the phenomenon of organic repression. It was Moll, however, who first classified the compulsive desire to touch a person of the opposite sex as '*Kontrektrationstrieb*' ('toucherism').[19]

Like Moll, Iwan Bloch (1872–1922), who coined the term 'sexology' in 1907, adopted a phylogenetic and anthropological approach to human sexuality. Freud was clearly well acquainted with Bloch's

Beiträge zur Aetiologie der Psychopathia sexualis (Contributions to the Aetiology of *Psychopathia sexualis*, 1902–3), in which the author maintained that under certain cultural conditions any sense organ could function as an erogenous zone. In his best-selling *Das Sexualleben unserer Zeit* (The Sexual Life of our Time, 1906), which was translated into numerous languages and appeared in a twelfth edition in 1919, Bloch dealt with the erotic function of the skin sense: 'It has been rightly said that the first deliberate touching of the skin of a beloved person is already half the sexual act, for this is confirmed by the fact that such intimate physical touchings quickly produce strong feelings of sexual arousal in places far removed from the genitalia.'[20] In this context Bloch refers approvingly to another German pioneer in the field of sexual research: 'Magnus Hirschfeld has correctly described the feelings of pleasure aroused by the skin sense as a point of transition, at which the power of self-control and resistance of drives converted into motions and actions by tactile perceptions most frequently weakens.' So, if they wished to escape being overwhelmed by the sex drive, Bloch's readers are advised to steer clear of such contacts as far as possible.

Freud was, however, even more strongly influenced by the then highly regarded writings of the sexual psychologist Henry Havelock Ellis (1859–1939). This is particularly evident in the case of the problem of infantile sexual development which features so prominently in the work of the founder of psychoanalysis. Ellis's *Sexual Selection in Man* (1906) is especially relevant to the history of the senses, for the book actually begins with a description of the sense of touch in general and the sexual skin centres in particular. The senses of smell, hearing and vision appear in second, third and fourth positions respectively. This 'natural order', as Ellis calls it, represents the privileged position of the sense of touch in sexual life, from the dawn of history to the present: 'The skin is the archaeological field of human and pre-human experience, the foundation on which all forms of sensory perception have grown up, and as sexual sensibility is among the most ancient of all forms of sensibility, the sexual instinct is necessarily, in the main, a comparatively slightly modified form of general touch sensibility.'[21] In this context Ellis also mentions the massage institutes, which were sprouting out of the ground like mushrooms in European cities at the turn of the century. His casual remark that these establishments were frequented by women in search of sexual satisfaction was grist to the mills of the apostles of rectitude in the medical profession, who crusaded against the sexually intoxicating effects of therapeutic massage.

The growing need for 'loving sex'

If it is true, as several recent studies have claimed,[22] that the mutual fondling of intimate places on the body has become a normal form of behaviour between sexual partners since the 1970s, this has undoubtedly had a good deal to do with the influence of Freud's pupil Wilhelm Reich. In 1927, Reich published the results of his pioneering study of *Genitality in the Theory and Therapy of Neurosis*. This revealed among other things that many men and women had no idea that the capacity to achieve orgasm was not restricted to the male sex. 'Genital sexuality', he explained 'is so anally encumbered that it is unable to connect with the pursuit of tenderness.'[23] Reich also noted that many people who had played with their genitals in childhood felt the need to touch them before the sexual act. Women in particular often had to resort to manual stimulation in order to achieve orgasm. In a much-quoted essay on the therapeutic significance of genital libido written in 1925, Reich described the apparent success of his treatment: 'In many cases of vaginal anaesthesia with existent clitoral eroticism, I was able to activate a vaginal orgasm by advising suppression of clitoral masturbation while allowing vaginal masturbation.'[24]

Coming from a doctor, this kind of advice would have been almost unthinkable a hundred years previously, when anti-masturbation devices were invented to frustrate the touching of the genitals. In 1816, one clinical marriage counsellor was in no two minds about how the married couple should cope with the tactile sense: 'As long as the master of the house is neither for nor against the act . . . there must be no intervening hand-play.'[25]

Around 80 per cent of the people who participated in a recent German survey stated that stroking was an important part of their sex lives. In addition to this, both sexes laid great stress on the physical appearance of their partners' hands, which they saw as indicators of the quality of their sexual performance. In another recent scholarly investigation, newly divorced partners complained that they most missed the physical contact of the marriage bed. In the aftermath of

President Clinton's affair with Monica Lewinsky, the American population was asked about its attitudes towards certain sexual practices, from which it also emerged that only 15 per cent of Americans regarded the stroking of erogenous zones as sex.

A woman's right to sexual gratification, of which Wilhelm Reich was an early outspoken supporter, is no longer seriously contested today, although things look somewhat different in practice in the American marital bed – and not only there. Just how much catching up still remains to be done in Germany is underlined by the numerous introductions to erotic partner massage that have appeared on the book market over the past two decades. In the 1970s there was a choice of ten titles on the subject. Twenty years later, there were twenty-one – all dangling the prospect 'of using sensitive massage to discover erogenous zones, whose sensitivity has for long been ignored.'[26]

Pedagogic stroking games

But the need to catch up on tactile sensations appears not to be confined to the realm of the erotic. Unlike in the early 1990s, it is now no longer possible to count on the fingers of one hand the number of exhibitions and museums inviting the visitor to enter the 'empire of the senses' and partake of a course of tactile training. 'Touch Me', an exhibition held in Basel in 1996, was devoted entirely to the sense of touch. To judge from one of the newspaper reports, this 'show of sense' was a big success:

> The visitors come in their hundreds at the weekend, turning the show into a spectacle. The acoustics of the main exhibition hall are like an indoor swimming pool, and the place echoes with shrieks of eeek! as yet another unsuspecting yet intrepid soul pokes his hand through one of these holes, encounters the aquarium, and quickly withdraws it to shake the slimy liquid from his fingers. Or when someone running his hand over sods of real grass comes upon the snake: a plastic slow-worm, as it turns out. Or again when someone happens to brush the hotplate when fondling a ceramic hob . . .'[27]

The gender-specific attractions included, predictably, a risk-free grope of the full breasts of the goddess Aphrodite (in plaster-cast form, of course) and the hands-on experience of an antique male torso.

Just one year later (1997), the German Museum of Hygiene in Dresden put on an exhibition entitled 'Paths of Feeling'. Nine artists had loaned stone, wood, metal, wax, paper and ceramic sculptures to be touched by visitors in a totally dark room. According to the brochure, this unusual approach to contemporary sculpture was intended 'to encourage the sighted to strengthen their haptic sense and to give them the opportunity to create a new world of experience for themselves.' The exhibition opened with the performance of a dance entitled 'From the Hands' Point of View'.

According to a report in the *Deutsches Sonntagblatt* of 9 September 1996, the Protestant Church has recently rediscovered the sense of touch as a way of getting people to go to church more often. Special blessing services are being held, during which the members of the congregation perform the act of laying on hands. As long ago as 1968, the World Council of Churches held a so-called sensuality seminar during its meeting in Uppsala. The regular church congresses of today are occasions of 'feeling' and physical proximity as well as reflection and meditation.

The training of the sense of touch has long been part of the curriculum of the Waldorf schools. According to their founder, Rudolf Steiner (1861–1925), the sense of touch – one of the twelve senses recognized by anthroposophical doctrine – represented 'the feeling of God'.[28] Ordinary schools and state educational institutions have experienced more problems with the provision of haptic experiences, as the controversy surrounding the 'Sexy Egg' in the state of Rhineland-Palatinate in 1997 clearly demonstrates. In collaboration with the State Centre for the Promotion of Health, students of design at the Institute of Higher Education in Mainz produced an egg that was one and a half metres wide and three-quarters of a metre high, and looked rather like an extra-terrestrial spaceship. Inside it was a bunch of 'keys', with which schoolboys and schoolgirls were supposed to unlock the senses. The *Frankfurter Allgemeine Zeitung* of 20 October 1997 wrote a very positive review of its approach to the sense of touch: 'Materials for feeling-games and tactile encounters in the form of feathers, pebbles, dough, massage oil and massage balls provide gentle experiences of feel and touch. A peep-show on the subject of "men", "women", "skin", "couples", "secrets" and "pleasure", a "feely-ball" containing hidden objects, a "foreplay" in the form of a game of charades and an array of scents are all intended to show that sex is an essential component of sensuality and of life as such.' But the 'Sexy Egg', which was intended to interest fourteen- to eighteen-year-olds in the pleasures of the senses, never saw active educational service. For this project of sexual enlightenment ran into political opposition, and the 'Sexy Egg' quietly vanished into the cellars of the Centre for the Promotion of Health. Even the entirely respectable Association of Catholic Youth was refused when it wanted to borrow it for the German Catholic Congress.

The state of Bavaria has a similar educational toy, though it is clearly more harmless and less likely to cause offence than its counterpart in the Rhineland-Palatinate. The Bavarian State Centre of Health (www.lzg-bayern.de/lzg/expo/sf_ausst.htm) owns and lends out a 'mobile experience for the development of the senses', based on the ideas of the artist and educationalist Hugo Kükelhaus. While the importance of sensory perception for the development of the capacity for sexual experience is not excluded from this creation, it is not the central subject of the various games of touching. So this particular multimedia educational resource for the training of the senses is unlikely to cause offence to anyone.

Haptic experiences on the Internet

But today's young people can turn to other media for their education in the sense of touch. The Internet site at <www.sport-thieme.de> offers all kinds of new games, including a stroking game, in which the players have to stroke each other and take proper notice of each other's presence. The same site also offers so-called foot-touching boxes for developing the sensitivity of the feet. In 1999, an American company called Immersion unveiled a new computer mouse with a sense of touch. According to the *Berliner Morgenpost* of 13 February 1998 (so this wasn't an April Fool's Day hoax!), it is now possible, for example, to test the softness of a mattress offered for sale on a home page by means of the impulses transmitted by the mouse. Provided the suppliers program their website correctly, the mouse could even be used to obtain a tactile impression of the textures of solid and liquid surface structures.

The surfer of the Internet is offered more than just a selection of stroking games and foot-touch mats. Among the more serious offers is a home page (www.autohuna.com/royart/drhpelo/haut.htm) containing an essay by a Dr H. Pelo. Its main subject is not the *Praise of the Skin* announced in the title but a rather vague treatment of 'tactility and desire'. In fact, this little U-certificate Internet tract hardly advances beyond banalities such as 'The skin is our real sex organ.' Somewhat more enticing, on the other hand, is a home page (minus the usual display material) called Feminat, which offers partner massages to couples in search of 'a "new" kind of erotic kick'.

A large number of the more than 80,000 websites listed by one of the large Internet search engines (Altavista) under the heading 'massage' are advertisements for explicitly sexual services. Besides pornographic images and texts, German websites include listings under the headword 'loving sex'. The number of men and women who place the accent on stroking, embracing and other forms of tactile tenderness is clearly increasing. The reader survey on the theme of 'sex in the dark' – supposedly a 'new' source of haptic pleasure – conducted in the December 1999 number of the on-line edition of the lubricious German magazine *Praline* was, therefore, very much in tune with the trend. As always, however, another magazine had got in first. A special edition of *Der Spiegel* (May 1998), now also available for consultation on the Internet, quotes no less a figure than Jean-Paul Sartre (1905–1980), who seems to have made no secret of his (dis-)pleasure: 'I had intercourse often, though always with a certain indifference. For me the essential emotional relation consisted in kissing, stroking and allowing my mouth to explore another body.' Who would have thought it? Jean-Paul Sartre, existentialist philosopher, husband of Simone de Beauvoir (1908–1986), and now prophet of loving sex!?

—— 12 ——

Tasting – or What Do Fast Food and Nouvelle Cuisine Have in Common?

Do you remember? Simply numbed by our paltry feelings, we ate little. If only we'd realized that it would all be over in five minutes, the Wellington roast beef would have tasted different, quite different.

Hans Magnus Enzensberger, *Short History of the Bourgeoisie* (1983)

'The taste of necessity'

In the 1930s, Filippo Tommaso Marinetti (1876–1944) and his Italian comrades-in-arms launched a new aesthetics of eating and drinking that became known as 'La Cucina Futuristica'. This futuristic art of cooking set out to create entirely new kinds of dishes and 'at last to bring about a state of harmony between the palate of man and his present and future life.'[1] In order to accomplish this aim, nourishment, the actual purpose of human nutrition, had to be relegated to the background. According to Marinetti, the priority accorded to nutrition had tied man too closely to animal life, making him eat like ants, cats or mice. In the kitchens of the future, meals would be prepared according to exclusively aesthetic criteria. The futurists therefore often loftily disregarded ordinary ideas of the edible and tasty and dreamed of an 'artistic cuisine', which they called 'the first human cuisine', since it raised a basic human need to the status of an art form.

But the revolution of taste did not take place in quite the way the Italian futurists had envisaged. 'The physiology of nutrition', writes the sociologist of medicine Nicolaus Heim, 'became involved in a "pacte de famine" with the rulers of the 1930s, who set about depopulating Europe by creating a home-made, artificial famine.'[2]

Once concentration-camp prisoners and the inmates of the mental homes of the National Socialist regime had been deliberately starved to death, and the Second World War began to intensify, it was again the turn of the civilian population to undergo the basic experience of hunger. In times of war and crisis, the nutritional consumption of a large part of the population is determined by what Pierre Bourdieu has called 'the taste of necessity'. Food rationing, which drastically altered the peacetime consumption patterns of not only the German people, produced a monotonous bill of fare which barely filled rumbling stomachs and became smaller and smaller as the war continued. Few escaped the dictatorship of hunger. In 1940, Ernst Günter Schenk, an expert dietician, and for many years nutritional adviser to the Reich Chamber of Physicians, issued the slogan: 'The basic necessities and nothing more'.[3] Artificial substitutes (e.g., for coffee) and inferior produce began to replace foods that were both tasty and highly nutritious: meat and fat gradually gave way to potatoes and pulses.

According to official statistics for the city of Essen, the ordinary rations of adult citizens there in the period between 1940 and 1945 fell from 124.2 to 113.5 kilos of bread per year, and from 26.2 to 8.1 kilos of meat. While bread, flour and potato rations were larger in Germany, meat and fat rations were appreciably smaller there than in Denmark, Sweden and Spain. The Germans also had to lose their predilection for sugar during these difficult times. According to a standard history of nutrition during the Third Reich, average German sugar rations 'fell well below Scandinavian, and just below Dutch and Belgian consumption levels, but remained on a par with the "great enemy" (i.e., England).'[4] Under these circumstances, consumption patterns were obviously determined by necessity rather than taste. The most vivid example of the 'taste of necessity' is provided by the 'Guidelines for Life under the Simplest Conditions', which the National Socialists had printed and distributed to district offices of public health just a few days before the end of the war. The brochure contains detailed instructions for the nutritional exploitation of tree bark, roots, lichen, chestnuts, beechnuts and acorns, as well as hints on how to catch frogs – whose legs would have appealed to no more than a handful of francophile gourmets under peacetime conditions.

So it is not surprising that in the immediate post-war period, when much of the German population was hungry, and the daily menu was, if anything, even more monotonous than during the difficult preceding years, people dreamed first and foremost of eating their fill for once. They also longed for the taste of 'good' butter and 'real' coffee. In August 1946, the *Nürnberger Nachrichten* published extracts from essays written by the sixth-formers of a school for girls. At a certain point in her essay, one girl declared that she wanted 'to really eat my fill for a change – to eat exactly what I please.'[5] So the war had brought no lasting changes to people's tastes.

It is a well-known fact that the recollection of fine-tasting, unappetizing and even revolting food remains deeply engraved on the long-term human memory. On 24 October 1996, the *Frankfurter Allgemeine Zeitung* carried an article about a Dutch olfactory psychologist who claimed that eating revived the memories of old people. The article quoted the example of the psychologist's ninety-year-old mother. When she ate red cabbage, this old lady was apparently able to recall the exact topic of family conversation when the same dish had appeared on the table at her parental home. Meanwhile, we do not (necessarily) need a historian of everyday life to tell us that the unbalanced diet and enduring aftertaste of the notorious 'winter of swede' of 1916–17 has remained lodged in the collective German memory. Members of the older generation still experience a slight wave of nausea when offered swede as a cleverly prepared delicacy in one of today's top nouvelle cuisine restaurants.

The 'wave of gluttony' and the 'new' taste

Once the worst period of hunger was over, and care packages were arriving from America in great numbers, the old tastes slowly began to revive. But new and hitherto largely unknown flavours were discovered at the same time. Among them was the pleasantly sweetish, peppermint taste of chewing gum, which was quickly adopted by children and teenagers, who had received this symbol of the American enjoyment of life from the soldiers of the occupation. The adult population, which bartered goods on the black market, soon got used to American cigarettes, which had a different and lighter taste than the 'oriental cigarettes' – made from Southern European or Near Eastern tobacco – that the Germans had always smoked before the war. Some of the tinned vegetables included in the care packages were likewise new to the German palate, but people soon began to get used to them too. Tinned sweetcorn, for instance, was considered something of a speciality by Germans in the years immediately following the war, as can be seen from an article in the *Süddeutsche Zeitung* of 30 July 1946: 'The corn in the can is ready to eat. It tastes sweet and many people see it as a "funny kind of novelty".'

The much-cited German 'wave of gluttony' got under way at the beginning of the 1950s in the wake of the currency reform. With regard to meat eating, it marked a return to old tastes and preferences after a long period of deprivation. On the other hand, it led to the 'conspicuous consumption' of foodstuffs which were luxury items at the time, or at least regarded as exotic. Oranges are one example. A decade later, the German Federal Republic had become the world's leading importer of citrus and tropical fruit! Before the wave of German tourism began, Hawaiian toast brought a little exoticism to German kitchens. The following ingredients for a serving for four people is taken from Clemens Wilmenrod, Germany's first television cook: four rounds of toasted bread, sixteen slices of thinly cut smoked ham, eight slices of tinned pineapple, four slices of processed cheese, some red pepper and four cocktail cherries. No one would have dared even to dream of such ingredients in the immediate post-war period, and when placed under a grill or cooked in an oven this tempting composition produced a taste that was initially strange to the German palate. Today, the dish is a fairly standard and relatively cheap item on the menu of restaurants with few pretensions to a Michelin star.

With the onset of the 'wave of gluttony', the advertisers began once more to extol the flavours of foodstuffs. In 1956, a German margarine firm launched a slogan that became famous: 'Rama ist die Vollendung des guten Geschmacks' (Rama is the perfection of good taste). Soft cheeses such as Milkana and Velveta transformed a modest slice of bread and butter into a delicate 'little canapé'. The advertisement appealed to the sense of taste, but also to a new feeling for life. As the contemporary historian Michael Wildt has observed, 'the promise embodied in new products such as Milkana and Velveta has more to do with the lifestyle their consumption implies than with cheese or the sense of taste. Their material substance is no longer the primary referent. The immediate, sensuous experience of tasting fades into the background.'[6]

This change of diet may be expressed statistically. At the beginning of the 1960s, people were buying only half as much flour as ten years previously. However, expenditures on bread, cakes and pastries, honey, confectionery, quark and tea doubled over the same period. The consumption of coffee and fresh citrus fruit also multiplied several times over. Sales of evaporated milk, another product recommended by the advertisers for the quality of its taste, increased at quite a dramatic rate, with average monthly consumption climbing from 206 grams in 1950 to 2 kilos in 1960. One of the main reasons for this sharp rise was the parallel increase in coffee consumption. An advertisement for Libby's evaporated milk dating from the early 1950s explains how other products also tasted better when laced with long-life tinned milk: 'Creamy Libby's milk makes biscuits light and tasty, improves the aroma of coffee, and gives body to cocoa. It enhances the flavour of puddings and desserts, soups and many main courses.'[7]

The intensive promotion of foodstuffs as especially tasty or conducive to the refinement of taste that has been such a feature of the advertising literature of the last fifty years is hardly an exclusively German phenomenon. A study of Dutch women's magazines covering the period between 1900 and 1985 shows that, over the last half-century, advertising strategists have made progressively greater use of this type of argument in their advertising copy.[8] In the 1950s, it saw service in slightly more than 60 per cent of all advertisements. This figure had increased to over 80 per cent just twenty years later. Compare this with the beginning of the twentieth century, when the proportion of advertisements of this kind was well below 20 per cent. What we also see here is how, in the course of the last fifty years, the 'taste of necessity', which Pierre Bourdieu portrays as 'the taste of the lower classes for food that is as nourishing as it is cheap',[9] has gradually yielded to 'the taste of luxury', typified by delicious meals and consumer choice. However, we need to beware of suggesting a linear trend. The 'democratization of good taste' (Karl Möckl) did not occur everywhere simultaneously, and there are regional as well as national fracturings, faultlines and differences. Nor should we overlook the phenomenon of 'new poverty' which affected the lives of millions of people in the Federal Republic alone. Their behaviour as buyers and consumers continues to be dominated by the 'taste of necessity'.

The spread of 'culinary pluralism'

In his fascinating cultural history of eating, the English historian Stephen Mennell maintains that the differences between the culinary arts of the professional elite and everyday domestic cuisine became steadily less pronounced in the closing decades of the twentieth century, and that the 'culinary pluralism' of the present shows a tendency to place variety above contrast.

There can indeed be little doubt that the differences between the eating habits of the various social groups are no longer so strongly marked as they still were at the beginning of the twentieth century and during the decade following the end of the Second World War. The editorial of a 1964 issue of the English trade journal *Hotel and Restaurant Management* shows just how early this levelling process began: 'Chi-chi writers sneering at caterers who provide simple inexpensive meals at the expense of traditional haute cuisine underestimate both public demand and changing taste. The brightly-lit, classless popular catering establishment is rapidly replacing the old dirty dingy "café round the corner".'[10] In England, as in other Western countries, going out to a restaurant is nowadays taken for granted, and no longer perceived as a luxury. The *Frankfurter Allgemeine Zeitung* of 16 March 1999 carried an article about a study entitled 'Who ate what, where and when?', from which it emerged that every German now eats out 3.2 times a week on average, representing a total spend of DM 121 billion (*c.*£40 billion). Twenty-eight of these billions found their way into the tills of restaurants offering German or regional cooking. A further DM 22 billion was spent in the numerous restaurants specializing in foreign cuisine, with most Germans apparently preferring to 'eat Italian'. Greek and Chinese restaurants came in second and third.

The recent interest in what is known as gourmet tourism is a further sign of advancing uniformity. This new form of tourism includes so-called feast weeks: introductory courses in the high art of regional or French cookery which are organized and hosted by leading chefs. An essential feature of gourmet tourism is its 'broad-based appeal and lack of social exclusiveness'.[11] Italy has had 'slow-food restaurants' for some years, and one Italian good-food guide now lists 1700 restaurants where the food is freshly prepared, inexpensive and consumed in a leisurely ambience. The guide, which marks these 'places of peace and enjoyment' with a snail symbol, has clearly joined battle against an increasingly rampant Italian fast-food culture.

The legacy of 'nouvelle cuisine'

'Nouvelle cuisine', which reached Germany as early as the 1970s, is no longer strictly for the well-to-do, for there are now many restaurants which offer fine French food at reasonable prices. The cookery enthusiast who doesn't have to watch every penny can now choose from among more than half a dozen works on 'nouvelle cuisine' and almost fifty collections of recipes for French dishes.

The name of this new and easy style of cooking was originally coined by Henri Gault and Christian Millau, whose names are associated to this day with the restaurant guide prized by every gourmet. The term cropped up occasionally in France at the end of the nineteenth century, but it was not until the 1960s that it acquired its present meaning. The distinguishing features of this form of cooking, as developed and perfected by the master chefs Paul Bocuse, Jean and Pierre Troisgros, Michel Guérard, Roger Vergé and Raymond Olivier, may be summarized as follows: no complicated cooking procedures; shorter simmering times to allow for the rediscovery of 'forgotten taste notes'; only absolutely fresh market produce and no second-rate ingredients; just a small selection of dishes on the menu to avoid the need to use pre-cooked ingredients; no rich or heavy sauces; innovative borrowings from regional cuisine; the use of the latest kitchen technology (ovens, food mixers, etc.); light meals in compliance with the most recent recommendations of nutritional-physiological science; and, finally, the creativity and inventiveness that is the hallmark of the recipes of these French master cooks (e.g., salmon with sorrel). 'Smell and taste', wrote the sociologist Eva Barlösius, 'became an experimental discipline devoted to the creation of new olfactory and gustatory experiences.'[12]

The German assimilation of 'nouvelle cuisine' was to a large extent the achievement of Eckart Witzigmann, the legendary chef of the 'Tantris' restaurant in Munich, who had learned his trade with Paul Bocuse and Paul Häberlin. He was the first German to be awarded the coveted three Michelin stars, and his ideal of light and fine-tasting cooking is encapsulated in the following words: 'A good meal should be as harmonious as a symphony and as finely constructed as a Gothic cathedral.'[13] The popularization of this 'combination of the modest and the luxurious to create a higher stage of gastronomic perfection' (Karl Möckl) is witnessed by numerous specialized periodicals, whose German market readership has climbed steadily since the 1970s. The periodical *Essen und Trinken* (Eating and Drinking) has appeared since 1972, *Der Feinschmecker* (The Epicure) since 1975 and *Gourmet* since 1976. The influence of nouvelle cuisine is most apparent in the case of the German taste in wine. In 1970s, dry wines, whether white or red, finally succeeded in conquering haute cuisine and other elevated repasts. Meanwhile, people continue to buy the delightful wines from the Rhine and the Mosel – for which Germany was once famous abroad – in the supermarkets.

The internationalization of the sense of taste

The lessening of contrasts has been accompanied by increasing variety and differentiation. The recipes in the cookery sections of journals, women's magazines, consumer periodicals and weekly newspapers such as *Die Zeit* are now longer and more varied. Nevertheless, with the exception of French and Italian cookery, foreign cuisine does not figure prominently in non-specialized German and English cookery books. This has much to do with the fact that a large part of the population is still put off by the characteristic smells and tastes of foreign cooking. The culinary arts of certain immigrant communities (Turkish, Mexican, Serbo-Croatian, etc.) are rejected as 'physically disagreeable, too strongly spiced, sensorially overstimulating and not very trustworthy'.[14] But this does not alter the fact that some of these dishes – doner kebabs or tacos, for example – have become very popular with the natives. However, many of these once exotic dishes now have little in common with the original recipes of their countries of origin, and have largely been adapted to suit German, English or American tastes. So here it is appropriate to speak of a creolization or hybridization of 'national dishes'. Whether the German doner still tastes Turkish or not is largely a matter of taste. At any rate, the important thing from the point of view of the consumer is that: 'Anyone eating a doner should believe that he is eating something

Turkish. Anyone biting into a pizza should feel that Italy is not far away, and anyone who orders tortillas should be convinced that he is about to partake of a piece of Mexico.'[15]

A further sign of the diversity and cosmopolitan character of food consumption is the polarization of the gastronomic market that has been a feature of the last two decades. It is not only the gourmet restaurants that are doing good business. All over the world, people are flocking to fast-food restaurants and snack bars in ever-increasing numbers. Although more and more young people are going to McDonald's, fried sausages and hot dogs are still among the most popular meat dishes consumed by Germans outside the four walls of the home. All the same, the Big Mac, a fried minced-beef hamburger squeezed between the two halves of a roll sprinkled with sesame seeds, and topped with pickled gherkin and a slice of American processed cheese, has come to epitomize fast-food culture as such. One German cultural critic has captured its flawlessly universal flavour in the following words: 'Take a hamburger made by one of the big meat firms, put it with a Coke, and the first thing that strikes you is the pure absence of taste.' Clearly no fan of fast food, he concludes: 'The hamburger is much more than a piece of fried meat loaf. It is a sensorially supersensory object. Its supersensory aspect is precisely its tastelessness.'[16] But the international community of consumers seems largely unperturbed by the withering judgements of the epicures. In the mid-1990s, 28 million customers, in more than 79 countries of the world, ate 26 billion dollars' worth of hamburgers and other fast foods at more than 15,200 branches of McDonald's. Can they *all* be suffering from the same disease of the taste buds?

The problem of the internationalization of taste is also highlighted by a beverage that is nowadays drunk throughout the world. It has many imitators (Afri-Cola, Pepsi-Cola) and a brand-name presence unequalled by any other food product. Since its arrival in Germany in the 1950s, Coca-Cola has become the non-alcoholic drink of choice for young and old. 'Coke' has been marketed on an international scale from a very early stage of its existence, and has permanently altered German taste by displacing regionally produced and natural-tasting fruit juices, and by using its market position to impose the uniform taste of global brands on German manufacturers of fizzy drinks (Sprite, Fanta). John S. Pemberton (1831–1888), who on 8 May 1886 introduced the American public to a refreshing drink with the exotic-sounding name of Coca-Cola, has proved to be a prophet. 'The special taste of Coca-Cola will appeal to every palate', he declared grandiosely at the end of the nineteenth century, and just look at what has happened.[17]

Artificial taste

Meanwhile, actual or alleged culinary variety now appears to be seriously under threat – at least if we are to believe what the nutritionists and restaurant critics tell us. 'Food design' has made great advances since the mid-1980s. The term refers to a method of industrial food production in which basic foodstuffs (milk, cereals, sugar, etc.) are no longer process-refined. Instead, essential substances are isolated from cheap vegetable raw materials (e.g., soya) and assembled by chemical synthesis into products with a considerably higher value. For, unlike agriculturally produced foodstuffs, their quality does not fluctuate. Thus, basic natural produce (maize, potatoes, cereals) now simply supplies the raw materials of food designed by market strategists and consumer researchers.

It has been evident for some time that the production methods of the modern food industry tend to rob foodstuffs of their characteristic aromas, or at least cause them to change. If the manufacturer is unwilling to wait for the consumer to get used to the difference, the 'genuine' or 'natural' flavour of the product has to be re-created by industrial aromatics. The sterilization of milk at ultra-high temperatures, cost-cutting curtailment of the maturation processes of cheese and wine, shorter baking times for bread and the transportation of concentrated fruit juices in weight-reduced, powdered form are just some of the technological interventions that affect the aromas of comestibles. In a letter to the *Frankfurter Allgemeine Zeitung*, one wine connoisseur wrote of the 'Americanization of the taste of wine' following the introduction of new oenological techniques in the USA. He also complained that Germany, too, was abandoning traditional viticulture in favour of industrially 'manufactured' wine.

The victorious march of aromatized basic and semi-luxury food seems unstoppable. Since the 1980s, the aromatics industry has produced a host of natural (concentrated) and quasi-natural (synthetic) aromas. Then there are the artificial aromatic substances identified by the letter 'E' on the lists of additives on product labels. The most common of these is ethyl vanillin, which tastes four times more strongly of vanilla than the natural vanillin contained in vanilla pods. Eva Barlösius sees obvious reasons for the growing demand for aromatic additives: 'Food aromas are used in the first instance to disguise the tastelessness and odourlessness of the raw materials, secondly to add spice to food and thirdly to compensate for the removal of "cooking smells" (e.g., the smell of baked bread or fried meat) by the rationalized methods of food production.'[18] The food industry now employs so-called flavourists, who have the job of putting taste into food. They use the latest technological and sensory-physiological research in order to test the sensorial qualities of manufactured foodstuffs.

The consequences of aromatization for the sense of taste are becoming increasingly evident. First, normal ideas of taste have been altered so radically by the massive use of artificial and quasi-natural aromas that consumers will often no longer accept a natural taste. Secondly, many naturally occurring variations of flavour – between different kinds of apple juice, for instance – have been supplanted by the generic smell of apple. And thirdly, the taste of many aromatized foodstuffs is no longer of primary importance. 'Soup-carton hallucinations' was the term used by the *Stuttgarter Nachrichten* (29 September 1999) to describe this phenomenon. Even the senses of professional tasters have been fooled by these concoctions: in one experiment they managed to mistake blue-tinted orange juice for blueberry juice. When Howard Hillmann, an American author of cookery books, dyed an artificially flavoured hamburger a poisonous shade of green his human guinea-pigs declared that it did not taste of hamburger, even though the dye had not actually altered its flavour. According to an article in the *Süddeutsche Zeitung* of 24 December 1997, the makers of items for nibbling are now exploiting the sensory-physiological discovery that not only smell but also sight and hearing play a part in the sensation of taste. It seems that the louder a potato crisp or pretzel stick crunches when we bite into it, the more intensely we savour its taste.

To summarize: at the beginning of the twenty-first century we face a development whose long-term consequences are unpredictable. While a large part of the world's population is threatened by hunger and forced – where fortunate – to make do with the 'taste of necessity', the tastes of those who can afford any amount of food are increasingly subject to manipulation and standardization. The upshot is that, in the age of the technical producibility of food, the sense of taste is being deadened, and may even have begun to degenerate. Both ordinary consumers and gourmets and epicures will experience more and more difficulty in finding fresh market produce that is authentically 'natural' and not genetically modified or otherwise tampered with. Such at least is the scenario suggested by the results of the sensory experiments conducted in the early 1980s at several German institutes of agricultural testing and research.[19] At that time, only slightly more than 75 per cent of those who took part in bread samplings were able to tell the difference between factory-baked bread and organic bread baked in an oven in the traditional way. In the case of 'alternative' apples, the average recognition rate was merely 51 per cent. As for those whose capacities of sensory discrimination were apparently still in excellent working order, 26 per cent thought that factory-produced bread tasted better, while 23 per cent preferred the organic variety; 30 per cent were unable to make up their minds. So must we conclude that it's all just a matter of taste?

— 13 —

Scenting – or From Deodorization to Reodorization

The ovens,/the stench,/I couldn't repeat/the stench. You/have to breathe./
You can wipe out/what you don't want/to see. Close your/eyes. You don't
want/to taste. You can/block out all the senses/except smell.

Barbara Hyett, *In Evidence* (1986)

The politics of smell: environmental protection

'Smells can still be agreeable or disagreeable', writes the French historian Annick Le Guérer, 'but they have lost their powers of life and death.'[1] And indeed, the miasmic 'stench of plague', the sign of a very real menace in pre-modern times, is nowadays just a rather worn metaphor for any kind of bad smell ('it smells like the plague'). Thanks to a hundred years of popular campaigning against billowing factory chimneys, stinking rivers and open sewers, smells have become an avoidable nuisance. At the beginning of the twentieth century the German Association of Public Health conducted a survey of all German towns with more than 15,000 inhabitants, which revealed that between a quarter and a fifth of the population was infected by the 'smoke plague',[2] as air pollution was then called. Since then, the improvement of the quality of the atmosphere and the reduction of smell pollution have become major issues in science and technology and local and environmental politics.

Since industry was slow to install air filters to deal with oppressive smells and dangerous but odourless emissions, and normally acted only in response to enormous pressure, the legislature was forced to intervene at an early stage. The Civil Code of 1900 expressly assured property owners that they were not obliged to put up with 'excessive' nuisance, which included smells (§907). All the same, an owner could only seek legal redress if the smell interfered seriously with the use of his property or exceeded 'normal local levels'. After 1915, the courts no longer took the average use of the property as their yardstick but 'what the residents of the area concerned regarded as normal'.[3] This implied a new, 'sensory' interpretation of 'local norms' which remained in force until 1959, when the passage referring to 'normal local levels' was amended. Since then, nuisances of any kind do not have to be tolerated 'if they may be prevented by measures for which those who are responsible may reasonably be expected to pay.'[4]

Translating all this into action was both crucial and difficult. The problem is highlighted by the so-called technical provisions of the 1895 trading regulations, which actually remained in force until 1964. The clean air provisions of these regulations deal with noise and smell pollution in very general terms and only specify limits in a few exceptional cases (such as sulphur emissions from glassworks). However, they did not preclude the prescription of limits in individual cases by competent licensing authorities. In the 1920s, for example, the municipal council of the city of Berlin considered the enactment of 'municipal air-protection regulations' to stem a rising tide of dissatisfaction with the much-lauded 'Berlin air'. In the event, the chief constable of Berlin found himself forced to drop this impractical legal device 'because it would be impossible to implement.'[5]

But by the beginning of the twentieth century it was not just smoking chimneys and car-exhaust fumes which were poisoning the air of urban conurbations and provoking ever more vociferous public protests. People had also had their noseful of the stenches issuing from rivers that had been turned into sewers, and were in search of some form of systematic control. In 1901, the Prussian government issued a decree intended to produce cleaner water and effective protection against air pollution: 'Clouded, discoloured, noxious and bad-tasting waters are aesthetically displeasing . . . and detrimental to hygiene.'[6] A particularly poignant case was the struggle of the people of Wuppertal to clean up the stinking Wupper – a river that found literary fame in a play of the same name by Else Lasker-Schüler. A government bill presented in 1928 called for the observation of a minimum degree of cleanliness, though merely 'to the extent of avoiding intrusive smells'.[7] The authorities wished to do as much as was feasible to get rid of the smell of the Wupper, short of actually cleaning it up. The Wupper Association was founded in 1930 for the specific purpose of supervising the gradual implementation of these

proposals. By 1944, the association was already operating four purification plants, although its successes in the campaign against the
increasing pollution of the water and the smells that accompanied it
were if anything rather modest during the period of National Socialist rule. The general confusion about who was responsible for what
during the Third Reich was one factor in this; others were the 'four-
year plan' of 1936, which was primarily concerned with stepping up
arms production, and the war economy established in 1939.

The monotonous, 'international' smell of car-exhaust fumes and
industrial effluvia hung over industrial urban areas until well into the
post-war period. Given that a large part of the population continued to
be preoccupied with everyday cares, it was some time before environmental awareness was again strong enough in Germany to compel
the attention of politicians. A similar phenomenon may be observed
during the period between the First and the Second World War.
'Over the longer term', writes the environmental historian Dietmar
Klenke, 'the growing prosperity of Western industrial societies and
the increasing exploitation of their natural resources also generated a
greater sensitivity to the negative aspects of this development.'[8] In
this context we might consider the election campaign fought by the
SPD (German Social Democratic Party) in North Rhine-Westphalia
in the 1970s, which promised the return of blue skies to the Ruhr.
The date 17 September 1970 is often seen as a watershed in environmental politics, for it was then that the new liberal-socialist coalition
introduced an immediate programme for the environment aimed at
the purification of air and water and the restriction of noise. By the
time Willy Brandt resigned as federal chancellor, three important
bills had cleared the parliamentary hurdles: the Leaded Petrol Act of
1971, the Waste Disposal Act of 1972 and the Federal Air Pollution
Act of 1974.

It was unrealistic to expect rapid results. The 1970s and 1980s
were a period of industrial resistance and administrative foot-
dragging, and almost two decades elapsed before a German minister
of the environment was able to demonstrate the improved quality of
the waters of German rivers by bathing in the Rhine under the carefully staged gaze of the media. The clean air legislation was also slow
to take effect.

A great deal has been achieved, however, and in industrial cities
smog alerts and driving bans are now issued only in extreme weather

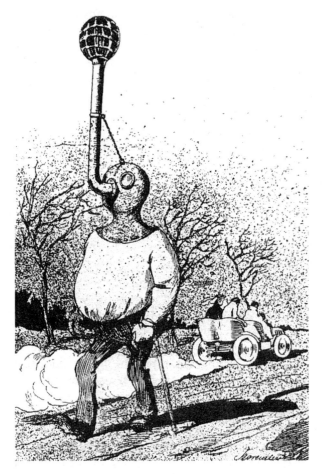

Figure 13.1   Fresh air for pedestrians; cartoon ('Old banger', 1904), from
Beiträge zur historischen Sozialkunde

conditions. It seems, therefore, that our sense of smell is no longer
taking as much punishment as it did just a few decades ago. Indeed,
people are now beginning to lament the 'odourlessness of our cities'.
According to the Viennese social- and cultural historian Peter Payer,
'people are beginning to realize that thorough deodorization not
only banished foul-smelling smog from the city but also got rid of
pleasant scents, which can now be savoured only in a few isolated

—— 268 ——

'smell reservations'.[9] So city planners are now beginning to 'reodorize' their cities by creating areas of greenery. The planning and development department of the city of Munich, for instance, is guided by a so-called scent map, on which such islands of fragrance are already marked out. The *Neue Zürcher Zeitung* of 4–5 September 1999 called for the creation of inner-city 'islands of scent, where we can fill up and sharpen our senses.'

The olfactory imagination

Olfactory perception became a political issue in the twentieth century, and not only in the context of environmental protection. The German-Jewish sociologist Georg Simmel rightly describes smell as a 'dissociating sense', for it not only creates 'much more repulsion than attraction' between individuals in everyday social life, but there is also something 'radical and non-negotiable' about its emotional judgements.[10]

Turning up one's nose at someone is hardly a new phenomenon, but is a behavioural gesture that may be encountered in almost all cultures throughout history. In the nineteenth and early twentieth centuries, for instance, the arch-enemies France and Germany 'couldn't stand the smell' of each other – which did not prevent the middle classes of both countries from scorning the 'stinking working class'. In the United States the notion that the blacks stank, and therefore had to be segregated, persisted even after the abolition of slavery. Supporters of apartheid in South Africa followed a similar path of reasoning.

In Germany the idea that Jews were dirty and spread a repellent smell (*foetor judaicus*) was not invented by Hitler. 'A bad smell is clearly an extension of the attribute of dirtiness', writes the American historian John Efron, 'and the copious testimony of popular culture allows us to conclude that the foul-smelling Jew was largely the creation of the "Christian olfactory imagination".'[11] An anti-Semitic Franconian proverb runs: 'Anständige Juden und Juden, die nicht stinken, / kannst du wohl suchen, aber nicht finden' (Decent Jews and Jews that don't stink / are harder to find than you think). Even children's rhymes played their part in carrying the negative stereotypes deep into the twentieth century: 'Der Jude Isaak Meyer / Der stinkt wie faule Eier' (Isaak Meyer, the dirty Yid / Smells just like a pile of shit; lit: 'The Jew Isaak Meyer stinks like a rotten egg') could be heard from the mouths of children during the Third Reich. The traditional prejudice acquired a new and lethal resonance when Hitler used it as one of the building blocks of his racial anti-Semitism. In *Mein Kampf* the future dictator claimed that the smell of an orthodox Jew would often turn his stomach during his years in Vienna. One of the consequences of this 'olfactory imagination' is now very well known: millions of Jews were murdered in gas chambers disguised as disinfection units.

Yet even though it was tackled with incredible bureaucratic energy and German precision, the 'final solution' failed to deliver the National Socialists from 'the smell of the Jew'. One of the most striking manifestations of the Nazi regime's obsession with the sense of smell was its attempts to conceal from the outside world the smell of burning flesh issuing from the chimneys of the ovens of Auschwitz and other death camps. Most of these efforts were futile. One Auschwitz doctor said later that his wife had been given the usual 'fiction' reserved for visitors: 'in such a large place it was inevitable that many people died, so that a crematorium was needed, and the smoke was due to the fact that it was not working properly.'[12] However, it was impossible to deceive the victims' sense of smell. As one Auschwitz survivor relates: 'And then of course immediately you realized what the unbelievable smell was . . . that you have been smelling . . . Somehow or other they [the inmates] were . . . already so inured.'[13] Even the murderers themselves had needed time to adjust to it, as an anonymous Auschwitz doctor admitted in an interview with the medical historian Robert Jay Lifton: 'When you have gone into a slaughterhouse, where animals are being slaughtered . . . the smell is also part of it . . . not just the fact that they [the cattle] fall over [dead] and so forth. A steak will probably not taste good to us afterwards. And when you do that [stay in the situation] every day for two weeks, then your steak again tastes as good as before.'[14]

So, for all their hankering after German perfection, not even the Nazis managed to find a way of disposing of corpses without creating a smell. Even in the murderous twentieth century, a monstrous and perfidious project of this kind could only be imagined as science fiction. Strangely enough, however, the idea actually appears as a theme in the work of a Jewish writer. In 1911, Salomo

Friedländer (1871–1946), under the pseudonym Mynona, published a grotesque entitled *Von der Wollust über Brücken zu gehen* (On the Delights of Walking over Bridges). The plot is reminiscent of a modern science-fiction novel. A German scientist named Dr van der Krendelen discovers a chemical formula for ridding the earth of bad smells. But few manage to survive in the perfectly pure air. Most people die and have to be cremated. And then something quite miraculous occurs: 'Furthermore, the corpses burned in the wonderful air of the early spring without giving off the faintest smell of decomposition.'[15]

Fighting mouth- and body odour

An openly anti-Semitic tract, with the pseudo-scientific title *Der Jude im Sprichwort der Zeitalter* (The Jews in the Proverbs of the Ages; Nuremberg, 1942), offers a 'racial-biological' explanation of why a non-Jew can also suffer from bad breath: 'He's been kissing a Jew.' In the 1920s, the Odol company was still innocently advertising its famous mouthwash with the text: 'Why doesn't he kiss me? Even the most beautiful woman is undesirable if she has bad breath.'[16]

The story of the Germans' preoccupation with bad breath – that most intimate of physical subjects – would make a gripping study of mental attitudes. It is inextricably entwined with the history of a global company whose name is still on everyone's lips: Odol. Today around 20 million Germans use a mouthwash daily; 70 per cent choose Odol, a brand with a hundred years of tradition and success.

Since the turn of the twentieth century, when Odol first became synonymous with mouthwash as such, bad breath has been a subject that could be talked about openly in Germany without giving rise to embarrassment. In England and the United States, on the other hand, people were still reluctant to talk about bad breath in the 1920s, so the advertising department of the Lambert Pharmaceutical Company had to find a scientific name for it. It quickly came up with the word 'halitosis', which proved to be a great success. Following the launch of a mouthwash named Listerine, the firm's turnover rose from $100,000 in 1920 to over $4 million in 1927. However, the German manufacturer Karl August Ferdinand Linger had not needed to resort to this sort of euphemistic wordplay in order to make his fortune with Odol at quite an early date. As early as the winter of 1900–01, the Dresden Chemical Laboratory founded by Linger was promoting itself as the world's largest producer of mouthwash. By 1924, the export share of product sales was already 60 per cent. This success on the international market is reflected in the purposely more elaborate text of one of the company's newspaper advertisements in the 1920s: 'Women of all races and nations pay tribute to Odol-Hygiene. We adore the blonde gentleness of the German woman, the cool elegance of the Scotswoman, the grace of the Frenchwoman, the bright freshness of Scandinavian femininity and the springy resilience of the women of the United States . . . But regardless of all differences of racial type, we adore a woman with a fresh mouth, beautiful, snow-white teeth and seductively pure breath' (see figure 13.2)[17]

Just a few years later, advertising copy of this kind would no longer have been considered politically correct – always assuming that it had not already succumbed to self-censorship. The Odol advertisements of the Third Reich tended to emphasize the blonde Nordic type. The woman of these images is no longer a vamp or seductress, but a housewife and mother, who is pictured looking up at her husband with a radiant smile: 'superb teeth and a fresh mouth, thanks to Odol'. This covert sucking up to National Socialist ideology did not appear to disturb even those whom the regime had compelled to emigrate, for they remained loyal to the brand in their countries of exile, unwilling to renounce their beloved mouthwash. Among the items on view at an exhibition organized by the German Museum of Hygiene in 1993 was a postcard which gives a striking illustration of product loyalty. It reached Dresden from the USA shortly after the end of the war, and its writer wishes to know whether he can now count on receiving his precious Odol again.

The development of mouthwashes into mass-produced articles and the fashioning of brands into 'household names' were not just the work of the advertisers. It is also necessary to take account of the general change of attitudes to oral health and hygiene following the publication, in 1883, of the pioneering research of the American dentist Willoughby Dayton Miller (1853–1907) into the micro-organisms of the oral cavity that cause caries and bad breath. What had been hitherto an occasional cosmetic option now became a medically recommended prophylactic. As early as 1890, Carl Röse (1864–?), another pioneer in the field of oral hygiene, had examined

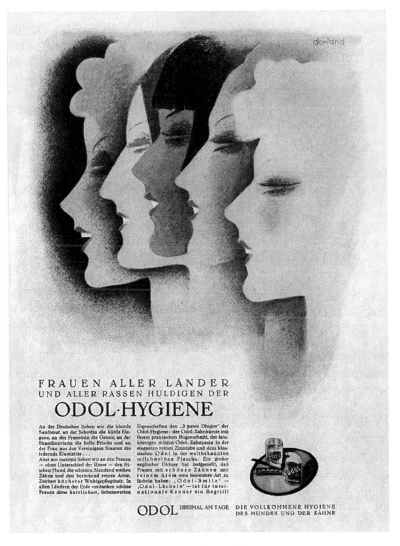

Figure 13.2   Newspaper advertisement for Odol (1920s)

Odol in his laboratory: 'Setting aside the extravagant manner in which it is advertised, I find that with respect to harmlessness, germicidal efficiency and pleasant taste Odol is the best mouthwash I have come across.'[18] To this day, there are very few advertisements for tooth-paste and mouthwash that do not include a scientific endorsement of the prophylactic effects of the product in question.

When you reach for a bottle of mouthwash such as Odol, you are not just following the disciplines of oral hygiene laid down by dentists. As the novelist Robert Walser (1878–1956) notes ironically in one of his prose pieces, pure, fresh breath has been a passport to civilized modern living for quite some time: 'Civilization is unthinkable with-out Odol. If you want to be regarded as a cultivated human being and not just a barbarian, you'd better get hold of a bottle of Odol without delay.'[19] Kurt Tucholsky (1890–1935) was also aware of the needs of the modern artist and intellectual: 'Tinte, Rotwein und Odol / sind drei Flüssigkeiten wohl – / Damit kann der Mensch schon leben' (With these three fluids, / Odol, ink and red wine, / I can get along just fine).[20] But the man or woman of the twenty-first century requires more than a mouthwash. Deodorants are now a scarcely less vital, if not indeed indispensable, article of hygiene. Fortunately, not everyone applies them with quite the zeal of the sixteen-year-old boy from Manchester, whose death in 1998 produced the following newspaper headline: 'Clean Youth Poisons Himself with Deodorant' (*Stuttgarter Nachrichten*, 16 November 1998). Obsessed about body odour, this young teenager had sprayed himself from head to foot with deodorant at least twice a day, explaining to his worried father that he wanted to smell pleasant. He finally died from what the post-mortem described as an overdose of propane and butane, the by no means harmless propellants used to spray the scent from the can onto the body. A representative of the British Association of Aerosol Manufacturers said at the time that she had never encountered a case like it.

Under normal circumstances, people are a little more sparing in their use of deodorants. According to an article in the *Frankfurter Allgemeine Zeitung* of 23 November 1998, only one in two French-men uses a deodorant – and this in a country which is one of the leading consumers of perfume. A non-representative survey conducted by the psychologist Ingelore Ebberfeld in 1998 revealed that people are particularly fond of smelling their partners just after they have emerged from the shower (61.6 per cent). If this percentage seems rather high, we should bear in mind that in Germany and Britain no less than 70 per cent of the population now baths or showers daily. The figure for France is said to be just 47 per cent. Rising expenditures on bodycare products suggest that the citizens of the Federal Republic are smelling better and attaching more importance to a clean appearance. Per capita spending in 1998 was DM 208, which was 3.9 per cent more than in 1997. The two major items were skin- and haircare products. In third place were toothpaste and dental products, followed by 'fragrances', on which women spent 3.5 per cent more in 1998 than in the previous year.

Body odour is definitely 'out' these days. Like almost everything else in our highly technologized and science-obsessed society, it has its own standard unit of measurement: 1 olf is the amount of air pollution produced by an adult in a sitting position with a hygiene rating of 0.7 baths per day.

Changing scent notes

In 1998, a new perfume appeared on the market almost every two days. Alcohol-based perfumes comprise one-quarter of the entire market. In France alone, the perfume industry now employs over 36,000 people. Perfume now has a 40 per cent share of the gift market, and the recipients have long since ceased to consist entirely of women. Competition is fierce in this expanding international market, despite growing demand. The market success of a perfume is determined not only by the way it is advertised but also by the prominence or otherwise of characteristics such as complexity, naturalness and artificiality.

Perfume fashions changed during the course of the twentieth century, though not as much as dress fashions. Women still use the great perfume classic Chanel No. 5, the legendary 'scent of a northern morning by a lake' first introduced in 1921 by the couturière Coco Chanel (1883–1971). Arpège, by Lanvin (1927), and Joy, by Patou (1935), are still popular brands. All the same, there have been certain noticeable changes in consumer attitudes. One of them was the change to musk, which first caught on in the United States. With their heavy emphasis of the physical element, perfumes with this base-note broke all the classical rules of perfume production. Scent compositions with the word 'musk' in their names were regarded as non-perfumes, or at least as highly unconventional. At the end of the 1970s, leading fashion designers sought market success with heavy perfumes (Classic, by Karl Lagerfeld, for example, or Opium, by Yves Saint Laurent). Towards the end of the 1980s, these heavy and bewitching scents made way for purer and clearer compositions. In the last decade of the twentieth century light perfumes finally prevailed. CK one, by Calvin Klein, became a market leader.

There have also been other developments during the last few decades. According to the perfume expert J. Stephan Jellinek, 'The last few years have seen the development of a new attitude towards perfume. Fragrances are now expected to be not only aesthetically pleasing but also capable of altering our mood and state of mind.'[21] In Japan perfumed pillows have been marketed as aids to recuperative slumber since the beginning of the 1990s. Meanwhile, the nose has been discovered by the sales managers of German supermarkets. According to a report in *Die Zeit* (8 July 1999), there are now shopping centres in which so-called scent columns emit electronically controlled fragrances, which are said to put customers into a buying mood. A study of more than a hundred shops, which was completed by Paderborn Polytechnic, found that customers tended to linger longer in supermarkets perfumed in this way. The willingness of customers to part with their money rose by 15 per cent, representing a 6 per cent increase in turnover.

Although condemned as manipulation by consumer protection organizations, the automatic fragrancing of spaces has already entered offices and factory floors in Japan. Managers at the Toyota car company claim that the scenting of the assembly areas with the smell of lemon has reduced conveyor-belt errors by as much as 30 per cent. When the miniature Smart car (originally a German-Swiss collaboration) was introduced to the public at the end of the 1990s, the ingenious advertising strategists came up with something special: the lemon yellow demonstration model had a pleasant lemony smell. It was a breach of the time-honoured code of the motor industry, which lays down that a new car must have a neutral smell. This is why car manufacturers all over the world employ highly paid olfactologists (professional 'sniffers') to test each new car for the unpleasant smell of plastic or rubber.

Going to the smellies

Although still a project of the future, the sensuous 'scented TV', with a remote control unit containing aromatic capsules activated by a radio signal, already haunts the nightmares of the critics of our media society, who fear that the five senses are gradually being monopolized by the multimedia. However, the sense of smell has in fact already entered the world of cinema. As the Constance media specialist Anne Paech has noted: 'In its pursuit of the ultimate illusion, cinema has already made several serious attempts to heighten certain visual effects for the spectator by introducing corresponding olfactory sensations.'[22]

The first film to appeal to the olfactory nerves of the audience was screened at the New York World Fair in 1940. Its title, *My Dream*, alluded to a perfume that was very popular at the time. Using the 'Odorated Talking Pictures' process developed by the Swiss Hans E. Laube, it first became possible to reproduce smells during the performance of a film using a fully automated system. A cinema of scent was a long-standing dream, and the reader may recall the synchronized olfactory experiences created by the famous 'scent organ' in Aldous Huxley's dystopian novel *Brave New World* (1932).

There was another successful attempt to appeal to the film-goer's sense of smell in 1960. The 'Aroma-Rama' process developed by Charles Weiss involved piping smells into the auditorium through the air-conditioning system, and was used in a film documentary about the Great Wall of China. However, owing to the 'olfactory chaos' (Anne Paech) produced by the relatively primitive technology, it found no immediate imitators.

In the same year, another 'smelly' made film history. This was Mike Todd Jr's thriller *Scent of Mystery*. The American producer had taken Hans E. Laube's process a stage further, renaming it 'Glorious-Smell-o-Vision'. However, this unique olfactory experience was available only to audiences at specially converted cinemas in Chicago, New York and Los Angeles, where the seats were connected to a system of tubes. A signal on the film's soundtrack triggered the emission of the appropriate smell in the auditorium at a given point in the action. This was then followed immediately by the release of a neutralizing scent, prior to the next sequence of smells. 'The olfactory information', writes Anne Paech, 'matched by and large the images on the screen, which were connected with things such as garlic, gunpowder, wine, peppermint, shoe polish, lemons, fish, bananas, pipe tobacco, perfume and more than twenty other smells.'[23] Despite all the expense, this state-of-the-art version of olfactory cinema was also only a modest commercial success.

The less elaborate process first used in 1981 by the American horror film producer John Waters, in a thriller entitled *Polyester*, is perhaps still the best known. To enable the members of the audience to savour the 'evil smells' described in the film's plot (which included the hallucinations of a glue-sniffer), Waters distributed scratch cards, which they were invited to smell when the numbers of the matching scenes appeared on the screen. The nauseating smells and brutal scenes of Waters's 'shocker' apparently turned the stomachs of some of the more sensitive spectators.

What looks like the last attempt – at least for the time being – to create a sophisticated cinema of scent took place in Paris in 1989. On this occasion the 'smelly' was a film about diving entitled *Le Grand Bleu* (The Great Blueness). The moment the blue sea appeared on the screen, the auditorium was pervaded by the tangy smell of sea salt, which was passed through the air-conditioning. So what does the future hold in store? The assault on the olfactory nerves is not the only one that devotees of the new visual medium have had to face since the 1950s. 'Commercial cinema', notes the American film historian Patricia Mellenkamp, 'bombards the senses of touch, taste and smell, as well as sight and hearing.'[24] Yet this does not necessarily mean that we are moving towards new 'sensuous' or even synaesthetic cinematic experiences.

Aromatherapy

The rediscovery of the sense of smell in the twentieth century was accompanied by the revival of an ancient form of therapy which acquired the special name of 'aromatherapy' only in the 1930s. In the meantime, the word has come to mean more than just a simple therapy of scent. Its implications are now more general, and it is often taken to refer to 'an integrated therapeutic method, which, with the assistance of essential oils, exercises an influence on both physical and mental processes.'[25]

Essential oils are known to have been used for medicinal purposes in antiquity. Nowadays they barely get a mention in official pharmacopoeias, which simply note their aromatic effects and limited usefulness in certain treatments (e.g., for flatulence). But for the highly promising therapeutic experiments conducted at the beginning of the twentieth century by the chemist René-Maurice Gattefossé (1881–1950) in the small town of Grasse, one of the bastions of the perfume industry, the exploitation of essential oils would have been confined largely to the perfume industry. It was Gattefossé who coined the term 'aromatherapy', which we hear all around us today.

Still controversial, this alternative medicinal therapy enjoyed an early period of florescence in France before the Second World War. With the trend towards alternative medicine that spread to almost all the countries of the West in the 1970s, aromatherapy became known outside France. Marguerite Maury, who together with her husband championed and organized courses in the therapy, was for many years one of its leading exponents. Nowadays, the chemist or drugstore that does not stock a wide selection of essential oils is a rare phenomenon. Regardless of the method preferred (burning the oils in an 'essential oil burner' or rubbing or massaging them into the skin), the aromatic substances released are supposed to have an immediate effect on the body, mind and spirit. And, for 'rapidly banishing unpleasant smells or negative vibrations [*sic*!] from the atmosphere of a room', one recently published handbook of esoteric therapies recommends the use of a room spray consisting of a mixture of essential oils (e.g., rose oil) and pure alcohol.

The signs are, therefore, that that process of deodorization, which the French cultural historian Alain Corbin has described as a product of the medical enlightenment and increasing hygienic awareness of the late eighteenth and early nineteenth centuries, is now giving way to a process of 'reodorization'. This transformation is marked by the more or less definitive suppression of stenches of any kind by the latest modern technology. So, regardless of where the nose pokes itself in, the only smells it encounters are fragrant. Viewing the long-term character of this development, Constance Classen, an American ethnologist and the author of a remarkable cultural sociology of smelling, poses the obvious question: 'As odours, like roses, have long-standing associations with both spirituality and sensuality, one wonders if this post-modern interest in smell is evidence of a quest for spiritual and/or sensual fulfilment.'[26] The use of pheromones – mysterious, sexually enticing substances secreted by the body – in the production of perfume may perhaps be regarded as part of this quest.

— 14 —
Listening Effects – or The Art and Power of Noises

hello i'm the ear.
can you hear me?
i imitate
the striking of the clock

and now
imagine you are in the street.
i'm a horse
and milk cart

my colleague
is lying on your arm
and is already asleep.

allow me
to withdraw
inside your alarm clock
        Ernst Jandl, *the ear* (1985)

(Post-)industrial soundscapes

In 1913, the Italian futurist Luigi Russolo published a manifesto entitled *The Art of Noises*, in which he introduced his orchestra of the future. This orchestra would be capable of producing all the noises that have become typical of the modern world. The six noise families which he thought would 'enrich mankind with a new and unsuspected pleasure of the senses' were: '1. Roars, thunderings, explosions, rattling bangs, booms; 2. Whistling, hissing, puffing; 3. Whispers, murmurs, mumbling, muttering, gurgling; 4. Screeching, creaking, rustling, humming, crackling, rubbing; 5. Noises obtained by beating on metals, woods, skins, stones, pottery, etc.; 6. Voices of animals and people, shouts, screams, shrieks, wails, hoots, howls, death rattles, sobs.'[1] Anyone who has spent a night in one of the inexpensive hotels on Times Square in New York will have vivid recollections of this kind of noise pattern. The American 'orchestra of the metropolis' plays night and day, leaving the musical ear with an impression of total cacophony.

The Berlin folklorist Wolfgang Kaschuba describes an acoustic scenario that is perhaps more typical of contemporary post-industrial society: 'The ringing of the microwave oven replies to the beeps of the washing machine, and then your girl friend phones to arrange how to get your kids and her kids to school or tennis lessons, while the clothes dryer, freezer programme, calorie scale and the kids' computer hum and tick along in between.'[2] There can be little doubt that the coming of the so-called second industrial revolution has profoundly altered the soundscape of our cities. 'Industrial machinery, railways, cars, aircraft, telephones, gramophones, radio, television, computers, have introduced new worlds of sound, tone and noise which it would be interesting to examine in the context of a historical-anthropological investigation of the process of civilization',[3] writes the Berlin cultural historian Christoph Wulf. By the beginning of the twentieth century, people had by and large become inured to the chugging of steam locomotives, the piercing whistles of platform guards, the loud roar of 'petrol coaches' (as the first cars were called), the heavy thump of steam hammers and the whirring of the rotating cogs of machines. These were now joined by new kinds of noise such as the sound of aircraft. Other noise sources suddenly took on an entirely new dimension. One of them was the so-called noise of leisure.

Aircraft noise

Judging from the number of anti-noise action groups, there can be little doubt that people in Germany feel more bothered by aircraft noise than anything else. A recently published directory lists over sixty such associations, distributed over the whole area of the Federal Republic. According to a still fairly recent questionnaire, half the German population feels disturbed by the noise of air traffic, and 16 per cent of those questioned stated that it was seriously affecting their lives. There are a number of reasons for this. 'Air traffic is particularly problematic', writes the social scientist Stephan Marks, 'because the noise it produces spreads through the air unimpeded. The sound of a single aircraft can blanket a whole area for several minutes, since it is not muffled by buildings or noise-protection walls.'[4]

Most modern air traffic involves the use of relatively noisy types of aircraft such as propeller aircraft and large jets. Noise prevention regulations have been in force in Germany since 1991, yet even when followed to the letter they still allow a single jet fighter to produce a noise of the order of 93 to 108 dB (A). The level recommended for propeller aircraft ranges from 64 to 106 dB (A). Compare also the 120 dB (A) of a pneumatic hammer with the 40 dB (A) of birdsong. Small wonder, therefore, that the writer Robert Gernhardt has included aircraft noise in his 'eleventh commandment' against noise: 'Thou shalt also not jet around the heavens, for sporting aircraft, ultra-light flying machines and helicopters are an offence to my ears.'[5] This popular author may be unusually sensitive to noise, but here he is merely expressing the way many Germans feel about the increasing congestion of their country's airspace.

Just how much times have changed is highlighted by a comparison with one of Gernhardt's literary predecessors. Although renowned for his biting criticisms of contemporary life, Kurt Tucholsky none-theless managed to derive a certain pleasure from the noise of aircraft. In a short prose piece written in 1931, he describes an experience at his holiday home in the south-east of England. Shortly before agreeing to rent this house, he asked the gardener: 'And is it quiet here too?' 'Absolutely quiet', replied the gardener, 'quite unusually and even awfully quiet. There's just . . . but no . . . that's not import-ant.'[6] What the gardener considered to be too negligible a noise to be worth mentioning was the then little-used flight path to the contin-ent, which passed right over the house. Tucholsky was unperturbed by this information and became curious: 'Little yapping dogs, ladies singing and playing the piano, someone still banging away at some-thing – but fliers . . . ? Fliers over the house? This was something new. So I rented the place.' Amused and intrigued, he spent the holiday waiting for the 'flying crates' to appear in the sky suddenly at certain times of the day and vanish over the horizon a few minutes later. Upon discovering that some of them were carrying mail rather than passengers, he jotted down his one and only comment about the noise:

'Letters surely don't make such a racket.' Otherwise, this German poet and journalist seems to have welcomed these strange noises in the sky as a distraction from the labours of his working holiday in Kent.

Tucholsky did not live to hear the ear-splitting sound of the giant squadrons of aircraft that crossed the English Channel in both directions just a few years later to unload their deadly bombs over German and British cities. Although there are periodic complaints about the loud droning of Nato transport aircraft and the thunder of low-flying jet fighters, the real sore point on both sides of the channel today is civil air traffic. In Britain, Germany and elsewhere the noise of passenger aircraft has increased to such an extent over the past forty years that what was once no more than an occasional disruption has become a permanent source of stress for many people. In the Federal Republic alone, air traffic has more than trebled since 1980. While it is true that the legislation enacted by the German parliament in 1971 provides for the creation of zones of protection against aircraft noise, it does not apply to all airports. Noisy locations such as helicopter landing-pads and regional and company airports are excluded from its terms of reference. Critics have faulted both the loopholes of this legislation and its method of calculating noise levels. For it does not start out from the highest noise levels, which are often between 30 and 50 dB (A) above the level normally taken as the average, and therefore does little to redress the situation.

Recreational noise

In the twentieth century, the sound of aircraft was joined by another source of noise, which, although not entirely new, had never existed in that particular form before: the noise of leisure. The rise of recreational noise is connected with the fact that, in post-industrial society, people are spending less time at work and have more free time on their hands than at any time in the past. In this context, listening to music, one of the most popular leisure-time pursuits, has become a major health hazard. Ear specialists have issued warnings about ear-splitting disco music and the unbelievably high phonal levels of rock and pop concerts, and cautioned against playing Walkman with the volume set too high. They have also drawn attention to the sometimes quite loud noises produced by toys (e.g., toy guns)

In June 1999, the scientific committee of the Chamber of Federal German Doctors issued the following statement about the problem: 'The incidence of hearing impairment among young persons who have never worked in noisy environments has risen to alarming levels. We assume that the cause must be exposure to high levels of sound during leisure periods.'[7] This body therefore urgently recommends the restriction of the sound levels of portable and other devices equipped with earphones to a maximum of 90 dB (A), and the prescription of levels not exceeding 95 dB (A) for discotheques. The present levels are still considerably higher than this. Sound-level measurements taken in discotheques average out at between 92 and 111 dB (A). The sound input of Walkmans can be as high as 120 dB (A), which is equivalent to the sound produced by a pneumatic hammer. Research has shown that hearing impairments cannot be excluded at levels in excess of 84 dB (A).

Questionnaires on leisure-time activities among young people show that the number at risk is by no means low. The information collected suggests that almost 80 per cent of those aged between eighteen and nineteen spend an average of 6.2 hours a week in a disco. The same percentage listens to loud music for much longer in other contexts. Here the average is 11.4 hours per week. On the basis of these (musical) listening habits, it is predicted that around 10 per cent of young people will have suffered a hearing loss of the order of 10 dB (A) or more in five years' time. In 1988, two-thirds of the disco-goers who took part in a study stated that they occasionally experienced symptoms such as tinnitus and temporary deafness.[8] Small wonder, therefore, that Robert Gernhardt's poetic 'anathema' also extends to this and other forms of recreational sound. 'Ye shall silence Walkmans in trams and trains: for know ye that the Walkman is an engine invented by the Devil for the confusion of the wits of man, making him believe that though he filleth his head with music, his neighbour heareth it not.'[9]

Noise in contemporary art and music

Besides doctors, artists were among the first to respond to the new soundscape of an increasingly technologized world. The trailblazers here were the futurist painters. The manifesto *The Painting of Sounds*,

Noises and Smells by Carlo Carràs (1881–1966) appeared simultaneously with Russolo's Art of Noises in 1913. Carràs's colleague
Umberto Boccioni (1882–1916) translated his appeal for a new kind
of pictorial art – which also fascinated the painters of the Blaue
Reiter (The Blue Rider) – into a synaesthetic painting entitled The
Sound of the Streets Invades the House (1911). However, when one
considers the way the viewer's gaze is manipulated by this picture, in
which the human figures are suspended in mid-air and the façades
of the houses look as though they are about to topple over, one is
inclined to wonder, like the art historian Doris Schuhmacher-Chilla,
'whether the iconographic execution does not in fact fail to match
the aura of the artist's visionary experience.'[10]

Although it is, in fact, a work in the neo-classical style that developed
around 1920 in response to modern musical impressionism and
expressionism, the symphony Pacific 231 (1923) by Arthur Honegger
(1892–1955) became a monument to the integration of new worlds of
sound into the music of the twentieth century. The famous American
steam locomotive has, so to speak, written musical history. The slow
piston stampings of the departing locomotive and its progress towards
top speed are imitated by the Swiss composer's rhythms. The effects
are achieved by means of expressive resources such as accelerando
and chorale-like forms. Luigi Russolo had already experimented with
noise-music ('bruitisme') a few years before Honegger, but it had
little impact, and found very few imitators outside futuristic circles.
One of Russolo's most important comrades-in-arms was Ballila
Pratella (1880–1955), who in 1911 declared that: '[Music] must represent the spirit of crowds, of great industrial complexes, of trains, of
ocean liners, of battle fleets, of automobiles and airplanes. It must
add to the great central themes of the musical poem the domain of
the machine and the victorious realm of electricity.'[11] Yet his own
music was rather conventional compared to that of Russolo, who
even invented special instruments for the creation of noise. The way
they sounded can be judged from a recording that was only rediscovered in the 1950s. Russolo's contemporaries were not very taken
with this applied 'art of noise', as he himself admitted. Most of the
audience left his concerts before the end, loudly protesting against
their sheer presumption.

The futurists' call for the musical incorporation of the sounds of
modern technology was not repeated until a few decades later, when

it was taken up by the proponents of what has become known as *musique concrète*. Its most important representative was the French sound engineer Pierre Schaeffer (1910–1984), who in 1948 began to edit and arrange tape-recorded real or 'concrete' sounds (din, noise, birdsong) into musical compositions. His first work was a piece entitled *Etude aux chemins de fer* (Etude for Railways, 1948), which, while bearing some thematic resemblances to Arthur Honegger's earlier work, adopted a much more radical approach to the conversion of the sounds of modern mass transportation into concrete tonal images. The first performance was held in Paris in 1950.

The rather loose association of composers calling itself the Groupe de musique concrète came into being at this time. Its sometime members include such famous composers as Olivier Messiaen, with his *Timbres-du-rées*, and Pierre Boulez, with his two *Etudes*. Another important figure in the reception of the movement was Luc Ferrari, whose *Visage 5* (1959) is full of mechanical sounds and strikingly (and hardly accidentally) reminiscent of the futuristic music of Russolo. Ferrari wanted to take concrete music out of an elite circle of enthusiasts and perform it before larger audiences – even to integrate it into popular music. 'My intention', said Ferrari, 'was to pave the way for amateur concrete music, much as people take snapshots during vacations.'[12] It was impossible to predict at the time that the youth culture of the 1970s, and above all the 1990s, would one day borrow heavily from this loudspeaker music, in which concrete sound materials were arranged into musical compositions by means of the latest modern technological resources (tape recorders, synthesizers, amplifiers).

The avant-garde music of the American composer John Cage (1912–1992) is essentially a part of this movement, for it too seeks to create aesthetic experiences using experimental noises and tonal alienation effects. This is nowhere more evident than in the case of Cage's *Railway Concerto*, which was performed as a kind of 'happening' at the Bologna music festival of 1978. The musicologist Manfred Mixner's description of this occasion is brief and to the point: 'On three of the evenings, the audience boarded a train specially equipped with loudspeakers and microphones, so the excursion turned into a journey through sound.'[13] This unusual 'concertante' event inspired the French philosopher of music Daniel Charles to write an essay aptly entitled 'Alla ricerca del silenzio perduto' (In Search of Lost

Silence). It recalls writings by Cage, in which the composer describes his attempts to exclude the subjective dimension of music and discover purely objective sounds. Hence, perhaps, his weakness for new technology. As long ago as 1942, Cage predicted that the synthesizer, which did not appear on the market until the beginning of the 1950s, would one day radically transform modern music: 'Many musicians have dreamed of compact technological boxes, inside which all audible sounds, including noise, would be ready to come forth at the command of the composer.'[14]

Cage refers explicitly to Russolo's *Art of Noises* in his musicological writings, but for him the real 'father of noise' in twentieth-century music is the American composer Edgar Varèse (1883–1965). Varèse refused on principle to produce scores of his music. Instead, he set off in pursuit of radically innovative tonal possibilities. The end products were *Ionisation* (1931), a work for thirty-one different percussion instruments, and *Déserts* (1954), which features strange noises played from a tape recorder.

From industrial music to techno

We have already hinted that the avante-garde composers who were trying to integrate the sounds of the industrial age into modern music were responding to social change on the basis of more or less strong political convictions. Jacques Attali, former advisor to the French president and author of numerous books, has perceived this connection most clearly. His book *Noise: The Political Economy of Music* (1985) is a Marxist account of the history of music. According to Attali, contemporary music represents the fourth stage of musical history, in which music loses its commodity character. Henceforth, music may be composed for the sheer joy of it. 'Listening to music', writes Attali, 'is listening to all noise, realising that its appropriation and control is a reflection of power; that it is essentially political.'[15]

In the original French edition of his book, which appeared in 1977, Attali had failed to take account of a musical trend which was at that time gradually becoming established in England, the United States and Germany. It came from outside the experimental studios and developed far away from the classical concert halls, where avant-garde music was occasionally performed before mostly small audiences. We are referring to so-called industrial music, which moved into the niche left unoccupied by hard rock and punk.

The term 'industrial music' probably goes back to the American performance artist Monte Cazazza, who created a sensation on the Californian music scene at the end of the 1970s with eccentric record albums such as *To Mom on Mother's Day*, which earned him a reputation with the critics as an 'art gangster' and a 'real sick guy'. Although largely unadvertised, his album *Something for Nobody* sold 3000 copies in a few weeks. One of the tracks on this LP ('Distress') consists largely of recorded gunfire and a squawky male voice – supposedly that of the popular British entertainer Max Bygraves.

Monte Cazazza's music strongly influenced a British group called Throbbing Gristle, whose recordings were marketed by an 'alternative' record company named Industrial Records, which also had other British bands (Cabaret Voltaire, ClockDVA) under contract. These bands delighted in experimenting with all manner of sounds, and sometimes consciously borrowed from both electronic E-music and *musique concrète*. The English cultural sociologist Jon Savage has described some of the other distinctive features of industrial music. First, these bands clung to their autonomy and refused to allow themselves to be co-opted by the big record companies. Second, they preferred to control their own publicity (they had their own mouthpiece in the form of a periodical called *Industrial News*). Third, they exploited the technological possibilities of the synthesizer to create so-called anti-music (noise, din). Fourth, they incorporated non-musical elements such as films and videos into their performances, which was something highly unusual in the rock and pop scene at the time. Finally, they deliberately set out to shock listeners and audiences, and thus ran the risk of having their concerts seriously disrupted or even broken up.[16] In the words of the British music historian Brian Duguid: 'As a response to society, noise is the apotheosis of many of industrial music's aims. Throbbing Gristle and Cabaret Voltaire may have mirrored the faceless anonymity of post-industrial society in their drab, grey-stained rhythms, but the noise elements in their music also reflected an anger, recognising their own alienation and loathing it deeply.'[17]

At almost exactly the same time in Germany, rock bands such as Tangerine Dream and, above all, Kraftwerk were experimenting with the tonal elements of synthetically produced music. By filtering, over-laying, compressing and shortening sine tones, they produced pulsat-ing rhythms that produced hypnotic effects when listened to over a long period of time. Kraftwerk even reached the American charts at this time and established the musical basis of what later became the trade-mark sound of techno music: 'bum bum bum bum' in four-four time. The unusual musical subjects and the socially critical character of the lyrics are already foreshadowed in the titles of successful albums such as *Autobahn* (1975) and *Menschenmaschine* (Human Machine, 1977).

The transition from industrial music to techno was fluid. It took place around the year 1989, which was a remarkable historical turn-ing point in Germany and above all in Berlin, where the musical youth culture has its base. Shortly before German reunification, the Bethanien Artists' House in the Berlin district of Kreuzberg put on an Atonal Festival, which featured disc jockeys rather than bands as the central attraction. The DJs served up a fascinating musical mixture of industrial and early techno to a young and dance-crazed audience. The event quickly gave birth to a rampant underground culture, which began to organize 'techno house parties' in strange places like old East German military bunkers and the cellars of condemned houses. An eye- (and ear)witness has described the new sound experiences of these round-the-clock parties as follows:

> The new thing about this music was that it no longer mattered whether you played the A or B side of a record, who the performer was, or who had written the music. All that mattered were the new sounds that went with it. You have to imagine it like this: you hear your favourite piece, and you just start dancing to it. You eventually reach a point where you realize that you've been dancing for hours.[18]

The youth of Berlin, not least the youngsters from the eastern part of the formerly divided city, were enraptured by the harsh basses and monotonous rhythms of techno, which they quickly learned to tell apart from Chicago house music, which is a blend of exported Ger-man hard rock à la Kraftwerk and black gospel music. Shortly after the Berlin Wall came down, odd groups of East Berliners danced themselves into a state of physical exhaustion at the UFO, a cult club in West Berlin, and began to throw communal 'techno parties', for which all they needed, besides an innovative DJ, was some powerful audio equipment, a dry-ice machine to make billowing white fog for the dance floor and a stroboscope for the flashing light. In 1991, over 6000 techno fans descended on Berlin from all over the Federal Republic. The German pioneers of techno-rock – the arty-sounding disc jockey Dr Motte and Jürgen Laarmann, editor of the magazine *Frontpage* – immediately became the cult figures of a new youth movement, which has since become thoroughly commercialized and is now being imitated in non-German-speaking countries. One million young people from Germany and other countries now flock to the annual Berlin Love Parade, the high-point of the techno-cultural year, with just one thing in mind: to experience mass ecstasy in the harmony of monotonous bass sounds, entering a sort of trance, in which the sole medium of communication is the universal language of the body. The Berlin cultural sociologist Dietmar Kamper is convinced that, in a still relentlessly visual post-modern industrial society, techno parties represent 'the ear's protest' against the omnipresent 'tyranny of the eye'.[19]

Radio: the medium of the new listening

Sound as the opposite of silence is not only a theme of the various trends within contemporary music. It also occasionally appears as the subject of modern plays for radio. In his radio play *Geräusch eines Geräusches* (Noise of a Noise, 1969), Peter Handke dispenses more or less completely with the spoken word, and focuses instead on the portrayal of sounds. According to Handke, the play is based on the notion that 'we are sitting alone in a large apartment, let's say on a winter afternoon. It is eerily quiet, and then the sounds around us begin to take on a quite extraordinary quality.'[20] The noises portrayed in this radio play are intended to trigger associations in the listener, causing him to reflect upon his own inner world. The play's lack of a plot or other frame of reference is thus all part of the dramatic intention.

With broadcast drama we come to a twentieth-century medium that has made a decisive contribution to the phenomenon of 'new hearing'. Small wonder that the contemporary composer Mauricio Kagel once described radio as the 'acoustic department' of the 'giant hospital' that was the modern world.[21] The first regular radio broadcasts began in the USA in 1920. In the same year, the main German radio station in Königswusterhausen transmitted the first broadcast of an orchestral concert. The official opening of German radio took place in Berlin on 29 October 1923. By the end of 1924, there were already fifteen stations. About 99,000 people owned radio sets at the time, making a total of around one million regular listeners. At the beginning of the 1990s, there were over 28 million radio receivers in the Federal Republic, which means that more than 91 per cent of German households own a radio. Transmission periods have also lengthened continually since the early days. Between them, German radio stations were on the air for 854 hours a day in 1991.

In the light of these figures, it is hardly surprising that the alteration of people's listening habits by the new medium has been the subject of much critical scrutiny. As early as 1924, when radio was still in its infancy, an article appeared in *Simplicissimus*, a magazine known for its acerbic commentaries on contemporary issues. A few years later, Bertolt Brecht described radio as a mere piece of technological gadgetry, bereft of substance. But there were other writers and artists in this early phase of radio who immediately recognized the new medium's attraction and potential. One of them was the film-maker Dziga Vertov (1896–1954), who referred to the still experimental new medium of sound radio as the 'radio-ear'. In 1916–17, Vertov had set up a 'laboratory of hearing', in which he used a phonograph to produce 'documentary compositions and musical and literary montages'.[22]

The new medium not only transformed the traditional listening habits of lovers of music and literature (today's talking books would probably have been inconceivable without the invention of the radio play), but also quickly acquired a role in the political domain that was to last until the advent of television. Politicians recognized the extraordinary potential of sound radio as a medium of mass propaganda at a very early stage of its existence. The broadcasting politics of the National Socialists and the pre- and post-war American presidential election campaigns are an eloquent testimony to this development.

The progressive 'regression of listening'

With the possible exception of the easily accessible 'techno-sound', modern music makes relatively strenuous demands on the sense of hearing. Observing that, thanks to modern technology, more music was being heard in the twentieth century than at any time in the past, the philosopher and musical theorist Theodor W. Adorno (1903–1969) set about classifying the various forms of musical listening. He was able to distinguish between expert listening, good listening, educational listening, emotional listening, 'resentful listening' (supposedly typical of Bach enthusiasts), listening for relaxation, and indifferent listening. The last applies above all to the functional background music we hear nowadays in almost every department store and restaurant – 'acoustic environmental pollution', as one critic (Wolfgang Welsch) has described it.

At the same time, according to Adorno, the new sound media (radio, cassette recorders, CD players), which are now exploited by both elite modern music and popular light music (be it jazz, rock, pop, punk, hip-hop or techno), have led to what he calls the 'regression of listening', or acoustic degeneration. In the light of this, there have been a number of initiatives in recent years to reconnect with 'proper' forms of listening and even to create a new 'culture of listening' (Wolfgang Welsch).

In 1991, a guide was published in Great Britain listing more than 400 shops, pubs and restaurants which refrained, on principle, from inundating their customers with music. In 1999, the Federal Republic was already celebrating its second 'Day for Silence – against Noise', which is the German version of the international 'Noise Awareness Day' first proclaimed in the USA in 1994.

The Baden School of Hearing was recently established in Rastatt. Its purpose is to help children and adults suffering from poor concentration and hyperactivity – as opposed to any actual hearing impediments – to restore their acoustic perception to good working order. The institution, which was founded by Günter Siegwarth, a music teacher and former head of the Baden-Baden School of Music, is called the Institute for the Promotion of Sensory Perception. In the same year, the *Stuttgarter Nachrichten* devoted almost a whole page in one of its editions (21 March 1999) to the 'Rediscovery of

Conscious Listening'. The article drew attention to the enormous demand for spiritual exercises and monastic 'silence seminars', the proliferation of adult-education courses in 'Good Conversation through Active Listening', and the current boom in the talking-book market. The growing popularity of talking books in particular seems to be a sign of a new willingness to learn how to listen again, since a talking book is unsuitable for 'background' consumption and normally requires the listener to pay attention and concentrate.

Earlier calls for a revival of the kind described tended to fall on deaf ears. In 1967, a non-fictional work entitled *Ear Cleaning* argued more or less in vain for a continual exercising of the sense of hearing for the sake of better all-round sensory perception and a consequent improvement in the quality of life. Richard Murray Schafer, the book's author, has also written a very readable cultural history of listening. Although now more than twenty years old, the issues he raises are still very much alive. He envisages the establishment of a new field of interdisciplinary study which he calls acoustic design. Its task would 'consist of documenting important features, of noting differences, parallels and trends, of collecting sounds threatened with extinction, of studying the effects of new sounds before they are indiscriminately released into the environment [in order] to use these insights in planning future environments for man.'[23]

Thus, at the beginning of a new millennium, the project of retrieving and enjoying the senses involves the restoration of the hereditary rights of hearing and the devotion of more care and attention to noises and sounds that have been buried under, or effaced by, the stimulatory inundation of a highly technologized, multimedia society. We are still a long way from the 'Science of Aural Reception' first contemplated by the German cultural philosopher Eugen Rosenstock-Huessy (1888–1973) some fifty years ago during the Second World War, when the soundscape of large areas of Europe and Asia was being fashioned by columns of marching soldiers, tanks, gunfire, exploding bombs and grenades, and the roar and howl of aircraft engines. Yet his appeal merits reconsideration, for, as the psychologist Karl-Josef Pazzini has remarked, 'it underlines the need for an ethics focused on hearing in order to forestall the emergence of a passive form of bondage, a bondage tantamount to feudal attachment and dependency.'[24]

— 15 —

Ways of Seeing – or The Human Rights of the Eye

Our society is characterized by a cancerous growth of vision, measuring everything by its ability to show or be shown and transmuting communication into a visual journey.

Michel de Certeau, *The Practice of Everyday Life* (1984)

'The society of spectacle'

According to Martin Heidegger (1889–1976), the process of rationalization began with Western philosophy's privileging of the sense of sight, which made existence predictable and culminated in modern technology. Heidegger himself thought of escaping the primacy of visually determined reason by returning to 'the ear of our thought'.[1] This critical attitude towards the visual sense is particularly pronounced in contemporary French philosophy. Georges Bataille's critique of voyeurism in his philosophical-pornographic novel *The History of the Eye* (1967) is one case in point. Michel Foucault's celebrated *Discipline and Punish* (1975) is likewise devoted to the microphysics of the power and omnipotence of seeing. The work of Michel de Certeau (1925–1986), whom we quote at the head of this chapter, should also be read against this background.

The most comprehensive settlement of scores with the omnipresent economy of seeing stems from the pen of the French cultural critic Guy Debord (1931–1994). The title of his book *The Society of the Spectacle* (1967) became a byword for the warped development of sense perception in the twentieth century. 'The spectacle cannot be understood either as a deliberate distortion of the visual world or as a product of the technology of the mass dissemination of images. It is far better viewed as a *Weltanschauung* that has been actualized, translated into the material realm – a world view transformed into an objective force.'[2] This is somewhat reminiscent of Martin Heidegger's dictum that, in the modern age, what was once a view of life has become an image of the world. Yet, as the following quotation suggests, Debord's critique of the primacy of seeing owes more to Karl Marx's theory of alienation than the phenomenological reflections of the author of *Being and Time*:

> The spectator's alienation from and submission to the contemplated object (which is the outcome of his unthinking activity) works like this: the more he contemplates, the less he lives; the more readily he recognizes his own needs in the images of need proposed by the dominant system, the less he understands his own existence and his own desires. The spectacle's externality with respect to the acting subject is demonstrated by the fact that the individual's own gestures are no longer his own, but rather those of someone else who represents them to him. The spectator feels at home nowhere, for the spectacle is everywhere.[3]

It is not the new visual technology that creates this 'spectacularistic society', but rather the other way round: society itself fashions the technology into an instrument of its purpose. 'The spectacle', continues Debord, 'is hence a technological version of the exiling of human powers in a "world beyond".'[4]

X-ray eyes

But what exactly are these special new technologies, which according to Debord were developed to satisfy the social needs of a modern society? And how is the new seeing manifested? The French cultural sociologist Jean-Claude Kaufmann has claimed that the beach is an ideal modern 'laboratory of advanced experimental research into the modernity of this gaze'.[5] For isn't the beach nowadays a place of spectacle, where the human body is put on display? It is here that we may observe how the gazes of the men are fixed on naked breasts, and how a preponderantly male group of openly curious participants is practising what Kaufmann aptly describes as 'the art of looking without seeing'.[6] The eyes that target the female body are X-ray eyes, so to speak: they convert it into a spectacle.

Modern technology has come up with a solution to those occasions when female modesty can be a hindrance to these 'inspections of flesh'. A short while ago, the newspapers warned women that a well-known Japanese firm had produced a new camcorder equipped with an infra-red light facility that made bathing costumes transparent. The public was highly indignant. Behind every harmless-looking pater familias filming holiday scenes with his video camera could lurk a lecher. Concerned about its good name, the company responded to this 'abuse' of its latest technology by immediately issuing a statement to the effect that, although the media had exaggerated the risk, steps would be taken to ensure that this voyeuristic option would be discontinued in future models.

Joking references to people with X-ray eyes reveal just how much the discovery of 'X-rays', as Wilhelm Conrad Röntgen (1845–1923) called the rays named after him, has contributed to the formation of the modern gaze. It implies an ability to look right through someone and to see what that person cannot see, or would like to conceal from prying eyes. On the threshold of the twentieth century, just a few years after Röntgen's pioneering experiments of 1895, the users of this new technology were already fully aware that they were witnessing a transformation of vision: 'The . . . importance of X-rays for research consists in their ability to break objects down to their individual constituents from a quite new perspective. . . . Using this point of view, we build up a three-dimensional perspective of the object as we look at it, which is something that was previously possible only after extremely laborious dissection and chemical analysis.'[7] The highly versatile X-ray process soon won recognition as one of the twentieth century's most prestigious technologies, and provided hospital patients at least with a graphic demonstration of the fundamental principle of the visual epoch: 'seeing is more certain than sensing' (Monika Domman).

The further development of the X-ray into a metaphor of seeing into the social body has much to do with spectacle in Guy Debord's sense or, more precisely, with what he calls 'The spectacle [which] is self-generated, and . . . makes up its own rules . . . And . . . makes no secret of what it *is*, namely, hierarchical power evolving on its own.'[8] It was not in the first instance the new and previously inconceivable possibility of diagnosing broken bones, gun-shot wounds or the degeneration of the human skeleton that changed the perception of the body, but the development of mass X-ray techniques, which made it feasible to 'screen' an entire population.

The first mass X-raying was carried out on French soldiers in 1901. Other armies also X-rayed their troops during the First World War. By the beginning of the 1930s, the debate in Germany about whether to extend the X-raying of soldiers of the German army to the population as a whole was long over, for in 1927 the German tuberculosis specialist Franz Redeker (1891–1962) had called for the creation of a national X-ray register, although it would be some years before his recommendations could be implemented. The project had to be delayed until the development of the cheaper and more practical X-ray process that was used all over the world after the mid-1930s.

Although the diagnostic value of mass X-ray screening was still a matter of contention during the period of the Weimar Republic, the debate soon turned to the strictly legal question of whether such examinations should be voluntary or made compulsory. One of the few critical voices heard at the time warned that 'the recommended periodic examination of all German citizens means the total social-ization of free individuality, the expropriation of the healthy person's right to the ownership of his body and mind.'[9]

A few years later, political conditions in Germany had altered dramatically. Things were now seen differently: through the eyes of the Führer, that is to say, and in the light of National Socialist health policies. 'These accusations of compulsion are derived from ideas of freedom which we no longer comprehend, now that it is taken for granted that self-serving notions and desires must bow to the neces-sity of the common good', explained one of the most respected German tuberculosis specialists in 1937.[10] The Führer state assumed the right to pronounce on anything and everything. Not even the body's interior was exempt from its gaze. This, then, was the ideo-logical backdrop to the first legally compulsory mass screening of the German people in the year 1939. By 1944, when the enterprise was abandoned owing to lack of money and materials, 20 million citizens of the German Reich had been screened. In the very literal sense, therefore, a large proportion of the people had been 'seen through' with the explicit approval of the National Socialist regime. The Gestapo and the notorious security service, of course, had their own 'diagnostic techniques' for seeing into the political hearts and minds of the people. It seems, therefore, that there is no essential difference between medical and metaphorical X-rays.

The art and deconstruction of the gaze

The X-ray gaze embodies just one aspect of the new form of seeing. It is, so to speak, the symbol of a new spatial dimension, namely the inner worlds of bodies which are suddenly revealed to the eye by means of rays. But the form of perception has changed as well. 'The new mode of seeing', writes Jean-Claude Kaufmann, 'tends to be floating, hypermobile, fleeting, and slippery.'[11]

This new and unusual mode of vision is already present in the art of the end of the nineteenth century, above all in impressionism. It is also evident in pointillism, a school of painting which appears to prefigure the 'mosaic-like concentrations of puntal elements', which the media theorist Vilém Flusser, writing in the 1980s, perceives as the distinguishing feature of 'technological images' as opposed to the analogical fluidity of 'traditional images'.[12] At the beginning of the twentieth century, cubism, Italian futurism and Russian constructivism continued this process by resolutely abandoning the single-point perspective that had dominated Western art for centuries. 'The object', write Hans-Georg Soeffner and Jürgen Raab, 'is deconstructed into a multiplicity of different angles of view and then reassembled as a collage, so that it no longer addresses a single angle of view but combines all the angles of view from which it could possibly be observed.'[13] The following instructive sentence is taken from the painter Paul Klee (1879–1940), who developed his own very distinctive style and produced works which are more to be decoded than viewed: 'The task of art is not to reproduce the visible but to make it visible.'[14] The eye of the viewer must learn to be mobile and abandon its fixed perspective. 'Vision in motion is a simultaneous grasp . . . a creative performance – seeing, feeling and thinking in relationship and not as a series of isolated phenomena', is how the Bauhaus artist Laszlo Moholy-Nagy (1895–1946) described this new form of seeing.[15] The new seeing had still to conquer Bauhaus art and architecture when the now rather neglected artist and film director Walther Ruttmann (1887–1941) was in the process of developing a theory of moving images. In 1919, he completed the scenario of a new form of art which he called 'painting with time'. It was 'a visual art form which differs from painting in that it is temporal (like music), so its artistic emphasis lies not, as in a painting, on the compression of a real or imagined event into a moment, but precisely on the development of that event in time.'[16]

The 'cinema-eye'

The 'cinema-eye' had penetrated modern art long before the multi-media video installation, with its mix of photographic, electronic and digital images, was added to the artistic repertoire. One early example is the synaesthetic work of art by Ruttmann entitled *Photodram Opus I* (1921). Interestingly enough, this work was not unveiled in a museum of art, but 'premiered' in a Frankfurt cinema. Painters and film directors were by then collaborating in experiments with the new visual technology. The most famous example of this type of collaboration is undoubtedly the film classic *Un Chien Andalou* (1928) by Luis Buñuel (1900–1983) and Salvador Dali (1904–1989). The film contains a scene showing an eye being sliced across the middle by a razor, which is still quite gruesome even by today's standards. The sequence is laden with significance, for it underlines the radical changes that have overtaken our sensory perception since the end of the nineteenth century, following the dissolution of central perspective in modern art and, above all, the coming of the variable gaze of the 'cinema eye' – a gaze that became even more mobile when the film camera itself began to move about and techniques of cutting and montage improved.

The notion that cinema and television have taught people to see 'faster' and 'more superficially' is now something of a cultural-historical platitude. But even in the days when cinema had only just learned to walk, there were already some who were quick to sense the new medium's by no means unproblematic tendency to instrumentalize the human gaze. Returning from a visit to the cinema in 1913, Franz Kafka wrote in his diary: 'Am quite empty and insensible, the passing tram has more living feeling.'[17] Three years before this, the editor-in-chief of *Licht-Bühne*, a professional journal of cinematography based in Berlin, had taken a journey through the German world of cinema. The scene in Cologne had left a lasting impression:

> Everything here smells of film. We live in the age of machine technology. We are no longer looking for things like personality and individuality, insights into the emotional lives of others, the contact between stage and audience, the vibration of sounds through the ears and into the heart, the language of poets. No. We just want to indulge our eyes. The emotions have to be condensed to the utmost brevity and rushed

past us like telegrams. The sound of our world is just the rattling of the soundless projector, even though now and again a gramophone is wound up as a sort of necessary evil. . . . Things will get much worse as cinemas increase in number. The 'see-sickness' will spare no one. We will end by forgetting how to read, and newspapers will be replaced by film journals. In prisons, the worst form of punishment will be withdrawal of cinema rations, and any mother refusing to give her children money for the flicks will be burned as a witch. – Yes. I can feel it. I need to get out of Cologne, which is just one big cinema. Otherwise I shall begin to have anxieties about the future.[18]

How might this cinema expert have phrased his forebodings had he been able to anticipate the coming of television, the 'cinema in the home'? Today we are used to hearing people claim that too much television has an adverse effect on concentration and dulls the faculties of perception, particularly those of children and young people. Yet the same reservations were expressed when the first permanent cinemas were opened in the big cities, and cinema gradually began to lose its stigma as an essentially proletarian form of entertainment. Artistically ambitious films, along with the latest developments in the vocabulary of cinema (montage, close-up), actually attracted large numbers of middle-class film-goers to the newly modernized auditoria at quite an early date. In 1913, the primary school teachers of Düsseldorf took part in a survey, which revealed that 59 per cent of all children of school age had been to the cinema at least once during the past year. Among the adverse effects listed by the teachers were 'poor concentration', 'loss of domestic application', 'thoughtlessness', 'overexcited imagination', 'disruption of the nervous system and sense of reality' and, last but not least, 'imitation of criminal behaviour' – pretty much the same black marks, therefore, as those handed out by today's teachers and media educationalists.[19]

Television as 'visual neo-culture'

The debut of the sound film at the end of the 1920s was 'a cinematic anticipation of television' (Siegfried Zielinski). Contemplating this extraordinarily rapid development, the trade journal *Der Deutsche Rundfunk* prophesied in 1930 that sound films would move into more intimate settings: 'families and smaller circles of people will sit listening to the story on the talking screen in the privacy of their own homes.'[20] The first experiments with the new medium of television had just begun at the time. In 1929, following the first successful test transmissions conducted by the German Post Office, the firms Robert Bosch GmbH, Baird Television Ltd in England, D. S. Loewe and Zeiss-Ikon set up a company named Fernseh-AG to drive the research project forward. In the spring of 1935, a sensational announcement appeared in the magazine *Fernsehen und Tonfilm*: 'Today [22 March 1935], the National Socialist Broadcasting Company, in co-operation with the Imperial Postal Service and German industry, has become the first broadcaster in the world to begin regular television transmissions.'[21] The intention was undoubtedly to score a propaganda victory over the British, for the reality was in fact rather more modest. It simply meant that, with the help of the German Post Office, a few privileged viewers could now watch experimental audio-visual programmes on three evenings a week. Nonetheless, the television makers were already dreaming of the hour when 'these few will have become thousands and hundreds of thousands of television-watching national comrades, until finally a whole people will be able to participate in the greatest visual feast on offer.'[22] It would take another fifty years for that moment to arrive. Today, more than 97 per cent of German households own at least one television set, and each German citizen now spends an average of 3 hours and 18 minutes a day in front of a television screen.

One of the great propaganda successes of the Nazi regime was the televising of the 1936 summer Olympic Games in Berlin, the first live transmission of a major sporting event. In the capital, more than 10,000 people a day could follow the games in twenty-six specially erected public television rooms and on two large screens in the city centre. It was the first time in the history of television that viewers had seen an ambitious live transmission of this kind. At other times, the nation's still tiny population of television viewers had to make do with more meagre fare, such as cinema films which had been hacked to pieces and 'adapted for television'. The 'television plays' that began to flicker across the tube soon afterwards had prosaic titles such as *Die Speisekarte* (The Menu) or *Frau Matschke greift ein* (Mrs Matschke Intervenes) and consisted for the most part of trivial scenes from everyday life.

Besides which, the 'feasts for the eyes' grandiosely promised by the Nazi regime were hampered by certain technical limitations. The new television standard (441 lines displaying twenty-five images per second), which matched the quality of 16 mm cine film, could not actually be introduced until 1938. But the poor quality of the pictures appears not to have affected the popularity of the medium, although this did not actually soar to undreamed of heights until after the Second World War. In 1939, the BBC advertised its television programming with the slogan 'You can't shut your eyes to it', at a time when television programming was still in its infancy. The advertisers of those times would therefore appear to have anticipated what today's media critics most deplore: the magical attraction of the television screen.

Television, like cinema, is an ideal means of instrumentalizing the human gaze. 'Seeing' is replaced by 'watching'. Unlike other visual media, television allows the viewer to be present at events occurring in different places (you go there 'live'!). After the 1936 Olympics, which were seen on television by relatively few people in the world as a whole, the new medium achieved its first successes in the mass-entertainment market with the coronation of Queen Elizabeth II in England in 1953 and the world football championship of 1954. In 1954 alone, when the German national side won the World Cup against all expectations and returned to Germany in triumph, the number of television subscribers leapt from 11,658 to 84,278.

The philosopher Günter Anders (1902–1992) was one of the few contemporaries to remain sober as television mania seized hold of large sectors of the German population. In 1956, he asked his readers to consider that: 'Besides the production of mass hermits and the conversion of the family into a miniature audience, the truly revolutionary achievement of radio and TV is that football matches, church services and atomic explosions visit *us*; the mountain comes to Mohammed, the world now comes to man, he does not go out to meet *it*.'[23] A few years later, the Fluxus artist Wolf Vostell (1932–1998) targeted television with a 'happening' entitled *TV-Begräbnis* (Television Funeral, 1963). The artist wrapped a television set in barbed wire and gave it a 'symbolic burial'. The video installations created by the Korean artist Nam June Paik in the early 1970s are not least a critical artistic response to a medium whose popularity was boosted by the invention of the video recorder. The sociologist Rolf Lindner adopted a more positive attitude towards the developing 'visual neo-culture' by portraying it as a challenge to conventional habits of seeing: 'Television addresses all the senses at once and is thus able to absorb them in quite a special way, which makes it a useful means of creating psychological distance from the working day.'[24] At exactly the same time, however, disciples of the critical theory of the Frankfurt school such as Oskar Negt and Alexander Kluge were subjecting the 'class medium of television' (Siegfried Zielinski) to a radical critique. During the 1970s, they explored the socio-economic and moral implications of life in a televisual world in the light of the theories of Marshall McLuhan.

The eye as weapon

Today's wars are not just broadcast on television, but actually take place on screen in the computer rooms of reconnaissance aircraft and centres of military command. 'The battlefield has been a field of vision from the very beginning', claims the media theorist Paul Virilio: 'For the warrior, the function of the eye merges with the function of the weapon.'[25]

The First World War marked a decisive break in the history of sensory perception in that it reduced the field of vision to the line of fire. In the summer of 1917, the distinguished art historian Fritz Saxl (1890–1948) described his experiences at the front to his hardly less distinguished colleague Aby Warburg (1866–1929): 'They gave my battery a terrible pounding. I watched it like some kind of film: the incredible tempest of fountains of earth, flying bits of stone, trees, etc.'[26] The contemporary literary historian Bernd Hüppauf has drawn attention to the way the visual media depicted the soldier in the final phase of the First World War: 'The whole face is centred in a penetrating gaze which often seems to be conquering an imagined object with bare aggression. These portraits do not represent the eye as a window through which an impression of the world is absorbed by the inner person, for the eye itself is active, trained on a target imagined as a weapon.'[27] Let us also mention in passing that, according to German army medical reports, 4 per cent of all soldiers wounded in the First World War were hit in the head, and that more than half of the troops went to the surgeries of military doctors complaining of damaged vision.

Meanwhile, military technology has continued to change, and visual perception on the battlefield has changed with it. 'Remote-controlled and self-guiding missiles', writes the German cultural sociologist Marie-Anne Berr, 'are equipped with various combinations of sensors and artificial eyes, whose gaze is directed towards varying perceptual configurations.'[28] In recent decades the electronic battlefield has developed into a battle of the sensors, for radar and thermal reconnaissance have rendered traditional optical camouflage practically useless. 'One of the signs of the limited perceptual performance of military sensors and the poor recognition and decision-making capacities of automatic systems', continues Berr, 'is the technological integration of the organic: *the direct use of the natural eye as a weapon.*'[29] Her examples are infra-red telescopes with low-light enhancement and the helmet visors developed for fighter-pilots by Israeli technologists, which enable a pilot to aim rockets and missiles at his target simply by looking in its direction.

Sexual curiosity

Sexual curiosity, particularly the male variety, is hardly a modern phenomenon. We need only recall the biblical story of Bathsheba, who was secretly watched in her bath by David. In his *Three Essays on Sexual Theory* (1904–5), Sigmund Freud included sexually accentuated looking among the perfectly normal variants of sexual behaviour: 'Visual impressions remain the most frequent pathway along which libidinal excitation is aroused.'[30] These visual sexual pleasures should not be confused with voyeurism, for in the case of voyeurism the pleasure of looking becomes the sole or dominant purpose of sexual arousal.

Although the voyeurism that Freud regarded as a pathological form of behaviour is relatively rare, the non-pathological, secret observation of sexual objects or situations has undoubtedly increased during the past few decades, as the word 'peep-show', which arrived in the 1960s, attests. According to the German Duden dictionary, this English loan word means: 'the display of a naked woman for the purpose of sexual arousal, viewable through a small window in a private cabin on the insertion of money into a slot.'[31] Although the word first appears in English in 1861, it then referred to what is known in

German as a 'Guckkasten', or 'peep-box', and it retained this meaning for quite some time. In modern Anglo-American usage, a 'peeper' is someone who secretly observes naked women or those in the act of undressing, or couples making love. In German, the devotee of this unusual sexual persuasion is commonly known as a 'Spanner'.

Although these modern peep-shows have been banned by numerous city authorities in Germany, they are still among the attractions of the red-light districts of such European metropolises as Amsterdam, Paris and London. These simple establishments are more or less the same everywhere: a woman on a revolving stage displays her body to the accompaniment of provocative music, while an exclusively male audience watches her through the peep-holes let into a series of small cabins arranged in a circle round the stage. The peep-holes are fitted with shutters, which spring open for a certain period of time upon the insertion of a coin. The glass of the peep-hole is so anti-reflective that it is impossible to see into the cabins from the stage.

Today's peep-show is an epiphany of male sexual voyeurism: a brazen looking without being looked at in return. German courts and municipal authorities have therefore banned these shows as morally offensive, arguing that their one-way eye contact depersonalizes the woman and turns her into a commodity and that they reduce the transaction of buying and selling to the insertion of a coin into a vending machine.

This 'vending-machine effect', as the German courts called it (Federal Administrative Court 64, 270, 279), was incompatible with human dignity. The woman was 'placed on display as a purchasable object of sexual stimulation and offered to each of the spectators in the individual cabins as nothing more than an aid to the gratification of sexual interests.'[32] The argument that the showing of pornographic films in video cabins should also be banned as immoral, since it too provided sexual stimulation and the opportunity for covert self-gratification, was rejected by the court on grounds that impinge on our history of the senses. The court ruled that in this case there was no 'vending-machine effect', for it involved the interposition of film as a mediating and constraining medium between the sexual object (naked men or women) and the 'user' paying in cash or by switchcard.

Meanwhile, technology has played another trick on the judiciary. Peep-show booths may have disappeared from most German cities, but their cheap thrills can now be delivered straight to the living room via the Internet. Typing the appropriate word into one of the large international search engines at the beginning of the year 2000 produced an impressive haul: over 68,000 websites worldwide! Clearly, the demand for this kind of visual material continues to rise, and not only in Germany. In its edition of 1 August 1999, the newspaper *Sonntag Aktuell* profiled a German operator who was making DM 150,000 a month with this type of sex package.

Just as in 'real' peep-shows, the women who undress in front of the running cameras are unable to see their customers on the screen. They merely receive instructions from their 'users', who convey these by mouse or keyboard to the girl of their choice via the Internet.

This exposure of the female body, which gratifies male desires while depersonalizing the woman and turning her into a sex object, contributed significantly to the growth of the women's movement. American feminists protested that the voyeuristic 'male gaze' was not confined to the peep-shows, but was part of the everyday reality of public spaces: beaches, places of work, restaurants, etc. Women in Germany are also protesting increasingly against the ubiquitous male stare. On one Internet page, for instance, a woman complains of the peep-show held every weekend at an (unnamed) East German discotheque, where more or less decently dressed young girls are stared at 'like raw meat on a hook' by the men standing round the dance floor.

The electronic panopticon

Just how omnipresent the principle of 'seeing without being seen' has become is highlighted by the video surveillance of whole cities and streets that is the norm in the USA and Britain, as well as in other countries. It all began with the use of video cameras in department stores, supermarkets and high-security buildings such as banks and embassies. Since then, the 'electronic panopticon' (Günther Ortmann) has spread to other areas as well, and has replaced the architectural panopticon dreamed up – and in some cases implemented – by Jeremy Bentham and other nineteenth-century (prison) reformers.

'Cameras on Every Corner and in Every Room – the Future has a Thousand Eyes', ran the headline of an article in *Die Zeit* (30 December 1998). This piece contained an extract from a book entitled *The Transparent Society* (1998) by the British non-fiction writer David

Brin, which claimed that, thanks to the latest surveillance technology, we are now all living in a kind of glasshouse. The question is
simply: who exactly controls all the cameras filming our everyday
lives? According to the article, the installation of 300,000 surveillance cameras in British cities over the last decade betokens the 'end of
privacy'. In the London borough of Newham alone, life in the streets
and in public places is exposed to round-the-clock surveillance by
150 cameras. The pictures are now being sifted by computers in search
of the faces of wanted criminals.

So has Orwell's bleak vision in *1984* ('Big brother is watching
you') at last become a reality – just two decades after it was first due?
David Brin, who has made a reputation for himself as a science-
fiction writer, thinks not. The future is not some sort of Orwellian
totalitarian police state but a 'transparent' society. Certainly, there
will be surveillance cameras everywhere, but the pictures they take
will be accessible to everyone. Only some such 'democratization' of
surveillance can guarantee freedom in the long run. But the price will
be high, for society will have to abandon all claim to a private sphere.

'Thanks to' commercial television, this vision of the future was
already a reality for a small group of people in the Netherlands (and
not only there). On a studio set somewhere near Amsterdam, a group
of young people were living in cramped conditions in a bungalow.
They were completely shut off from the outside world and observed
night and day by twenty-four cameras. Not even the toilet and bedroom were camera-free, so they did not have a moment of privacy.
Similar programmes are broadcast daily at peak viewing times and
the producer alone decides what is going to be shown. For the sake
of financial gain, and perhaps for other motives as well, many people
are clearly prepared to make a spectacle of themselves by exposing
the intimate details of their lives. There is no shortage of contestants
for such programmes, which have been cloned by many TV stations
all over the world. The original Dutch programme was called, appropriately, 'Big Brother'. When asked in an interview in *Der Spiegel*
(1 November 1999) why he thought the programme had been such
a phenomenal success, Paul Roemer, the inventor of this reality TV
show, answered in just one word: 'voyeurism'.

― 16 ―

Psi Phenomena – or The Exploration of Extra-Sensory Perception

When I am in a deep hypnotic trance, all my senses are closed. Not only that: they have been surrendered to the hypnotist so completely that I can feel a pinch of *his* ear, taste the salt or sugar on *his* tongue and hear the ticking of a pocket watch placed against *his* ear. I also feel a burning sensation when a lighted match is held against *his* fingers.

Maria Reyes de Zierold, a Mexican clairvoyant (1923)

The origins of a fringe science

Parapsychology is still a very recent and controversial science. It deals with human experiences and behavioural manifestations that elude our normal explanatory frameworks (causality, coincidence) and are lumped together under the umbrella term 'psi' (named after the twenty-third letter of the Greek alphabet). Psi phenomena are divided into two groups: extra-sensory perception (ESP) and psychokinesis, or the ability to influence physical systems 'directly' by psychic means (e.g., causing tables to levitate).

The apparent ability of some people 'to give or receive information outside all known sensory channels'[1] merits some consideration in the context of a history of the senses. Official scientific terminology divides this gift into three types: 1) telepathy – the 'direct' transcription of psychic events such as feelings, images and thoughts; 2) clairvoyance – the 'direct' acquisition of information about things which no one else knows about; and 3) precognition – inexplicable foreknowledge of events. In everyday language, however, the word 'clairvoyance' has always had wider connotations and is often used as a synonym for the legendary 'sixth' sense.

Unlike the traditional five senses, which have been a subject of empirical scientific investigation since the early nineteenth century, the sixth sense did not come under quantitative scientific scrutiny until the twentieth century, although there had been a good deal of scientific interest in extra-sensory perception in Europe and the United States since the 1870s. However, it is now generally accepted that ESP research began in earnest in 1882 with the founding of the Society for Psychical Research (SPR) in England. The initiative came from Sir William Barrett (1844–1925), who had been interested from an early date in the phenomenon of thought communication during hypnosis. In addition to its first president, Professor Henry Sidgwick (1838–1900) of the University of Cambridge, the society's founding members included the physicist Lord Rayleigh (1842–1919), the scholar Edmund Gurney (1847–1888) and the classical philologist Frederic Myers (1843–1901), to whom we are indebted for the word 'telepathy'. 'From 1882 onward', writes D. Scott Rogo, 'psychical research was no longer to be a seance-room cops-and-robbers affair, not a pseudoscientific occultist study, but a rigorous and disciplined experimental and descriptive science organized by some of the best minds of the era.'[2] The SPR formulated the first exact criteria of extra-sensory perception, developed methods of research and built up a collection of cases, focusing on the various forms of extra-sensory perception (particularly clairvoyance) in preference to telekinetic phenomena. In 1885, a similar association was founded in the United States which later gave birth to the American Society for Psychical Research.

Similar organizations were also formed in Germany. The independent scholar Carl du Prel (1839–1899) and the doctor and hypnotist Albert von Schrenck-Notzing (1862–1929) played an important part in the establishment of the Munich Psychological Society in 1886. In 1888, the Society of Experimental Psychology was founded in Berlin. Among its leading lights were the psychologist Max Dessoir (1867–1947), the psychiatrist Albert Moll (1862–1939) and the philosopher Eduard von Hartmann (1842–1906). Around the turn of the twentieth century, the activities of these societies, which all studiously distanced themselves from spiritualistic circles and associations of mesmerists and magnetopaths, had generated a flow of important publications.

Although eminent British, American and German scientists had participated in these experiments with persons supposedly gifted with extra-sensory perception and telekinesis, the universities were slow to respond. Many regarded 'scientific occultism' as a suspect discipline. University-based psychologists remained sceptical and treated the pioneers of the new discipline with reserve. One of their sharpest German critics at the end of the nineteenth century was the philosopher, physician and founder of experimental psychology Wilhelm Wundt (1832–1920). Wundt was particularly critical of the physicist Karl Friedrich Zöllner (1834–1882), who had conducted telekinetic experiments with the English 'medium' Henry Slade (1840–1904?) – whom many suspected of fraud – and published his results in a work entitled *Transcendentale Physik* (Transcendental Physics, 1879), which had been very well received. Wundt was also sceptical of attempts to include evidence acquired from hypnosis in the new science (to which Max Dessoir gave the still common name of 'parapsychology' in 1889), objecting that such procedures were not subject to scientific verification.

By the end of the 1890s, the leading German scientists of the discipline had largely dissociated themselves from the 'experimental metaphysics' of which Wundt and others had accused them and had begun to interpret paranormal perception as a form of suggestion. Notwithstanding his long interest in the theory and practice of spiritualism, Albert Moll was perhaps the staunchest scientific 'materialist' in their ranks and certainly a lifelong stranger to spiritualistic experience. In his autobiography, which appeared in 1936, he states his scientific credo with characteristic verve: 'In common with many others, I believe that we must demand 100 per cent proofs, that we cannot be satisfied with approximations and probabilities, and that, just as we asked Röntgen for a 100 per cent proof of the existence of his hitherto unknown rays, so we must now require exactly the same from the occultist.'[3]

Photography and statistics in the service of parapsychology

The first attempts to obtain photographic records of occult phenomena took place in Germany and France at the end of the nineteenth century. Among the pioneers was the French doctor Hippolyte Baraduc (1850–1909). Following Röntgen's discovery of X-rays, Baraduc experimented for a time with thought photography, which he described as the 'human form of X-ray photography'. At about the same time, the French army major Louis Darget (1847–1921) produced his photographs of ectoplasmic emissions, which were recently rediscovered. The case studies amassed by the various scientific societies towards the end of the nineteenth century had long ceased to count as material proofs. Albert Moll, the Berlin 'soul doctor', was not the only scientist to warn against expecting too much in the way of hard facts from the material painstakingly assembled by the London Society for Psychical Research during the 1880s. To gain official recognition as science, 'scientific occultism' needed 'tangible' proofs of the existence of the phenomena under examination. With the discovery of X-rays in 1895, the conviction grew that photography would at last supply this proof, since it was an 'absolutely passive tool, whose verisimilitude was beyond dispute',[4] as one French doctor declared in 1909.

It is thus hardly surprising that the collection of the controversial scientific occultist Baron Albert von Schrenck-Notzing, which is now housed in the Freiburg Institute for Fringe Areas of Psychology and Mental Health, should consist of copious photographic documentation of occult phenomena. Most of the latter are concerned with telekinesis (the movement of objects at a distance) and materialization, and there is relatively little material on thought photography, which played a more significant role in developments in France. Albert Moll's autobiography contains a withering critique of Schrenck-Notzing, who was the author of a standard work entitled *Grundfragen der Parapsychologie* (Fundamental Questions of Parapsychology, 1929): 'I have never read anything so utterly unscientific.'[5] Not even the Munich doctor Rudolf Tischner (1879–1961), a distinguished author of histories of occult research and homeopathy, and one of Schrenck-Notzing's former collaborators, could refrain from commenting that, with all due respect and good will, the latter had been slow to adopt 'more rigorous experimental criteria'.[6] Tischner was referring to the experiments that Schrenck-Notzing, assisted by the Berlin engineer Fritz Grunewald (1885–1925) and the Munich 'animal psychologist' Karl Krall (1863–1929), had carried out in his well-appointed private laboratory.

Albert Moll, who had grown up watching the tricks of conjurers and magicians, was equally sceptical of the Frenchman Charles Richet (1850–1926). This eminent physiologist, who won the Nobel prize for medicine in 1918, had tried in 1884 to track down occult phenomena using statistical methods. However, besides being methodologically controversial even at the time, the results produced by his experiments with playing cards were not very significant.

The first statistical investigations of extra-sensory perception to comply with modern scientific standards were completed in the 1920s at the University of Groningen in the Netherlands, where one of the professors of psychology had encountered a student with remarkable telepathic abilities. The obvious next idea was to subject this psi phenomenon to controlled experimentation. The subject was blindfolded and taken into one of the rooms of the institute, where he was seated in front of a specially prepared chequerboard with forty-eight lettered and numbered squares. The idea was for the experimenters, who were in a room on the floor above, to guide the student's hand 'telepathically' towards a randomly chosen square.[7] In just the first series of tests, the student achieved thirty-two out of a possible eighty correct responses, which was statistically an extremely significant result. The other tests also produced astonishing results. A score of four out of a possible 187 would have conformed to the laws of probability. In this case, however, the student guinea pig achieved a score of sixty.

The additional physiological measurements taken during these tests by Professor Henri Johan Brugmans (1884–1961) and his colleagues, as well as their careful exclusion of all 'natural' sense perception, mark the beginning of a new era of parapsychological research. 'The Groningen experiments', writes D. Scott Rogo, 'illustrated another step forward in ESP research, that is the gradual shift of research from organized psychical research societies to the university campus.'[8] In 1921, Brugmans presented his sensational results to the First International Congress of Psychic Research in Copenhagen. During the period between the wars, conferences of this kind were an important forum for what was then just a handful of serious European parapsychologists. Further meetings were held in Warsaw in 1923 and in Paris in 1927.

Parapsychological research in the universities

The fledgling science of parapsychology was first accepted into the academic fold in the USA. Funded by a private foundation, Leonard Thompson Troland (1889–1926) had developed a new method of testing at Harvard University in 1916–17. His experimental subjects had to look into a sort of peep-show box and predict which side of the interior would be lit up by a switch connected to a random generator. A few years later, at the same university, George Estabrooks (1895–?) performed experiments with ordinary playing cards. For this experiment, the subjects and experimenters were placed in separate rooms. A red light told the subject when to make the guess. After a total of eighty-three experiments, the number of correct hits was one hundred more than that predicted by the law of chance. Estabrooks was also the first to notice that, under strict experimental conditions, the so-called psi-blank makes its appearance: in other words, the subject's score tends to fall after each additional experiment.

The definitive breakthrough of quantitative research in clairvoyance and telepathy (and thus of modern parapsychology as such) did not occur until a few years later, and then at another university. At the end of the 1920s, at Duke University in North Carolina, Joseph B. Rhine (1895–1980), his wife Louisa (1891–1983) and the psychologist William McDougall (1871–1938) had begun a systematic investigation into extra-sensory perception. 'It was Rhine's idea to start a large-scale ESP research project, carry it out at length so enough data could be amassed for an impressive analysis to be made, and repeat the experiments under the most stringent controls.'[9]

The experiments in clairvoyance carried out by Rhine and his colleagues at the beginning of the 1930s also made use of cards (see figure 16.2). These were not ordinary playing cards, however, but a deck of twenty-five cards, five suits of five cards consisting of simple geometric figures – star, circle, cross, wavy lines and rectangle (later changed to a square). The experimental team concentrated their thoughts on the card the subject was supposed to guess. The laws of chance predict an average of five hits in these circumstances, with the possibility of strong variations between shorter and longer series of experiments. In 1934, Rhine published the results of his pioneering research in a book entitled *Extra Sensory Perception*, which immediately – and predictably – ran into opposition. However, the criticisms of Rhine's statistical methods proved to be quite unfounded, since he had from the beginning employed eminent mathematicians to analyse the results of the experiments. More serious, on the other hand, were the criticisms of the manner in which he had ordered and arranged the experiments. He had, for instance, failed to exclude the possibility

Die wissenschaftliche Erforschung des Uebersinnlichen.

Blick in ein parapsychisches Laboratorium.

Von Dr. Alfred Gradenwitz (Berlin).

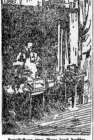

Versuchsstation einer Wage durch darüber gehaltene Hände.

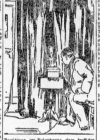

Vorrichtung zur Aufzeichnung einer sinnlichen Erscheinung, der sogenannten Klopftöne.

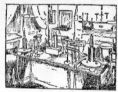

Prüfung der außersinnlichen Lichtphänome durch Spektralapparate.

Figure 16.1   The scientific investigation of the supersensory; undated newspaper report

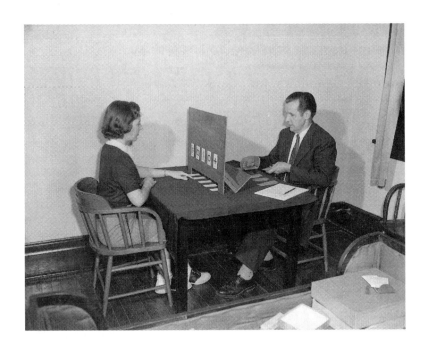

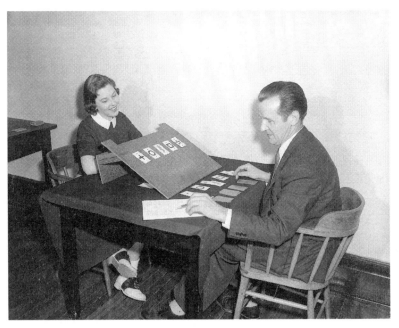

Figure 16.2 Clairvoyance experiments with ESP cards at the Rhine Institute

that the experimental subject might infer the correct card by rational means. So in 1935 Rhine adopted the practice of not informing his subjects of the statistical results of their choices.

The two decades between 1930 and 1950 saw the establishment at Duke University of the principles of experimental research that would shape work in the field of parapsychology for a long time to come. Today's ESP research is dominated by newer approaches and methods (e.g., remote viewing experiments). When Rhine looked back to the early phase during an address to the annual conference of the renowned American Psychological Association in the 1960s, he described the year 1951 as a watershed. By this point in its history, the still young science was already on the way to becoming established: 'The basic claims of the field had been verified experimentally and independently confirmed. These findings rested upon no single research center, or school, or profession, or even country.'[10] Rhine could be proud of his achievement. His life's work survived his death. Since 1965 the former Rhine Laboratory has continued its work as the Institute for Parapsychology, with the support of a foundation. In 1969, the international professional association (the Parapsychological Association) founded by Rhine in 1957 was accepted as a member of the prestigious American Association for the Advancement of Science.

Parapsychological research in the Federal Republic of Germany

Along with the USA and Great Britain, Germany has meanwhile become a centre of university-based parapsychological research. The Institute for Fringe Areas of Psychology and Mental Health was founded at the University of Freiburg in 1950 by the doctor and psychologist Hans Bender (1907–1991). The inaugural address was given by none other than Professor Rhine from the USA. The theme of his lecture was programmatic: 'The Science of Parapsychology Today'. The newly appointed director of the institute (who was awarded a chair in 1954), on the other hand, used the solemn moment to deliver a lecture entitled 'Okkultismus als Problem der Psychohygiene' (Occultism as a Problem of Mental Health), in which he laid down an agenda for future research. According to Bender at that time, the task of 'mental health' was: '*enlightenment*, the imparting of knowledge about the various forms in which we may encounter the unusual; the creation of a classificatory scheme intelligible to ordinary people which will enable them to find a name for things they find disturbing.'[11]

Not unexpectedly, therefore, the projects of the early phase of the Freiburg Institute focused on a subject which seemed in urgent need of enlightenment, namely the phenomenon of medical occultism (spiritual or faith healing). With the co-operation of the outpatients' department of the University of Freiburg Hospital, the institute invited 650 patients who had had contact with faith healers to participate in a study. From this, it emerged that it was above all else a patient's positive attitude towards the future that made him feel that his health was improving.

Another research project undertaken during the early days of the Freiburg Institute deserves mention here. In the 1950s, Bender and his colleagues collected more than a thousand spontaneous reports of paranormal experiences, which they then analysed and classified exhaustively. The experimenters made a careful study of the authors' personality structures, and set up a control group. This exercise laid the basis of later studies of 'the occult-directed personality', which the scientific literature of the time described as unstable, aggressive, easily confused and prone to projecting its feelings onto others. The case collection also distinguished between different 'forms of experience', separating dreams from premonitions and hallucinations. The categories of visions, inner voices, illusions, messages and consciousness of invisible presences were added to the list later.

To obtain more such spontaneous reports, the Freiburg team even took material from a series of articles in the popular daily *Bild-Zeitung* entitled 'Your sixth sense'. These articles had been put together from over 2000 readers' letters, and the analysis of the material revealed that around two-thirds of them were accounts of personal experiences of paranormal phenomena. Of these, 50 per cent related to telepathy and clairvoyance, 39 per cent to premonitions and 7 per cent to psychokinesis.

The extent to which these early investigations at the Freiburg Institute reflect not only the mood of those times, but also attitudes still prevalent among the population today, is demonstrated by the representative survey conducted in 1958 by the Opinion Research

Institute in Allensbach, and also by more recent surveys. In 1958, 53 per cent of those questioned thought it highly probable that there was some extraordinary source of information about the present and future; 36 per cent thought there was no such thing, while 11 per cent were undecided. Those who had answered in the affirmative were also asked if they had had any personal experience of the sixth sense. One in five adults claimed that they had. Although a third of the participants thought that the existence of extra-sensory perception had been proved conclusively, they were unable to refer to any experiences of their own.

There was little widespread belief in ghosts at the time, and this remains true of the present. While a good half of the West German population of 1958 were convinced of the existence of a sixth sense, only 18 per cent believed in ghosts, with 12 per cent claiming personal experience of them. At the end of the 1960s, following a heated media discussion of mysterious events at the office of a lawyer in Rosenheim, Bender and a physicist from Munich travelled to Rosenheim to investigate the ghostly phenomena. It was this investigation that first brought the Freiburg Institute to the attention of the world at large. In one of its early publications, the institute insisted that 'no known physical cause could be found' for the derangements of their measuring instruments.[12]

Besides adding to their stock of reports, Bender and his colleagues undertook their own qualitative investigations. One of the most famous of these was the series of experiments with the Dutch psychic Gerard Croiset (1910–1980), which took place in adult education colleges in the Lower Palatinate. In the presence of the director of the experiment, the clairvoyant, who was in Neustadt, stated the name of the person who would occupy the chair bearing the number 73 in the seating plan of an event due to take place that evening in Pirmasens. He also described the external appearance and personal circumstances of this individual. 'The method used during this "chair test" was developed further afterwards', wrote the Freiburg parapsychologist: 'the choice of test subjects and seats was later left to chance, the clairvoyant's statements were offered for comment to all participants in the experiment and the degree of "specificity" calculated from the number of confirmations. This was then factored into a quantitative evaluation.'[13] Dutch and American scientists also did a series of experiments with Croiset and came to the conclusion that he was clearly able to make telepathic contact with the experimental subjects. The Dutch clairvoyant's fame spread as his extraordinary abilities began to attract the attention of the television companies (Süddeutscher Rundfunk, 1955; BBC London, 1967).

In 1967, the Freiburg Institute completed its first quantitative-statistical experiments. These were financed by the Deutsche Forschungsgemeinschaft (German Research Council), which was itself a sign of Hans Bender's growing reputation in the scientific community. The team used a method developed by Joseph B. Rhine, which involved asking subjects to predict a randomly created sequence of cards (twenty-five cards consisting of five sets of geometric symbols or pictures). A new kind of calculator was brought into service on this occasion. The idea was to simplify the experimental process and to eliminate such common sources of error as the shuffling of a pack of cards by hand. In a paper published in 1987, two members of the institute who had worked on the project noted that 'only the telepathic tests produced significant overall results.'[14] However, the development of automatic testing devices, in which the Freiburg Institute played a leading role, was in some ways more important than the results of the research. The 'Psi-Recorder 70' was one such device. At the beginning of the 1970s, it was used to conduct experiments in extra-sensory perception with up to nine persons simultaneously, the results of which were then stored automatically on punch cards.

Despite strenuous efforts to explore paranormal phenomena on a strictly scientific basis, the Freiburg Institute has occasionally been accused of furthering the cause of occultism. At the end of the 1970s it was even suspected of being the victim of a hoax. But Hans Bender and Johannes Mischo, who later succeeded Bender as director, managed to disprove the allegations circulating in the press. An impassioned and systematic attack on parapsychology by Wilhelm Gubisch (1890–1972), which appeared in book form in 1961, also failed to inflict lasting damage on the fledgling 'fringe science'. The high international reputation of the specialist journal founded by Hans Bender in 1957 is further witness to the scientific community's recognition of the Freiburg Institute's pioneering work in extra-sensory perception. In 1981, the founding of a registered society named the Scientific Society for the Promotion of Parapsychology also helped to disarm sceptics within the academic community. This was again an initiative of the Freiburg chair of psychology and border areas of psychology, as was the Parapsychological Advice Centre established in Freiburg by Walter von Lucadou. The inclusion of Hans Bender's special parapsychological collection in the Deutsche Forschungsgemeinschaft's library support programme of 1973 further underlined the Freiburg Institute's standing in the eyes of the scientific community.

Nevertheless, parapsychology experienced many difficulties in gaining general acceptance in Germany as just one science among many others. Its marginal position was highlighted by its slow recognition as a science, its lack of institutional presence, its struggles to find funding and its slowness to acquire the professional disciplines of scientific enquiry. Meanwhile, the situation has improved considerably. Since the mid-1990s, the Freiburg Institute has enjoyed generous funding from a foundation and can afford to take a more optimistic view of the future. It now employs a staff of thirty and has opened several new sections. Collaborations with other German and foreign research institutions have also increased sharply.

This positive development is due not least to the fact that public interest in the question of the existence of extra-sensory perception remains undiminished, and has perhaps grown even stronger. Otherwise it would be difficult to explain the enormous success in German cinemas of the Hollywood film *The Sixth Sense*. In this film Bruce Willis, who is perhaps best known for his action films, plays the role of Malcom Crowe, a sensitive child psychologist, to whom an eight-year-old boy named Cole (played by Haley Joel Osment) is sent for treatment. The young patient is firmly convinced that he has supernatural abilities and can communicate with the dead. We shall not give away the surprising and dramatic conclusion of this parapsychologically and psychiatrically fascinating case history. What is worth noting, however, is its rather reserved and sometimes even hostile reception by German critics: 'an absurd blend of sentimental thriller and detective story', wrote the film critic of the *Stuttgarter Nachrichten* (30 December 1999). All the same, the film drew enormous audiences in the USA, earning the producers the fantastic sum of $300 million at the box office. You may not require a sixth sense for making money, but you certainly need a good nose!

Prospects

— 17 —

Cyberspace and the
Future of the Senses

Zira: 'There's nothing nicer than the sea breeze on your skin ... Can
technology create something like that? ... What do you think?
Spectator: 'No, I hate technology!'
Zira: 'But technology's here to stay ... You switch the light on, don't
you?'

Dialogue from *Grenzen von Utopia* (Borders of Utopia),
interactive film, MultiMediale Karlsruhe, 1995

Science fiction and cyberpunk

Even before the First World War, Italian futurists were dreaming
of multiple bodies and the progressive dematerialization of physical
existence. 'Cyberspace' and 'virtual reality' had not even been thought
of at the time. The bold visions of the early twentieth century that
now seem to be in the process of becoming real were essentially the
work of a few experimental writers and artists who were prepared to
give rein to their imaginations.

Shortly after the First World War, the German-Jewish writer Salomo
Friedländer, who published under the pseudonym Mynona, described
in one of his literary grotesques the invention of a 'telefeeler'. In the
age of cyberspace, Mynona's imaginary construction has long since
become a reality (headword 'Data glove'). This unjustly neglected
author already had his doubts about such inventions:

> But I can only touch and taste my nearest and dearest if they are right
> close up to me (which heaven forbid!). Anyway it all seems to imply
> that when someone asks me where I am, he is really asking where I can
> be felt. For he could be seen, heard and smelled somewhere else too.

Yes, feeling is a rather clod-hopping sort of thing! We need to prize it out, thaw it, wire it up and despatch it like a long-distance telegram. How simple![1]

This passage immediately brings to mind the 'data suits' bristling with wires and sensors that are now used in experiments with cybersex or for tactile adventures (sexual or otherwise) in virtual space.

Mynona was clearly inspired by the English novelist H. G. Wells (1866–1946), notably by his social allegory *The Time Machine* (1895). This famous story describes how, with the aid of a machine capable of shifting the axis of time forwards and backwards, people are able to leap across millennia while remaining in the same place. 'What good is Wells', remarks Mynona's first-person narrator ironically, 'if he can't come up with something like this [i.e., a telefeeler]?'[2] Several decades were to elapse before Mynona's bizarre idea was taken up again: this time by the cyberpunk writers of the late twentieth century.

The term 'cyberpunk' first appeared in 1983 in a story by the American writer Bruce Bethke.[3] The following year it was used by a literary critic of the *Washington Post* to describe a new trend in the science-fiction literature of the 1980s, in which sensory experience is replaced by digital simulation and abused by evil powers. Soon after this it became a term for a new direction in music, a kind of high-tech variant of hard rock (computer-generated hammering rhythms and electronically produced sound patterns) inspired by the sounds of the urban and industrial world. 'Cyberpunk' is now also used to describe interactive computer-musical compositions in which the human body is interfaced with machines. A piece composed by Tod Machover, head of the Department of Experimental Media at Massachusetts Institute of Technology (MIT), illustrates what all this involved in practice. At the beginning of the 1990s, Machover designed and performed experiments with a data glove that already seems 'antediluvian'. He used it to control a tonal sequence produced by two musicians playing electronic and acoustic guitars. All three performers were wired to each other and plugged into a computer-controlled 'hyperinstrument', which responded in real time to the sounds produced by the two human instrumentalists. In this way, it was possible to influence the tonal colours of the instruments with a wave of the 'conductor's' hand.

—— 325 ——

The porous term 'cyberspace', whose inflated use is now quite unstoppable, first appears in a story by the American cult author William Gibson, which was published in America in the early 1980s. This story tells of two computer hackers who, having managed to get inside the world-wide computer network via a sensory interface, temporarily lose control of their own sense perceptions. But the word only became a shimmering metaphor for virtual space as such with the publication of Gibson's science-fiction novel *New Romancer* (1984), which rapidly acquired cult status in America and the world at large. Since the success of *New Romancer*, cyberpunk literature has been littered with brain implants, artificial limbs, and cloned or biotechnologically engineered body organs.

So far, this space, which Gibson and other science-fiction authors portray as a place where the body is abandoned by the mind, and only streams of data are real, is a mere figment of the imagination. All the same, more and more people are living in a computerized world that disembodies human beings and is increasingly replacing their reality. But for the time being, at least, the cyberworld of the future as conceived in the mid-1990s by Hans Moravec, a leading American specialist in robotics, is still largely a vision:

> Try to imagine some advanced future state. It is as though you are in some sort of cocoon. Optical, acoustic, mechanical and electrical devices stimulate your senses and take precise readings of all your movements. The machine supplies pictures for your eyes, sounds for your ears and sensitivity to touch and temperature. It activates your muscles and provides smells for your nose and tastes for your tongue. Telepresence is what occurs when all these inputs and outputs are fed into and processed by a remote humanoid robot. When you reach for something on the screens, the robot senses what you are doing and provides your muscles and skin with exactly the right amount of heaviness, form, texture and heat, so you have the illusion that you are inside the body of the robot. Your conscious perception seems to have migrated to the robot. You are having a genuinely 'extra-corporeal' experience.[4]

Apart from isolated recent developments such as telemedicine, in which remote-controlled robots perform operations under the direction of surgeons, this 'remote robot' does not yet exist. In virtual reality, its role is still performed by computer simulation.

Cyber artists

The terms 'cyberspace' and 'virtual reality' are nowadays often used interchangeably, although there is a fine distinction between them. 'Virtual reality' refers essentially to the hardware and software that make it possible for virtual bodies to interact in cyberspace in the first place. The media theorist Achim Bühl describes it as a form of technology 'which enables the human being to be integrated immediately into computer-generated worlds', creating an interface between man and machine 'that engages several human senses simultaneously, . . . giving the user the impression that the computer-generated environment is actually real.'[5] Small wonder, therefore, that these new technological resources soon began to attract the attention of artists. One early example of virtual art is an installation entitled *Telematic Dreaming* (1992) by the British video artist Paul Sermon, who now teaches in Leipzig. This work uses a video-conference link to produce the impression that two real people, a man and a woman, are virtually sharing the same bed. We see their eyes meet and their hands reach out in search of each other, exactly as though they were together in a real place. However, it is nothing more than an encounter in virtual space. But since everything is happening in real time, our own perception is deceived and we begin to wonder where the boundaries of our bodies are really drawn. Derrick de Kerckhove describes the effect as follows: 'Two people in a virtual no man's world make physical contact by means of simulated trembling feelings transmitted to phantom limbs.'[6]

The ability of telepresence technology to simulate immediate physical contacts between persons is demonstrated by a performance work by two Canadian artists, which took place in Paris and Toronto simultaneously in 1986. As the title, *Transatlantic Wrestling*, suggests, the event consisted of a virtual wrestling match. By today's standards, the technology used in this performance was decidedly primitive. Two iron bars, one on each side of the Atlantic, were fitted with pressure sensors, which were linked to each other by a computer and modem. The motors fixed to the two iron bars responded via remote data transmission to changes of leverage, and thus to the amount of force applied. So spectators on both sides of the Atlantic received the impression that they were watching a real test of strength between the two artists, who were locked in physical combat across a distance of almost 4000 miles.

But it was the performance artists who produced the earliest and most radical visions of the future of the senses in cyberspace. The most celebrated performance artist of the present time is undoubtedly Stelios Arcadious, an Australian of Cypriot descent whose stage name is Stelarc. His appearance at the Pompidou Centre in Paris in 1995 caused a sensation. The centre of attention in this performance was the naked body of the artist, which was plastered with electrodes from head to foot and plugged into a computer. From various locations around the world, Stelarc's assistants triggered a series of electric shocks over the Internet, which threw the artist's body into wild and uncontrolled convulsions: 'entirely involuntary and unremembered movements', said Stelarc afterwards.

For more than thirty years this artist has sought to express the separation of the body from consciousness, to divert attention to the progressive estrangement of the body from itself in the post-modern age. At the beginning of his career, Stelarc's main concern as an artist was to discover ways of representing the impoverishment of sensory perception in a world of advanced technology. In 1979, for instance, he had himself clamped between two boards and his eyelids and lips sewn together as a graphic illustration of temporary sensory deprivation. At the end of this three-day exhibition, he said the most uncomfortable part had been not being able to yawn. In 1985, he created a stir in Copenhagen, when he had himself pierced with high-grade steel hooks and winched into the air. For several minutes he was suspended naked above the audience: extremely painful for the artist, strangely thrilling for the audience.

For the last few years Stelarc has been producing dazzling demonstrations of ways in which the human body has been extended by recent technology. Since 1996, his spectacular performances have invariably included his 'third hand', a kind of claw-arm operated by the muscles of his stomach and thighs. Stelarc brandishes it on stage and writes words on a blackboard with three hands. His eyes emit laser beams and he is connected by sensors to an industrial robot (see figure 17.1). Using small movements of his muscles, he is able to make the robot go into a dance, which can be viewed – and also altered interactively – at another level of reality on a video screen. In 1993, Stelarc turned his stomach into a work of art by passing a

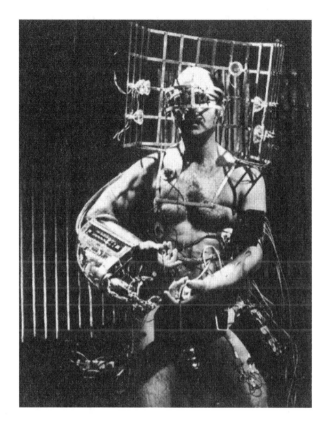

Figure 17.1   Stelarc with laser eyes, third hand and amplified body

flare into his digestive tract through a tube and filming the event with a tiny video camera. Looking at the monitor, the audience saw his stomach turn into a luminous body, to the accompaniment of little bleeping sounds from his abdomen.

At the beginning of the twenty-first century, Stelarc confidently predicts that, given the current rate of progress in nanotechnology, it will become possible not simply to interface the body with machines connected to it externally but also permanently to colonize its entrails and bloodstream with the products of technology. The human being, argues Stelarc, is increasingly able to ingest technology (artificial heart valves, pacemakers, etc.). The cyber artist, who has devoted twenty years to transcending the boundaries of the body, has quite specific ideas about its future shape: 'As I've been performing, I have begun to ask myself about the design of the human body. The more work I do, the more I believe that the human body is obsolete.'[7]

Artists such as Stelarc have the distinction of being the first to remind us that computers and robots are entirely separate from us, existing only in the outside world, but that they are externalizations and projections of our own existence. 'The epistemological follow-up to virtual reality', says Derrick de Kerckhove, 'must be a careful reconsideration of the meaning of thinking, and of the ways in which senses other than sight play a role in determining the way we perceive and organize reality.'[8] By taking the new technologies comprising 'virtual reality' as the theme of their highly physical art, performance artists have made us aware that in a high-tech world, in which electronic prostheses, stimulators, sensors, brainchips and virtual-reality interfaces are pushing the boundaries of the body ever further outwards, sensory perception has acquired new meanings and dimensions.

Seeing, hearing, tasting, smelling and touching are, thus, well on the way to becoming digitalized, computer-controlled processes that will progressively complement or even replace impressions traditionally supplied by the five 'natural' organs of sense. But today's virtual reality is still a long way from constructing an imaginary world which would fully integrate other senses besides hearing, vision and touch. We have still not emerged from the phase of sensory 'deconstruction', to use a word popular with literary theorists. How this will affect the perceptions and cognitive thought of the future remains to be seen. All the same, it is time at this point to ask how far the engineers and scientists who work with virtual reality and artificial intelligence have succeeded in developing computer-generated and computer-controlled tactile, olfactory and gustatory stimuli.

The spare-parts division of the senses

As long ago as the beginning of the nineteenth century, the American author Ralph Waldo Emerson (1803–1882) dreamed of detaching himself from natural sensation by turning into a 'transparent eyeball'.[9] A few decades ago, a sort of face mask or 'head mounted display' (HMD) was invented which provided highly realistic, three-dimensional images. The device was developed in 1966 by the American Ivan Sutherland. Owing to the cathode ray tubes still in use at the time, this helmet was so heavy that it had to be supported by a mechanical arm to avoid damaging the user's spinal column. With the advent of space research, however, this technology was quickly improved. In 1981, the general public was first introduced to the new liquid crystal display (LCD), which was less demanding on the eyes and is now used in laptop computers and other visual equipment. In combination with a technique known as VIVED (virtual visual environment display), digital images can now be projected onto the entire visual field by means of a special system of lenses. In addition to their military use (e.g., in the helmet visors of fighter-pilots), these simulations of a virtual space lying outside the natural visual field soon entered cyber art and consumer electronics.

Meanwhile medical scientists and biotechnicians are already at work on an artificial eye that will enable blind people to see again. There have been a number of successful experiments involving the implantation of tiny electrodes into the visual cortex. Electrical contact with a signal-processing computer is established via tiny wires in the scalp. In this way, the visual cortex can be stimulated in a manner that will enable a blind person to distinguish again between light and darkness. The American scientist William A. Dobelle believes that in the near future it will probably be possible to insert a miniature camera into an artificial eye, which would then be connected to the eye muscles. A pair of spectacles fitted with a battery-powered microprocessor will translate the camera images into phosphenes (bright spots deriving from an inadequate stimulation of the visual organ), which will then be communicated to the electrodes implanted in the visual cortex. This idea is as yet still a 'concrete' utopia, but research teams all over the world are working to turn it into a reality.

The Swiss Federal Institute of Technology in Zurich recently developed a computer chip with characteristics similar to the retina of the human eye. Unlike the natural retina, which consists of five separate cell layers, this artificial retina contains just three types of cell (photoreceptors and horizontal and bipolar cells). Using a new type of technology (high bandwidth channel), the signals produced by these cells, which would normally be transmitted to other cells via neuronal connections, can be transmitted alternately through just a few channels. These artificial retinas are already being used in laboratory experiments. A robot developed by the Zurich Institute of Neuro-Information Technology, for instance, uses it to distinguish between various colours and shapes. But it will be some time before it can be used in humans.

There is, however, already a technologically much simpler device on the market which helps blind people to differentiate between contrasting types of light. LumiTest, as the invention is called, measures luminous intensities, recognizes contrasts and converts them into tone signals, enabling a blind person to tell quickly whether the sky is cloudy or clear, or whether an item of clothing has a light or dark pattern.

Meanwhile the cyber artist Stelarc is planning to treat himself to a 'third ear'. Plastic surgery and modern microchip technology (hearing implants) have developed to a point where this sort of 'extension of the body in keeping with the times' (Stelarc) is well within the bounds of possibility. Over the last few years more than 1000 electronic prostheses for the improvement of the performance of the inner ear have been implanted by the Medical University of Hannover alone. The sound waves are received by a microphone and converted into electrical impulses. Provided that the auditory meatus is still intact, these are transmitted to the implant and reach the brain via the direct stimulation of the auditory nerve. Unlike traditional hearing aids, which merely amplify sound, cochlear implants can teach deaf people to hear.

Scientists at the University of Tübingen recently announced the development of a completely implantable hearing system for patients suffering from impairment of the inner ear. The report was published in the internationally respected British medical journal *The Lancet*. Although clearly superior to conventional hearing aids as far as tonal fidelity and linguistic audibility are concerned, the partially implantable hearing aids mentioned above were regarded as stigmatizing, since their components have to be worn externally, either on the head or somewhere on the body. The first implantation of a new and completely implantable type of hearing system for impaired inner ears took place recently at the ear, nose and throat clinic of the University of Tübingen under the direction of Professor Hans-Peter Zenner. The apparatus receives sound through the intact membrane of the acoustic meatus via a microphone installed near the ear drum. A multi-channel, digitally programmable audio processor implanted under the skin processes the signal and relays it to the incus of the ear via a piezoelectronic modifier in the mastoid process of the temporal bone. The energy is provided by an implantable, rechargeable battery. Patients equipped with a fully implanted hearing aid of this type can recharge the battery externally, more or less unobserved, and without the use of a cable. So when recharging the battery, the patient appears to an outsider to be just listening to a Walkman.

Television technology has been with us for more than seventy years, but we are still awaiting the appearance of a proper 'telesniffer'. Even the very latest modern multimedia technology has so far failed to simulate, let alone replace, the sense of smell. Cyberspace experts rightly deplore the fact that virtual erotic play or cybersex still lacks the vital sensorial ingredient of smell. On the other hand, artificial noses capable of identifying smells have been in use for years. British scientists have developed a device capable of smelling certain illnesses. It uses chemical sensors resembling those in the human nose. At the moment, this medical 'diag-noser' is still in the experimental stage. Scientists at the Karlsruhe Centre of Research have constructed a similar apparatus. On the basis of the smells which its forty highly sensitive sensors pick up and identify, it is able to diagnose numerous metabolic disorders of the human body. Still more ambitious is a research project – again involving the participation of the University of Tübingen – that was recently awarded the Körber Foundation prize for European science. This is the so-called Modular Sensor System, which is the same size as a stereo system and capable of identifying millions of smells.

The car- and foodstuff industries have a special interest in artificial noses, and the same applies to the chemical industry. Electronic tracker noses have the advantage of being able, for instance, to detect certain poisonous gases which humans are normally unable to smell. However, there are limits to what these sensor-equipped, high-tech apparatuses can achieve in the area of sensory perception, as Wolfgang Göpel, a scientist involved in one of these research projects, freely admits: 'The human nose will always have the edge when it's a question of the feelings associated with smells like wine and perfume.'[10]

The new generation of industrial robots is now also equipped with tactile sensors, which enable their grasping hands to be controlled with greater precision. Nevertheless, the sense of touch continues to be a headache for scientists working in virtual reality and robotics, since this sense is not located in a particular organ but spread over the whole body. The experiments conducted so far have concentrated largely on the transmission of the sense of pressures by means of data gloves with small inflatable balloons inside them. But it is impossible to recognize surface structures in this way. Another process uses little needles or tacks which press against the surface of the skin. The disadvantage here is that it is impossible to use them to simulate movements on the skin.

Despite such shortcomings, the invention of the 'sensing glove' by Scott Fisher in 1985 was an important milestone on the way to cyberspace. With it, hand movements, or rather the feeling, grasping and moving of objects, could be simulated as virtual reality for the first time. A simple and inexpensive version of this glove is now available as a computer toy. The 'data suit', with its armoury of pressure- and temperature-sensitive sensors, represents a further development of the glove. Although this suit has so far not been put to any practical use, it is occasionally worn by cyber artists. It comes in handy not least in experiments with cybersex, whose essential attraction is 'copulation without bodily contact'.[11] But, as reported recently in the American news magazine *Time*, even cybersex is not much fun without bodily contact. Which is why we need a data suit like this. It fits the body snugly like a second skin and is electronically equipped to pass on tactile erotic stimuli. Howard Rheingold describes the practice of 'teledildonics': 'You run your hand over your partner's clavicle and, 6000 miles away, an array of effectors are triggered, in just the right sequence, at just the right frequency, to convey the touch exactly the way you wish it to be conveyed.'[12] For many futurologists, the exchange of intimacies through a data suit is not the end of the story. 'Physical closeness', writes the German cyberspace expert Florian Rötzer, 'will soon no longer be a question of spatial proximity but of interfacing with cyberspace, which, while allowing people to touch each other, simultaneously blurs the distinction between body and machine, reality and simulation.'[13]

However we judge such erotic experiments and tele-affairs, there can be little doubt that in the age of cyberspace, whose birth pangs we are now experiencing, the tense of touch is once more high on the agenda.

Only the sense of taste seems so far to have eluded computer simulation. The Internet contains few references to such experiments. The taste nerves and the chemo-receptors of the tongue are one of the greatest challenges to simulation technology. So far, therefore, we have been spared the artificial tongue. We shall simply have to go on appearing at wine tastings in person, rather than mouse-clicking onto the Internet department store – a consoling thought for those with anxieties about the future.

Cyborgs and other hybrids

Our traditional image of the body is still largely intact, although the American feminist Donna Haraway thinks that the meteoric progress of medical technology over the past two decades has led to the mutation of the human body into a 'cyborg': 'Late twentieth-century machines have made thoroughly ambiguous the difference between natural and artificial, mind and body, self-developing and externally designed, and many other distinctions that used to apply to organisms and machines. Our machines are disturbingly lively, and we ourselves frighteningly inert.'[14] But does this development imply that we have broken out of the confines of the body irrevocably, and that the ontological categories of the past are no longer valid?

The term 'cyborg' was coined as long ago as 1960 by the American space scientist Manfred Clynes. It combines the words 'cybernetic' and 'organism' and means more than just a symbiotic relationship between humans and computers. A cyborg is a machine body controlled by artificial intelligence, and is therefore capable of existing without the assistance of human intelligence. However, it is questionable whether we shall ever reach a point where humans will be indistinguishable from computers. In an essay published in *Der Spiegel* at the beginning of the new millennium, the writer Hans Magnus Enzensberger had words of encouragement for all who had nightmares at the thought of these biotechnological fantasies of the future: 'The body's inertia will not let us down. Toothache is not virtual. We can't eat simulation. Our own death is not a media event. So, yes, we may rest assured that there is still life on this side of the digital world: the only life we have.'[15]

Notes

CHAPTER 1   APPROACHING THE SUPRAHISTORICAL

1 Barbara Duden, *Geschichte unter der Haut: ein Eisenacher Arzt und seine Patientinnen um 1730* (Stuttgart, 1987), p. 18.
2 Karl E. Rothschuh, *Physiologie: der Wandel ihrer Konzepte, Probleme, Methoden vom 16. bis 19. Jahrhundert* (Freiburg and Munich, 1968), p. 33.
3 Ibid., p. 27.
4 Karl Marx and Frederick Engels, *Collected Works* (London, 1975), vol. 3, pp. 299–300. See also Klaus Ottomeyer and Peter Anhalt, 'Leib, Sinnlichkeit und Körperverhältnis im Kontext der Marxschen Theorie', in Hilarion Petzold (ed.), *Leiblichkeit: philosophische, gesellschaftliche und therapeutische Perspektiven* (Paderborn, 1985), pp. 229–58.
5 Marx and Engels, *Collected Works*, vol. 3, pp. 301–2.
6 Sidney W. Mintz, *Sweetness and Power: The Place of Sugar in Modern History* (Harmondsworth, 1985).
7 See Bernd Busch, 'Eine Frage des Dufts', in Kunst- und Ausstellungshalle der Bundesrepublik Deutschland (ed.), *Das Riechen: von Nasen, Düften und Gestank* (Göttingen, 1995), pp. 10–22.
8 Walter Benjamin, *Illuminations*, trans. H. Zohn (London, 1973), p. 237.
9 Jonathan Crary, *Techniques of the Observer: On Vision and Modernity in the Nineteenth Century* (Cambridge, MA, and London, 1990).
10 Lucien Febvre, *Das Gewissen des Historikers*, ed. Ulrich Raulff (Frankfurt am Main, 1990), p. 85.
11 See Edward Shorter, *From Paralysis to Fatigue: A History of Psychosomatic Illness in the Modern Era* (New York, 1992); Joachim Radkau, *Das Zeitalter der Nervosität: Deutschland zwischen Bismarck und Hitler* (Munich, 1998).

12 Febvre, *Gewissen des Historikers*, p. 94.
13 *The Standard Edition of the Complete Works of Sigmund Freud* (London 1953–66), vol. 21, p. 99, n. 1.
14 Alain Corbin, *Time, Desire and Horror: Towards a History of the Senses*, trans. Jean Birrell (Cambridge, 1995), pp. 181–92.
15 Diane Ackerman, *A Natural History of the Senses* (New York, 1990).
16 See the bibliography in Barbara Duden and Ivan Illich, 'Die skopische Vergangenheit Europas und die Ethik der Opsis: Plädoyer für eine Geschichte des Blickes und Blickens', *Historische Anthropologie* 3 (1995), pp. 203–21.
17 See the bibliography in Kunst- und Ausstellungshalle der Bundesrepublik Deutschland (ed.), *Welt auf tönernen Füßen: die Töne und das Hören* (Göttingen, 1994).
18 See the bibliography in Kunst- und Ausstellungshalle der Bundesrepublik Deutschland (ed.), *Das Riechen*.
19 See the bibliography in Kunst- und Ausstellungshalle der Bundesrepublik Deutschland (ed.), *Tasten* (Göttingen, 1996).
20 See the bibliography in Kunst- und Ausstellungshalle der Bundesrepublik Deutschland (ed.), *Geschmacksache* (Göttingen, 1996).
21 Eckart Scheerer, 'Die Sinne', in *Historisches Wörterbuch der Philosophie* (1995), vol. 9, cols. 825–69.
22 See Chu-Tsing Li, 'The five senses in art: an analysis of its development in northern Europe' (PhD dissertation, University of Iowa, 1955); Sylvia Ferino-Pagden (ed.), *Immagini del sentire: i cinque sensi nell'arte*, exhibition catalogue (Cremona, 1996).
23 William F. Bynum and Roy Porter (eds), *Medicine and the Five Senses* (Cambridge, 1993).
24 Historisches Archiv der Stadt Köln, Chroniken und Darstellungen 50, f. 32v.
25 See Peter Dinzelbacher (ed.), *Europäische Mentalitätsgeschichte* (Stuttgart, 1993), p. xxv.
26 Jacques LeGoff, 'Eine mehrdeutige Geschichte', in Ulrich Raulff (ed.), *Mentalitäten-Geschichte* (Berlin, 1987), pp. 18–32 (p. 23).
27 Roger Chartier, *Cultural History: Between Practices and Representations*, trans. Lydia G. Cochrane (Ithaca and New York, 1988), p. 13.
28 Marx and Engels, *Collected Works*, vol. 1, p. 173.

CHAPTER 2   CONCEPTIONS: THE SENSORIUM

1 Unless indicated otherwise, the descriptions of ancient Indian sensory physiology which follow are based on Reinhold F. G. Müller, *Grundlagen*

altindischer Medizin (Halle/Saale, 1942); the same author's *Grundsätze altindischer Medizin* (Copenhagen, 1951); Hans Gerlach, 'Die Kenntnisse der alten Naturvölker von den gesunden und kranken Sinnesorganen auf Grund ihrer Anschauung von der Heilkunde', *Sudhoffs Archiv für die Geschichte der Medizin und der Naturwissenschaften* 29 (1937), pp. 271–88; Kuno Lorenz, 'Sāṃkhya', in Jürgen Mittelstraß (ed.), *Enzyklopädie Philosophie und Wissenschaftstheorie*, vol. 3 (1995), pp. 669–74.

2 Quoted from the translation in Müller, *Grundsätze altindischer Medizin*, p. 36 [trans. JL].

3 For the *tridoṣa* doctrine in Indian medicine, see Reinhold F. G. Müller, 'Über die Tridosa-Lehre in der altindischen Medizin', *Sudhoffs Archiv für die Geschichte der Medizin und der Naturwissenschaften* 32 (1939), pp. 290–314.

4 Quoted from the translation in Müller, *Grundsätze altindischer Medizin*, p. 45 [trans. JL].

5 See Manfred Porkert, *Die theoretischen Grundlagen der chinesischen Medizin* (Wiesbaden, 1973), p. 8ff.

6 Quoted by Paul U. Unschuld, in *Medicine in China: A History of Ideas* (Berkeley, 1985), p. 283.

7 Joseph Needham, *The Shorter Science and Civilisation in China*, an abridgement of his original text, ed. Colin A. Ronan (Cambridge, 1978), vol. 1 (vols. 1 and 2 of the major series), p. 147.

8 Unschuld, *Medicine in China*, p. 290.

9 Quoted by Needham, *Science and Civilisation in China*, p. 156.

10 Ibid., p. 164.

11 Unschuld, *Medicine in China*, p. 285.

12 Ibid., p. 286.

13 See Elisabeth Hsu, 'Figuratively speaking of "danger of death" in Chinese pulse diagnostics', in Robert Jütte, Motzi Eklöf and Marie C. Nelson (eds), *Historical Aspects of Unconventional Medicine: Approaches, Concepts: Case Studies* (Sheffield, 2000), pp. 193–210.

14 Unschuld, *Medicine in China*, p. 326.

15 Quoted in Needham, *Science and Civilisation in China*, p. 116.

16 See Yu-Lan Fung, *A History of Chinese Philosophy*, trans. Derk Bodde, 2 vols. (Princeton, 1952), vol. 1, p. 218.

17 Ibid., p. 303.

18 Needham, *Science and Civilisation in China*, p. 170.

19 Unless otherwise stated, the following descriptions of the senses in the pre-Socratics are based on Eckart Scheerer, 'Die Sinne', in *Historisches Wörterbuch der Philosophie* (1995), vol. 9, cols. 824–69, and John Isaac Beare, *Greek Theories of Elementary Cognition from Alcmaeon to Aristotle* (Oxford, 1906).

20 See Kurt von Fritz, 'Die Rolle des NOUS', in Hans-Georg Gadamer (ed.), *Die Begriffswelt der Vorsokratiker* (Darmstadt, 1968), pp. 246–363 (p. 353).

21 Xenophanes of Colophon, *Fragments*, a text and translation with a commentary by J. H. Lesher (Toronto, 1992), p. 102.

22 Gerlach, 'Die Kenntnisse der alten Naturvölker', p. 279.

23 George Malcolm Stratton, *Theophrastus and the Greek Physiological Psychology before Aristotle* (Amsterdam, 1964), p. 41.

24 G. S. Kirk and J. E. Raven, *The Presocratic Philosophers* (Cambridge, 1957), p. 422.

25 Ibid., p. 424.

26 Fritz, 'Die Rolle des NOUS', p. 349.

27 All the following quotations from Plato are taken from Plato, *The Complete Works*, ed. John M. Cooper (Indianapolis and Cambridge, 1997).

28 Unless otherwise stated, the following remarks are based on Clemens Bäumker, *Des Aristoteles Lehre von den äussern und innern Sinnesvermögen* (Leipzig, 1877); J. Neuhäuser, *Aristoteles' Lehre von dem sinnlichen Erkenntnisvermögen und seinen Organen* (Leipzig, 1878); John Isaac Beare, *Greek Theories of Elementary Cognition from Alcmaeon to Aristotle* (Oxford, 1906); Richard Sorabji, 'Aristotle on demarcating the five senses', *Philosophical Review* 80 (1971), pp. 55–79; P. Webb, 'Bodily structure and psychic faculties in Aristotle's theory of perception', *Hermes* 110 (1982), pp. 25–50. All quotations from Aristotle are from *The Works of Aristotle Translated into English*, ed. W. D. Ross (Oxford, 1910–52).

29 On the development of theories of vision since antiquity, see Huldrych M. Koelbing, 'Zur Sehtheorie im Altertum: Alkmeon und Aristoteles', *Gesnerus* 25 (1968), pp. 5–9; Wolfgang Münchow, *Geschichte der Augenheilkunde* (Stuttgart, 1984); Julius Hirschberg, *Geschichte der Augenheilkunde*, 2 vols. (Leipzig, 1899–1905); Gudrun Schleusener-Eichholz, *Das Auge im Mittelalter*, 2 vols. (Munich, 1985); David C. Lindberg, *Theories of Vision from Al-Kindi to Kepler* (Chicago and London, 1976).

30 Conrad Gesner, *De anima liber* (Zurich, 1563), p. 929.

31 On the development of theories of hearing since antiquity, see Hans Werner, *Geschichte des Taubstummenproblems bis ins 17. Jahrhundert* (Jena, 1932); Alan Towey, 'Aristotle and Alexander on hearing and instantaneous change: a dilemma in Aristotle's account of hearing', in Charles Burnett, Michael Fend and Penelope Gouk (eds), *The Second Sense: Studies in Hearing and Musical Judgement from Antiquity to the Seventeenth Century* (London, 1991), pp. 7–18; Charles Burnett, 'Sound

and its perception in the Middle Ages', in Burnett et al., *The Second Sense*, pp. 42–70.

32 Hieronymus Fabricius de Aquapendente, *De visione, voce, auditu* (Venice, 1600), p. 10.
33 Galen, *On the Doctrines of Hippocrates and Plato*, ed. and trans. Phillip de Lacy, 2nd edn (Berlin, 1984), p. 463.
34 See Jost Benedum, 'Das Riechorgan in der antiken und mittelalterlichen Hirnforschung und die Rezeption durch S. Th. Soemmering', in Gunter Mann and Franz Dumont (eds), *Gehirn – Nerven – Seele: Anatomie und Physiologie im Umfeld S. Th. Soemmerings* (Stuttgart, 1988), pp. 11–54; Karl Kassel, *Geschichte der Nasenheilkunde*, 2 vols. (Würzburg, 1914–22); Klaus Seifert, 'Geschichte und Bibliographie der Erforschung des peripheren Geruchsorgans', *Clio Medica* 4 (1969), pp. 305–37.
35 Johann Mauricius Hoffmann and Bernhard Matthias Franck, 'De gustu, atque experimentis & observationibus novissimus circa illum habitis' (MD dissertation, Altendorf, 1689), p. 36, from the German translation by Michael Ernst Weidemann in his 'Anschauungen über Bau und Funktion der Zunge in Dissertationen des ausgehenden 17. und der ersten Hälfte des 18. Jahrhunderts' (MD dissertation, Gießen, 1994), p. 86.
36 See Peter Theiss, *Die Wahrnehmungspsychologie und Sinnesphysiologie des Albertus Magnus: ein Modell der Sinnes- und Hirnfunktion aus der Zeit des Mittelalters: mit einer Übersetzung aus De anima* (Frankfurt am Main, 1997), pp. 78–9.
37 St Thomas Aquinas, *Commentary on Aristotle's 'De anima'*, trans. Kenelm Foster, OP, and Silvester Humphries, OP, rev. edn (Notre Dame, IN, 1994), p. 187.
38 See Max Wellmann, *Die pneumatische Schule bis auf Archigenes in ihrer Entwicklung dargestellt* (Berlin, 1895), pp. 142–3.
39 For Galen's theory of perception, see Rudolph Siegel, *Galen on Sense Perception* (Basel and New York, 1970).
40 Galen, *On Anatomical Procedures: The Later Books*, trans. W. L. H. Duckworth, ed. M. C. Lyons and B. Towers (Cambridge, 1962), p. 188.
41 Quoted in David C. Lindberg, *Theories of Vision from Al-Kindi to Kepler* (Chicago and London, 1976), p. 200.
42 Georg Harig, *Bestimmung der Intensität im medizinischen Systems Galens* (Berlin, 1974), p. 81.
43 For an exhaustive description of Plotinus' theory of perception, see Eyjólfur Kjalar Emilsson, *Plotinus on Sense Perception: A Philosophical Study* (Cambridge, 1988).
44 Nemesius Emesenus, *De natura hominis: Graece et Latine*, ed. Christian Friedrich Matthaei (Halle, 1802; repr. Hildesheim, 1967), chap. 6, p. 47 [trans. JL].

45 Ibid., p. 47. See also Boleslaw Domanski, *Die Psychologie des Nemesius* (Bonn, 1900), p. 80ff.
46 See Ulrich Wienbruch, *Erleuchtete Einsicht: zur Erkenntnislehre Augustins* (Bonn, 1989).
47 Lindberg, *Theories of Vision*, p. 89.
48 Aurelius Augustinus, *De genesi ad litteram*, ed. Joseph Zycha (Vienna, 1894), p. 23.
49 Aurelius Augustinus, *De trinitate*, vol. 2 of *The Select Library of the Nicene and Post-Nicene Fathers of the Christian Church*, ed. Philipp Schaff (Buffalo, 1887), p. 146.
50 Quoted in S. Landauer, 'Die Psychologie des Ibn Sînâ', *Zeitschrift der Deutschen Morgenländischen Gesellschaft* 29 (1876), p. 388 [trans. JL].
51 See Harry Austryn Wolfson, 'The Internal Senses in Latin, Arabic and Hebrew Philosophical Texts', *Harvard Theological Review* 28 (1935), pp. 69–133.
52 Quoted in Landauer, 'Psychologie des Ibn Sînâ', p. 388 [trans. JL].
53 Quoted in Jörg Alejandro Tellkamp, *Sinne, Gegenstände, Sensibilia: zur Wahrnehmungslehre des Thomas von Aquin* (Leiden, 1999), p. 67 [trans. JL].
54 Quoted in Theiss, *Die Wahrnehmungspsychologie und Sinnesphysiologie des Albertus Magnus*, p. 161 [trans. JL].
55 Quoted ibid., p. 162.
56 Quoted ibid., p. 278f.
57 Quoted ibid., p. 55.
58 See Tellkamp, *Sinne, Gegenstände, Sensibilia*, p. 194f.
59 Quoted ibid., p. 197.
60 Ibid., p. 207.
61 See Th. Dewender, 'Sensus communis II: Mittelalter', in *Historisches Wörterbuch der Philosophie*, vol. 9 (1995), cols. 634–9.
62 See Eckart Scheerer, 'Die Sinne', in *Historisches Wörterbuch der Philosophie*, vol. 9 (1995), cols. 824–69 (col. 842).
63 Tommaso Campanella, *Metafisica*, ed. G. di Napoli (Bologna, 1967), p. 140.
64 See Philipp Melanchthon, *De anima liber unus* (Lyons, 1555), p. 138.
65 René Descartes, *Treatise on Man* (Cambridge, MA, 1972), pp. 68–73. See also Alistair C. Crombie, 'Early Concepts of Senses and the Mind', *Scientific American* 210 (1964), pp. 108–16 (p. 116).
66 Johannes Kepler, *Weltharmonik*, ed. Max Caspar (Munich and Berlin, 1939), p. 214. Johannes Kepler, *Harmony of the World*, trans. E. J. Aiton, A. M. Duncan and J. V. Field (Philadelphia, 1997), p. 423.
67 Scheerer, 'Die Sinne', col. 845.

CHAPTER 3   CLASSIFICATIONS: THE HIERARCHY OF THE SENSES

1 Jacques Paul Migne, *Patrologiae cursus completus*, Latin series, 221 vols. (Paris, 1844–65), vol. 111, col. 143 [trans. JL].

2 *Deutsches Wörterbuch von Jacob und Wilhelm Grimm*, 16 vols. (Leipzig, 1854–1971 [repr. Munich, 1984]), vol. 10.1, col. 1142.

3 Albertus Magnus, *De anima* [trans. JL].

4 Leopold George, *Die fünf Sinne: nach den neueren Forschungen der Physik und der Physiologie dargestellt als Grundlage der Psychologie* (Berlin, 1846), p. 74.

5 See David Kaufmann, *Die Sinne: Beiträge zur Geschichte der Physiologie und Psychologie im Mittelalter aus hebräischen und arabischen Quellen* (Leipzig, 1884), p. 41.

6 Ibid., p. 43, n. 21.

7 Both quotations are taken from the *Deutsches Wörterbuch* (1910), vol. 10.1, col. 1144.

8 Quoted ibid., vol. 10.1, col. 1145.

9 Immanuel Kant, *Anthropology from a Pragmatic Point of View*, trans. Victor Lyle Dowdell, ed. Hans H. Rudnick (London, 1978).

10 Jean-Anthelme Brillat-Savarin, *The Physiology of Taste, or Meditations on Transcendental Gastronomy*, trans. M. F. K. Fisher (New York, 1949).

11 All quotations are taken from the *Deutsches Wörterbuch* (1910), vol. 10.1, col. 1143.

12 *Lexikon der christlichen Ikonographie*, ed. Engelbert Kischbaum, SJ, 8 vols. (Freiburg/Breisgau, 1986), vol. 2, col. 459.

13 See Kaufmann, *Die Sinne*, p. 13.

14 Wolfgang Welsch, *Aisthesis: Grundzüge und Perspektiven der Aristotelischen Sinnenlehre* (Stuttgart, 1987), pp. 64–5.

15 See S. Landauer, 'Die Psychologie des Ibn Sînâ', *Zeitschrift der Deutschen Morgenländischen Gesellschaft* 29 (1876), pp. 335–418 (p. 388).

16 Charles Bouvelles, *Que hoc volumine continentur: liber de intellectu, liber de sensu, liber de nichilo, ars oppositorum: liber de generatione, liber de sapiente, liber de duodecim numeris, epistole complures* (Paris, 1510), p. 31. See also Joseph Dippel, *Versuch einer systematischen Darstellung der Philosophie des Carolus Bovillus neben einem kurzen Lebensabrisse* (Würzburg, 1865), p. 208.

17 Peter Theiss, *Die Wahrnehmungspsychologie und Sinnesphysiologie des Albertus Magnus* (Frankfurt am Main, 1997), p. 264 [trans. JL].

18 See Kaufmann, *Die Sinne*, p. 13.

19 See Welsch, *Aisthesis*, pp. 64–5.

20 See Dippel, *Versuch*, p. 210.

21 See Marshall McLuhan, *The Gutenberg Galaxy* (Toronto, 1962), p. 29ff.; Constance Classen, *Worlds of Sense: Exploring the Senses in History and Across Cultures* (London and New York, 1993), p. 5; Alfred Krovoza, 'Gesichtssinn, Urbanität und Alltäglichkeit', in Kunst- und Ausstellungshalle der Bundesrepublik Deutschland (ed.), *Sehsucht* (Göttingen, 1995), pp. 43–52.

22 Thomas Tomkis, *Lingua, or The Combat of the Tongue and the Five Senses for Superiority* (London, 1607), act 5, scene 19.

23 Quoted from the translation by Richard Zoozmann in Friedrich R. Lehmann, *Rezepte der Liebesmittel: eine Kulturgeschichte der Liebe*, 2nd edn (Heidenheim, 1959), p. 48 [trans. JL].

24 Quoted from the German translation in Wilhelm Kühlmann and Robert Seidel, 'Askese oder Augenlust? Sinnesvermögen und Sinnlichkeit bei Jakob Balde SJ und Barthold Heinrich Brockes', in Wilhelm Kühlmann and Wolf-Dieter Müller-Jahncke (eds), *Iliaster: Literatur und Naturkunde in der Frühen Neuzeit* (Heidelberg, 1999), pp. 131–66, esp. p. 162.

25 See Florentine Mütherich, 'Ein Illustrationszyklus zum Anticlaudianus des Alanus ab Insulis', in *Münchner Jahrbuch der Bildenden Kunst*, 3rd series, vol. 4 (1951), pp. 73–88 (p. 73ff.); Elizabeth Sears, 'The iconography of auditory perception in the early Middle Ages: on psalm illustration and psalm exegesis', in Charles Burnett, Michael Fend and Penelope Gouk (eds), *The Second Sense: Studies in Hearing and Musical Judgement from Antiquity to the Seventeenth Century* (London, 1991), pp. 19–42 (p. 29ff.).

26 See Gudrun Schleusener-Eichholz, *Das Auge im Mittelalter*, 2 vols. (Munich, 1985), vol. 1, p. 211, n. 112.

27 See Kaufmann, *Die Sinne*, p. 45.

28 Quoted ibid., p. 140, n. 2.

29 Ovid, *Metamorphoses*, trans. Mary M. Innes (Harmondsworth, 1955), p. 31.

30 See the examples cited by Schleusener-Eichholz, *Das Auge im Mittelalter*, vol. 1, p. 203.

31 See *Sententiae*, I, 13: de sensibus carnis, in Migne, *Patrologiae cursus completus*, PL 83, cols. 563–4.

32 Hildegard von Bingen, *Welt und Mensch: das Buch 'De operatione Dei'*, trans. from the Geneva Codex, with explanatory notes, by Heinrich Schipperges (Salzburg, 1965), p. 107.

33 Quoted in Horst Wenzel, *Hören und Sehen: Schrift und Bild: Kultur und Gedächtnis im Mittelalter* (Munich, 1995), p. 31.

34 Quoted ibid., p. 61.

35 See Margaret Ruth Miles, *Image as Insight: Visual Understanding in Western Christianity and Secular Culture* (Boston, 1985), p. 66. On the

overemphasis of looking in popular medieval religiosity, see Bob Scribner, 'Das Visuelle in der Volksfrömmigkeit', in Scribner (ed.), *Bilder und Bildersturm im Spätmittelalter und in der frühen Neuzeit* (Wiesbaden, 1990), pp. 9–20.

36 Quoted in Kaufmann, *Die Sinne*, p. 140, n. 2.

37 Leonardo da Vinci, *Tagebücher und Aufzeichnungen*, ed. Theodor Lücke, 2nd edn (Leipzig, 1932), p. 119 [trans. JL]. For further treatments of the dissemination of this idea in the literature of the sixteenth and seventeenth centuries, see Anat Feinberg, 'The infinite vexation: mind, appearance and reality in selected Jacobean and Caroline plays' (PhD dissertation, University of London, 1978), p. 42; David Summers, *The Judgement of Sense: Renaissance Naturalism and the Rise of Aesthetics* (Cambridge, 1994), p. 32ff.; Alex Aronson, *Shakespeare and the Ocular Proof* (New York, 1995), p. 1ff.

38 Quoted in Thomas Kleinspehn, *Der flüchtige Blick: Sehen und Identität in der Kultur der Neuzeit* (Reinbek, 1989), p. 92.

39 See Ernst von Dobschütz, 'Die fünf Sinne im Neuen Testament', *Journal of Biblical Literature* 48 (1929), pp. 378–411 (pp. 396–7); Hans Joachim Kraus, 'Hören und Sehen in der althebräischen Tradition', *Studium Generale* 19 (1966), pp. 115–23 (pp. 119–20).

40 See Kaufmann, *Die Sinne*, p. 143.

41 Franz Pfeiffer (ed.), *Meister Eckart* (Leipzig, 1857).

42 Conrad von Megenberg, *Das Buch der Natur*, new High German edn by Hugo Schulu (Greifswald, 1897), p. 9.

43 See Kaufmann, *Die Sinne*, p. 155.

44 See Jean-Pierre Albert, *Odeurs de sainteté: la mythologie chrétienne des aromates* (Paris, 1990).

45 See Kaufmann, *Die Sinne*, p. 155.

46 See Ute Frackowiak, *Der gute Geschmack: Studien zur Entwicklung des Geschmacksbegriffs* (Munich, 1994), p. 24ff.

47 Ibid., pp. 27–8.

48 Aquinas, *Commentary on Aristotle's 'De anima'*, trans. Kenelm Foster, OP, and Silvester Humphries, OP, rev. edn (Notre Dame, IN, 1994), p. 187.

49 Ibid., p. 152.

50 Ibid.

51 See the passages quoted by Kaufmann, *Die Sinne*, pp. 188–9.

52 See Marjorie O'Rourke Boyle, *Senses of Touch: Human Dignity and Deformity from Michelangelo to Calvin* (Leiden, 1998); Sander L. Gilman, 'Touch, sexuality and disease', in William F. Bynum and Roy Porter (eds), *Medicine and the Five Senses* (Cambridge, 1993), pp. 198–224.

CHAPTER 4   REPRESENTATIONS: ALLEGORIES

1 Roger Chartier, *Cultural History*, trans. Lydia Cochrane (Cambridge, 1988), p. 8.
2 Quoted in *Deutsches Wörterbuch*, vol. 10.1 (1905), col. 1155.
3 See Ludwig Schrader, *Sinne und Sinnesverknüpfungen: Studien und Materialien zur Vorgeschichte der Synästhesie und zur Bewertung der Sinne in der italienischen, spanischen und französischen Literatur* (Heidelberg, 1969), p. 199.
4 For the sources of the following examples, see Ernst von Dobschütz, 'Die fünf Sinne im Neuen Testament', *Journal of Biblical Literature* 48 (1929), p. 383.
5 For the the sources of the following examples, see David Kaufmann, *Die Sinne: Beiträge zur Geschichte der Physiologie und Psychologie im Mittelalter aus hebräischen und arabischen Quellen* (Leipzig, 1884), pp. 10–26.
6 Ibid., p. 19.
7 Karl Rahner, 'Le début d'une doctrine des cinq sens spirituels chez Origène', *Revue d'ascétique et de mystique* 13 (1932), pp. 113–45 (pp. 143, 145).
8 See Elizabeth Sears, 'The iconography of auditory perception in the early Middle Ages: on psalm illustration and psalm exegesis', in Charles Burnett, Michael Fend and Penelope Gouk (eds), *The Second Sense: Studies in Hearing and Musical Judgement from Antiquity to the Seventeenth Century* (London, 1991), pp. 19–42 (p. 27); Gudrun Schleusener-Eichholz, *Das Auge im Mittelalter*, 2 vols. (Munich, 1985), vol. 1, p. 215, n. 125.
9 Heinrich von Seuse, *Deutsche Schriften*, ed. Karl Bihlmeyer (Stuttgart, 1907), p. 316.
10 For the sources of the following examples, see Schleusener-Eichholz, *Das Auge im Mittelalter*, vol. 1, p. 215, n. 125, and Schrader, *Sinne und Sinnesverknüpfungen*, pp. 65, 184.
11 Tilo von Kulm, *Von siben Ingesigeln*, ed. Karl Kochendörfer (Berlin, 1907), 5073ff. [trans. Ian Cooper].
12 Quoted in Chu-Tsing Li, 'The five senses in art: an analysis of its development in northern Europe' (PhD dissertation, University of Iowa, 1955), p. 108, n. 36.
13 See Carl Nordenfalk, 'Les cinq sens dans l'art du Moyen Age', *Revue de l'Art* 34 (1976), pp. 17–28 (p. 18), and Li, 'The five senses in art', pp. 18–19.
14 See Carl Nordenfalk, 'The five senses in late medieval and Renaissance art', *Journal of the Warburg and Courtauld Institutes* 48 (1985), pp. 1–22 (p. 1f.).

15 For a detailed discussion of Calderón's play, see Schrader, *Sinne und Sinnesverknüpfungen*, p. 76ff. For an illustration and interpretation of Escalante's painting, see Sylvia Ferino-Pagden (ed.), *Immagini del sentire: i cinque sensi nell'arte*, exhibition catalogue (Cremona, 1996), p. 284f.

16 B. Knipping, *De iconografie van de Contra-Reformatie in de Nederlanden* (Hilversum, 1939), vol. 1, p. 51ff.

17 Ignatius von Loyola, *Briefe und Unterweisung*, trans. Peter Knauer (Würzburg, 1993), p. 298 [trans. JL].

18 Werner Kutschmann, *Der Naturwissenschaftler und sein Körper: die Rolle der 'inneren Natur' in der experimentellen Naturwissenschaft der frühen Neuzeit* (Frankfurt am Main, 1986), p. 59.

19 Hans Kauffmann, 'Die fünf Sinne in der niederländischen Malerei des 17. Jahrhunderts', in Hans Tintelnot (ed.), *Kunstgeschichtliche Studien* (Breslau, 1943), pp. 133–57 (p. 143ff). See also Li, 'The five senses in art', p. 70ff.; Louise Vinge, *The Five Senses: Studies in a Literary Tradition* (Lund, 1975), p. 122; Carl Nordenfalk, 'The five senses in Flemish art before 1600', in G. Cavalli-Björkman (ed.), *Netherlandish Mannerism* (Stockholm, 1985), pp. 135–54 (p. 149ff.); Ferino-Pagden, *Immagini del sentire*, p. 198ff.

20 For illustrations of the still-life paintings mentioned here, see Ferino-Pagden, *Immagini del sentire*, p. 242ff.

21 For detailed discussion and illustrative texts, see Wilhelm Kühlmann and Robert Seidel, 'Askese oder Augenlust?', in Wilhelm Kühlmann and Wolf-Dieter Müller-Jahncke (eds), *Iliaster* (Heidelberg, 1999), p. 142ff.

22 Georg Philipp Harsdörfer, *Vollständig vermehrtes Trincirbuch von Tafeldecken trinciren, Zeitung der Mundkoste, Schauessen und Schaugerichten, benebens XXIV Gast- oder Tischfragen* (Nuremberg, 1652 [repr. Leipzig, 1976]), p. 140. See also Ulrike Zischka, Hans Ottomeyer and Susanne Bäumler (eds), *Die anständige Lust: von Eßkultur und Tafelsitten* (Munich, 1993), p. 110.

23 For the exact sources, see P. Wilpert, 'Auge', in *Reallexikon für Antike und Christentum*, vol. 1 (Stuttgart, 1950), cols. 957–69, and Schleusener-Eichholz, *Das Auge im Mittelalter*.

24 For further examples, see Herbert von Einem, 'Das Auge, der edelste Sinn', *Wallraf-Richartz-Jahrbuch* 30 (1968), pp. 275–86 (pp. 276–7).

25 See Arthur Henkel and Albrecht Schöne (eds), *Handbuch zur Sinnbildkunst des XVI. und XVII. Jahrhunderts* (Stuttgart, 1996), col. 1692ff.

26 See, among the numerous works on the subject, Siegfried Seligmann, *Der böse Blick und Verwandtes*, 2 vols. (Berlin, 1910), and Thomas Hauschild, *Der böse Blick* (Hamburg, 1979).

27 Reproduced in Henkel and Schöne, *Handbuch zur Sinnbildkunst*, col. 1359.

28 Thomas Hobbes, *Leviathan*, ed. C. B. Macpherson (Harmondsworth, 1968), p. 85.

29 Henkel and Schöne, *Handbuch zur Sinnbildkunst*, col. 1006.

30 Unless otherwise stated, the sources for these examples are *Deutsches Wörterbuch* (1887), vol. 7, cols. 1225–68, and Franz Mayr, 'Wort gegen Bild: zur Frühgeschichte der Symbolik des Hörens', in Robert Kuhn and Bernd Kreutz (eds), *Das Buch vom Hören* (Freiburg/Breisgau, 1991), pp. 16–37 (p. 16ff.).

31 See Hans Werner, *Geschichte des Taubstummenproblems bis ins 17. Jahrhundert* (Jena, 1932), p. 73.

32 For the physiognomy of the ear in the early modern era, see Johann Baptista Porta, *De humana physiognomia libri iii* (Hanover, 1593), p. 140.

33 For other depictions, see *Lexikon der christlichen Ikonographie*, ed. Engelbert Kischbaum, SJ (Freiburg/Breisgau, 1974), vol. 4, col. 430.

34 See illustration 6 in Elizabeth Sears, 'The iconography of auditory perception', p. 36.

35 Richard Palmer, 'In bad odours: smell and its significance in medicine from antiquity to the seventeenth century', in William F. Bynum and Roy Porter (eds), *Medicine and the Five Senses* (Cambridge, 1993), p. 61.

36 See Manfred Tietz, 'Nicht-verbale Überzeugungsstrategien bei François de Sales', in Volker Kapp (ed.), *Die Sprache der Zeichen und Bilder* (Marburg, 1990), pp. 90–101 (p. 93).

37 See Arnold Angenendt, *Heilige und Reliquien: die Geschichte ihres Kultes vom frühen Christentum bis zur Gegenwart* (Munich, 1997).

38 See Ernst Lohmeyer, 'Vom göttlichen Wohlgeruch', *Sitzungsberichte der Heidelberger Akademie der Wissenschaften*, philosophical-historical section, article 9 (1919), pp. 1–52.

39 Quoted in Horst Wenzel, *Hören und Sehen, Schrift und Bild: Kultur und Gedächtnis im Mittelalter* (Munich, 1995), p. 177.

40 See Jay Geller, '(G)nos(e)ology: the cultural construction of the Other', in Howard Eilberg-Schwartz (ed.), *People of the Body: Jews and Judaism from an Embodied Perspective* (New York, 1992), pp. 243–82. See also the same author's 'The aromatics of Jewish difference; or, Benjamin's allegory of aura', in Jonathan Boyarin and Daniel Boyarin (eds), *Jews and Other Differences* (Minneapolis and London, 1997), pp. 202–56.

41 See, for instance, the examples cited by Albert Wesselski in his *Der Sinn der Sinne: ein Kapitel der ältesten Menschheitsgeschichte* (Leipzig, 1934), p. 15.

42 Kaufmann, *Die Sinne*, p. 156.

43 Porta, *De humana physiognomia libri iii*, p. 227.
44 See Edward Shorter, *From Paralysis to Fatigue* (New York, 1992), p. 122.
45 Valentin Groebner, 'Das Gesicht wahren: abgeschnittene Nasen, abgeschnittene Ehre in der spätmittelalterlichen Stadt', in Klaus Schreiner and Gerd Schwerhoff (eds), *Verletzte Ehre: Ehrkonflikte in Gesellschaften des Mittelalters und der Frühen Neuzeit* (Weimar and Vienna, 1995), pp. 361–80 (p. 371).
46 Unless otherwise stated, the following examples are taken from *Deutsches Wörterbuch* (1954), vol. 16, col. 586ff.
47 Porta, *De humana physiognomia libri iii*, p. 227.
48 See Kaufmann, *Die Sinne*, p. 171.
49 See V. Kahn, 'The sense of taste in Montaigne's essays', *Modern Language Notes* (1980), pp. 1269–91.
50 See also the examples given in Ute Frackowiak, *Der gute Geschmack* (Munich, 1994), p. 148ff.
51 See Gabriel Josipovici, *Touch* (New Haven and London, 1996).
52 My full-text search in the Global Jewish Database at Bar Ilan University produced exactly 1974 examples, in contrast to the word *ayn* (eye), which occurred just 970 times. Compare this with Silvia Schroer and Thomas Staubli, *Die Körpersymbolik der Bibel* (Darmstadt, 1998), p. 171, which, for reasons I am unable to explain, gives a lower figure (1600) for the word *jad* (hand).
53 See figures 15 and 16 in Ilsebill Barta Fliedl and Christoph Geissmar (eds), *Die Beredsamkeit des Leibes: zur Körpersprache in der Kunst* (Vienna, 1992).
54 See Dobschütz, 'Die fünf Sinne im Neuen Testament', p. 388.
55 Sander L. Gilman, *Sexuality: an Illustrated History Representing the Sexual in Medicine and Culture from the Middle Ages to the Age of AIDS* (New York, 1989), p. 206.
56 Hans Peter Duerr, *Der erotische Leib: der Mythos vom Zivilisationsprozeß* (Frankfurt am Main, 1997), p. 107.
57 See also the numerous examples in Marjorie O'Rourke Boyle, *Senses of Touch: Human Dignity and Deformity from Michelangelo to Calvin* (Leiden, 1998), p. 110 and *passim*, and in Gilman, *Sexuality*, p. 148.
58 See Robert Jütte, 'Aging and body image in the sixteenth century: Hermann Weinsberg's (1518–1597) perception of the aging body', *European History Quarterly* 18 (1988), pp. 259–90.
59 See the illustrations in Ferino-Pagden, *Immagini del sentire*, pp. 203, 213. For Brouwer, see Konrad Renger, *Adriaen Brouwer und das niederländische Bauerngenre 1600–1660* (Munich, 1986), plate 7.
60 See the illustration and comments in Ferino-Pagden, *Immagini del sentire*, p. 138f.

CHAPTER 5 PRACTICES: THE SENSES AND THEIR AILMENTS

1 Quoted in Hans Gerlach, 'Die Kenntnisse der alten Naturvölker von den gesunden und kranken Sinnesorganen auf Grund ihrer Anschauung von der Heilkunde', *Sudhoffs Archiv für die Geschichte der Medizin und der Naturwissenschaften* 29 (1937), pp. 271–88 (p. 273); see also Wolfhart Westendorf, *Erwachen der Heilkunst: die Medizin im Alten Ägypten* (Zurich, 1992), pp. 224–5.

2 See Georg Harig, *Bestimmung der Intensität im medizinischen Systems Galens* (Berlin, 1974).

3 Lissa Roberts, 'The death of the sensuous chemist: the "new" chemistry and the transformation of sensuous technology', *Studies in the History and Philosophy of Science* 26 (1995), pp. 503–29.

4 Hippocrates, *In the Surgery*, trans. E. J. Withington, in *Hippocrates*, 5 vols. (London and Cambridge, MA, 1948), vol. 3, p. 59.

5 Samuel Gottlieb Vogel, *Kranken-Examen* (Vienna, 1797), p. 194.

6 See Christa Habrich, Frank Marguth and Jörg Henning Wolf (eds), *Medizinische Diagnostik in Geschichte und Gegenwart: Festschrift für Heinz Goerke zum 60. Geburtstag* (Munich, 1978); Volker Hess, *Von der semiotischen zur diagnostischen Medizin: die Entstehung der klinischen Methoden zwischen 1750 und 1850* (Husum, 1993).

7 Quoted in Wolfgang Eich, *Medizinische Semiotik (1750–1850): ein Beitrag zur Geschichte des Zeichenbegriffs in der Medizin* (Freiburg/ Breisgau, 1986), p. 50.

8 See *Lexikon für Theologie und Kirche*, 2nd fully rev. edn, ed. Josef Höfer and Karl Rahner, 14 vols. (Freiburg/Breisgau, 1986), vol. 6 (1961), cols. 585–91.

9 See the *Rituale Romanum*, ed. Pope Paul V (Mechelen, 1845), p. 88ff.

10 See Adolph Franz, *Das Rituale des Bischofs Heinrich I. von Breslau* (Freiburg/Breisgau, 1912).

11 Johann Heinrich Zedler, *Grosses Vollständiges Universal-Lexicon*, 64 vols. (Leipzig, 1732–50 [repr. Graz, 1993–8]), vol. 25, col. 741 [cited as *Zedler's Universal Lexicon* in all subsequent references in the text].

12 See E. W. M. Olfers, *Pastoralmedicin: die Naturwissenschaft auf dem Gebiet der katholischen Moral und Pastoral: ein Handbuch für den katholischen Clerus*, 2nd rev. and expanded edn (Freiburg/Breisgau, 1893), p. 128.

13 See August Stöhr, *Handbuch der Pastoralmedizin mit besonderer Berücksichtigung der Hygiene*, 5th rev. edn (Freiburg/Breisgau, 1909), p. 528.

14 Geiler von Kaysersberg, 'Dis büchlin wiset wie sich ein yeglicher Cristen mensch schicken soll zuo einer gantzen volkomne[n] vnd gemeiner beycht',

in *Die ältesten Schriften Geilers von Kaysersberg*, ed. Leon Dacheux (Freiburg/Breisgau, 1882), pp. 133–58 (p. 138) [trans. JL].

15 See Benedikt Kranemann, *Die Krankensalbung in der Zeit der Aufklärung: Ritualien und pastoralliturgische Studien im deutschen Sprachgebiet* (Münster, 1990), p. 327ff.

16 See Susan C. Karant-Nunn, *The Reformation of Ritual: An Interpretation of Early Modern Germany* (London and New York, 1997), p. 166.

17 Immanuel Kant, *Werke*, ed. Wilhelm Weischedel (Frankfurt am Main, 1968–), vol. 10, p. 454.

18 Christian Friedrich Richter, *Die höchst-nöthige Erkenntniß des Menschen sonderlich nach dem Leibe und natürlichen Leben, oder deutlicher Unterricht von der Gesundheit und deren Erhaltung . . .* , 3rd edn (Leipzig, 1710), p. 232.

19 Felix Platter, *Observationes: Krankheitsbeobachtungen in drei Büchern*, rev. Günther Goldschmidt, ed. Heinrich Buess (Bern and Stuttgart, 1963).

20 Marcus Tullius Cicero, *Tusculan Disputations*, V, 116.

21 *Zedler's Universal Lexicon*, vol. 37 (1743), col. 1697.

22 Leonardo da Vinci, 'Treatise on painting', in *The Literary Works of Leonardo da Vinci*, comp. and ed. from the original manuscripts by Jean Paul Richter, 3rd edn, 2 vols. (London, 1969), vol. 1, p. 40.

23 See Michael Tschoetschel, 'Die Diskussion über die Häufigkeit von Krankheiten bei den Juden bis 1920' (MD dissertation, University of Mainz, 1990), p. 219.

24 See Thilo von Haugwitz, *Augenheilkunde im 20. Jahrhundert: Ergebnisse und Ereignisse im deutschsprachigen Raum* (Stuttgart, 1991), p. 64.

25 See Wolfgang Münchow, *Geschichte der Augenheilkunde* (Stuttgart, 1984), p. 262f.

26 Celsus, *De medicina*, trans. W. G. Spencer, 3 vols. (London and Cambridge, MA, 1961), vol. 3, p. 351.

27 See Gudrun Schleusener-Eichholz, *Das Auge im Mittelalter*, 2 vols. (Munich, 1985), vol. 1, p. 514ff.

28 *Lexikon der christlichen Ikonographie*, ed. Engelbert Kischbaum, SJ (Freiburg/Breisgau, 1974), vol. 8, cols. 77–9.

29 Ibid., vol. 7, cols. 415–20.

30 See Barbara Schuh, *Jenseitigkeit in diesseitigen Formen: sozial- und mentalitätsgeschichtliche Aspekte spätmittelalterlicher Mirakelberichte* (Graz, 1989); Jürgen Jansen, *Medizinische Kasuistik in den 'Miracula sancte elyzabet': medizinhistorische Analyse und Übersetzungen der Wunderprotokolle am Grab der Elisabeth von Thüringen (1207–1231)* (Frankfurt am Main, 1985), p. 98.

31 Quoted in Ruth Wendel-Widmer, *Die Wunderheilungen am Grabe der Heiligen Elisabeth von Thüringen* (Zurich, 1987), p. 36.

32 See Otto Weinreich, *Antike Heilungswunder: Untersuchungen zum Wunderglauben der Griechen und Römer* (Gießen, 1909), p. 189ff.

33 See Monika Helbling, *Der altägyptische Augenkranke, sein Arzt und seine Götter* (Zurich, 1980), p. 66ff.; Axel Küster, *Blinde und Taubstumme im Römischen Recht* (Cologne, 1991), p. 11ff.

34 See Münchow, *Augenheilkunde*, p. 368.

35 See Schleusener-Eichholz, *Das Auge im Mittelalter*, p. 358ff.

36 Quoted in Münchow, *Augenheilkunde*, p. 204.

37 Lorenz Heister, *Chirurgie* (Nuremberg, 1763 [repr. Osnabrück, 1981]), p. 581.

38 'An account of persons who could not distinguish colours', *Philosophical Transactions of the Royal Society of London* 67 (1777), p. 262.

39 See Patrick Trevor-Roper, *The World Through Blunted Sight* (London, 1997), p. 85.

40 Quoted in Münchow, *Augenheilkunde*, p. 173. For a copiously illustrated general history of spectacles, see Annamarie Klotz, *Die Brille: Ausstellung zum 100. Todestag von Carl Zeiss in der Württembergischen Landesbibliothek Stuttgart 26. 10.–23. 12. 1988* (Stuttgart, 1988).

41 The precise sources of the following quotations from the 'Weinsberg Book' are given in Robert Jütte, 'Aging and body image in the sixteenth century', *European History Quarterly* 18 (1988), pp. 259–90.

42 Elisabeth Charlotte, Herzogin von Orléans, *Briefe aus den Jahren 1676–1722*, ed. Ludwig Holland, 6 vols. (Tübingen, 1871–81 [repr. Hildesheim, 1988]), vol. 4, p. 342.

43 See Paul Ingendaay, 'Ein Teufelsgezücht ist die Brillenschlange', *Frankfurter Allgemeine Zeitung*, 10 March 1999, p. 56.

44 Quoted in Thomas Kleinspehn, *Der flüchtige Blick: Sehen und Identität in der Kultur der Neuzeit* (Reinbek, 1989), p. 197.

45 See Thomas Stichnoth, *Taubstummheit: die medizinische Behandlung der Gehörlosigkeit vom 17. Jahrhundert bis zur Gegenwart* (Cologne, 1985), p. 65.

46 Kant, *Werke*, vol. 10, p. 455.

47 Conrad H. Rawski (ed.), *Petrarch's Remedies for Fortune Fair and Foul: A Modern English Translation of* De remediis utriusque fortunae, *with a Commentary* (Bloomington and Indianapolis, 1991), vol. 3, p. 240.

48 Quoted in *Deutsches Wörterbuch von Jacob und Wilhelm Grimm*, vol. 21 (Leipzig, 1935), col. 164.

49 See Küster, *Blinde und Taubstumme im Römischen Recht*, p. 40.

50 See Hans Werner, *Geschichte des Taubstummenproblems bis ins 17. Jahrhundert* (Jena, 1932), p. 106.

51 Unless otherwise indicated, the following diagnostic descriptions are indebted to Harald Feldmann, *Die geschichtliche Entwicklung der*

Hörprüfungsmethoden: kurze Darstellung und Bibliographie von den Anfängen bis zur Gegenwart (Stuttgart, 1960).

52 See Brian Grant, *The Quiet Ear: Deafness in Literature* (London, 1987), p. 210. For the period after 1800, see Nicholas Mirzoeff, *Silent Poetry: Deafness, Sign and Visual Culture in Modern France* (Princeton, NJ, 1995).

53 Quoted in Werner, *Geschichte des Taubstummenproblems*, p. 28.

54 Augustine, *De Magistro*, trans. George G. Leckie (New York and London, 1938), pp. 9–10.

55 See Jonathan Rée, *I See a Voice: A Philosophical History of Language, Deafness and the Senses* (London, 1999), p. 129ff.

56 See H. J. Zimmels, *Magicians, Theologians and Doctors: Studies in Folk-Medicine and Folk-lore as Reflected in the Rabbinical Responsa (12th–19th Centuries)* (London, 1952), p. 47.

57 *Zedler's Universal Lexicon*, vol. 10 (1735), col. 1206.

58 Quoted in Karl Kassel, *Geschichte der Nasenheilkunde*, 2 vols. (Würzburg, 1914–22), vol. 1, p. 244.

59 For medicinal smells, see Annick Le Guérer, *Scent: The Mysterious and Essential Powers of Smell*, trans. Richard Miller (London, 1993), pp. 63–101.

60 See Kassel, *Geschichte der Nasenheilkunde*, vol. 1, p. 51.

61 See Hans J. Rindisbacher, *The Smell of Books: A Cultural-Historical Study of Olfactory Perception in Literature* (Ann Arbor, 1992); Rolf Brüggemann (ed.), *Das Schnüffelbuch* (Stuttgart, 1995).

62 Wilhelm Sternberg, *Geschmack und Geruch: physiologische Untersuchungen über den Geschmackssinn* (Berlin, 1906), pp. 4–5.

63 *Zedler's Universal Lexicon*, vol. 8 (1734), col. 1228.

64 See Johannes von Fick, Paul Richter and Rudolf Spitzer, *Geschichte der Dermatologie, geographische Verteilung von Hautkrankheiten, Nomenklatur* (Berlin, 1928), p. 112, n. 3.

65 See Renate Wittern, 'Die Lepra aus der Sicht des Arztes am Beginn der Neuzeit', in Christa Habrich et al. (eds), *Aussatz, Lepra, Hansenkrankheit: ein Menschheitsproblem im Wandel* (Ingolstadt, 1982), vol. 1, pp. 41–50 (p. 45).

66 See Franz-Josef Kuhlen, *Zur Geschichte der Schmerz-, Schlaf- und Betäubungsmittel im Mittelalter und Früher Neuzeit* (Stuttgart, 1983), p. 184.

67 Ibid., p. 190.

68 *Zedler's Universal Lexicon*, vol. 8 (1734), cols. 1028–9.

69 See Marjorie O'Rourke Boyle, *Senses of Touch* (Leiden, 1998), p. 118.

70 *Zedler's Universal Lexicon*, vol. 9 (1735), col. 2231.

71 Platter, *Observationes*, p. 83.

72 Jansen, *Medizinische Kasuistik in den 'Miracula sancte elyzabet'*, pp. 180–1.
73 Paul Hoffmann and Peter Dohms (eds), *Die Mirakelbücher des Klosters Eberhardsklausen* (Düsseldorf, 1988), p. 459.

CHAPTER 6   PHILOSOPHICAL SENSUALISM IN THE
AGE OF SENSIBILITY

1 Jean Paul Marat, *A Philosophical Essay on Man* (London, 1773).
2 Immanuel Kant, *Critique of Pure Reason*, trans. Werner S. Pluhar (Indianapolis and Cambridge, 1996), p. 772.
3 For Locke's influence on sensualism, see Antoinette Stettler, 'Sensation und Sensibilität: zu John Lockes Einfluß auf das Konzept der Sensibilität im 18. Jahrhundert', *Gesnerus* 45 (1988), pp. 445–60.
4 John Locke, *An Essay Concerning Human Understanding*, ed. Peter H. Nidditch (Oxford, 1975), p. 105.
5 On Berkeley, see D. W. Hamlyn, *A History of Philosophy of Perception* (London, 1961), p. 104ff.
6 David Hume, *A Treatise of Human Nature*, with an introduction by A. D. Lindsay (London and Toronto, 1977), p. 71.
7 See Maurice Mandelbaum, *Philosophy, Science and Sense Perception: Historical and Critical Studies* (Baltimore, 1964), p. 135.
8 Roy Porter, 'Gefährlicher Ideenandrang', in *Frankfurter Allgemeine Zeitung*, 25 September 1999, supplement, p. iv.
9 *Encyclopédie, ou Dictionnaire raisonné des sciences, des arts et des métiers*, selection in 2 vols. (Paris, 1986), vol. 1, p. 77.
10 *Encyclopédie, ou Dictionnaire raisonné des sciences, des arts et des métiers* (Neuchâtel, 1751–98 [repr. Stuttgart, 1993]), vol. 15, p. 38.
11 Condillac, *Treatise on the Sensations*, trans. Geraldine Carr (London, 1930) [trans. JL].
12 Ibid., p. 289.
13 Ibid., p. 290.
14 J. L. Carr, 'Pygmalion and the philosophers', *Journal of the Warburg and Courtauld Institute* 23 (1960), pp. 239–55 (p. 239ff.).
15 Quoted in Klaus Völker (ed.), *Künstliche Menschen: über Golems, Homunculi, Androiden und lebende Statuen* (Frankfurt am Main, 1994), p. 329.
16 Condillac, *Treatise on the Sensations*, p. 101.
17 Moses Mendelssohn, *Die Bildsäule: ein psychologisch-allegorisches Traumgesicht*, in *Kleinere Schriften*, ed. Alexander Altmann (Stuttgart, 1981), vol. 1, pp. 74–87.

18 See Bernhard Dotzler, Peter Gendolla and Jörgen Schäfer, *Maschinen Menschen: eine Bibliographie* (Frankfurt am Main, 1992); Joachim Gessinger, *Auge & Ohr: Studien zur Erforschung der Sprache am Menschen 1700–1850* (Berlin and New York, 1994), p. 419ff.

19 Quoted in Völker, *Künstliche Menschen*, pp. 178–9.

20 See Michael J. Morgan, *Molyneux's Question: Vision, Touch and the Philosophy of Perception* (Cambridge, 1977); William R. Paulson, *Enlightenment, Romanticism, and the Blind in France* (Princeton, 1987); Marjolein Degenaar, *Molyneux's Problem: Three Centuries of Discussion on the Perception of Forms* (Dordrecht and Boston, 1996).

21 See Friedrich Dreves, '. . . *leider zum größten Theile Bettler geworden* . . .': *organisierte Blindenfürsorge in Preußen zwischen Aufklärung und Industrialisierung (1806–1860)* (Freiburg/Breisgau, 1998), p. 83.

22 Condillac, *Treatise on the Sensations*, p. 264.

23 See Louis Gayral et al., 'Les premières observations de l'enfant sauvage de Lacaune (dit "Victor" ou "le sauvage de l'Aveyron"): nouveaux documents', *Annales médico-psychologiques* 2 (1972), pp. 465–90.

24 Quoted in Harlan L. Lane, *The Wild Boy of Aveyron* (Cambridge, MA, 1976), p. 37.

25 Georg Friedrich Daumer and Anselm von Feuerbach, *Kaspar Hauser: mit einem Bericht von Johannes Mayer und einem Essay von Jeffrey M. Mason* (Die Andere Bibliothek, ed. Hans Magnus Enzensberger) (Frankfurt am Main, 1995), p. 21.

26 Reprinted in Peter Tradowsky (ed.), *Kaspar Hauser: Arztberichte* (Dornach, 1985), p. 132.

27 *Archiv für homöopathische Heilkunst* 11 (1832), pt 3, p. 13. See also Philipp Portwich, 'Kaspar Hauser, naturphilosophische Medizin und frühe Homöopathie', *Medizinhistorisches Journal* 31 (1996), pp. 89–119.

28 Reprinted in Tradowsky, *Kaspar Hauser*, p. 132.

29 See Hermann Hesse (ed.), *Blätter aus Prevorst: eine Auswahl von Berichten über Magnetismus, Heilungen, Geistererscheinungen aus dem Kreise Justinus Kerners und seiner Freunde* (Berlin, 1926 [repr. Frankfurt am Main, 1987]), p. 46ff.

30 See Otto-Joachim Grüsser, *Justinus Kerner 1786–1862: Arzt – Poet – Geisterseher* (Berlin, 1987), p. 212.

31 See Arnold Angenendt, *Heilige und Reliquien* (Munich, 1997), p. 278.

32 Johann Peter Eckermann, *Gespräche mit Goethe in den letzten Jahren seines Lebens*, ed. Ernst Beutler (Munich, 1976), p. 318.

33 Dorothea Christina Leporin, *Gründliche Untersuchung der Ursachen, die das weibliche Geschlecht vom Studiren abhalten (1742): mit einem Nachwort von Gerda Rechenberg* (Hildesheim and New York, 1977), p. 31.

34 See Londa Schiebinger, *The Mind Has No Sex? Women and the Origins of Modern Science* (Cambridge, MA, 1989).

35 See Johanna Borek, *Sensualismus und Sensation: zum Verhältnis von Natur, Moral und Ästhetik in der Spätaufklärung und im Fin de Siècle* (Vienna, Cologne and Graz, 1983); Lieselotte Steinbrügge, *The Moral Sex: Women's Nature in the French Enlightenment* (New York and Oxford, 1995); Anne C. Vila, *Enlightenment and Pathology: Sensibility in the Literature and Medicine of Eighteenth-Century France* (Baltimore and London, 1998).

36 P. J. G. Cabanis, *Rapports du physique et du morale de l'homme* (Paris, 1815), vol. 2, p. 297.

37 Gustav Carus, *Physis: zur Geschichte des leiblichen Lebens* (Stuttgart, 1851), p. 88.

38 Quoted in Friedrich Schlegel, *Theorie der Weiblichkeit*, ed. Winfried Menninghaus (Frankfurt am Main, 1983), p. 160.

39 Ibid., p. 129.

40 Jean Anthelme Brillat-Savarin, *The Physiology of Taste*, trans. M. F. K. Fisher (New York, 1949), p. 155.

41 See Karin Hausen, 'Die Polarisierung der "Geschlechtscharaktere": eine Spiegelung der Dissoziation von Erwerbs- und Familienleben', in Heidi Rosenbaum (ed.), *Seminar: Familie und Gesellschaftsstruktur*, 4th edn (Frankfurt am Main, 1988), pp. 161–91 (p. 162).

42 Quoted in Völker, *Künstliche Menschen*, p. 161.

CHAPTER 7   THE SENSES AND AESTHETICS

1 George Stubbes, *A Dialogue in the Manner of Plato on the Superiority of the Pleasures of Understanding to the Pleasures of the Senses* (London, 1734).

2 See *Historisches Wörterbuch der Philosophie*, ed. Joachim Ritter (Darmstadt, 1971–), vol. 8 (1992), col. 1370.

3 Ibid., col. 1371.

4 Ibid.

5 *Encyclopédie, ou Dictionnaire raisonné des sciences, des arts et des métiers* (Neuchâtel, 1751–98 [repr. Stuttgart, 1967], vol. 2, p. 178.

6 Denis Diderot, *Oeuvres choisies*, ed. François Tullon (Paris, 1983), vol. 1, p. 45.

7 See Nicholas Mirzoeff, *Silent Poetry: Deafness, Sign and Visual Culture in Modern France* (Princeton, 1995), pp. 108, 210.

8 Quoted in Anne C. Vila, *Enlightenment and Pathology: Sensibility in the Literature and Medicine of Eighteenth-Century France* (Baltimore and London, 1998), p. 41.

9 Johann Jakob Breitinger, *Critische Dichtkunst* (Stuttgart, 1966 [facsimile of 1740 edn]), vol. 1, p. 112.

10 Alexander Gottlieb Baumgarten, *Aesthetica*, 2 vols. (Frankfurt an der Oder, 1750–8 [repr. Hildesheim, 1961]).

11 *Historisches Wörterbuch der Philosophie*, vol. 1, col. 557.

12 Walter Benjamin, *Illuminations*, trans. Harry Zohn (London, 1992), p. 212.

13 Moses Mendelssohn, 'Über die Empfindungen', in *Gesammelte Schriften*, ed. Fritz Bamberger (Berlin, 1929), vol. 1, pp. 41–123 (p. 51).

14 Ibid., p. 58ff.

15 Quoted in Karl Vorländer, *Philosophie der Neuzeit* (Reinbek, 1967), vol. 5, p. 237.

16 Ibid., p. 238.

17 Johann Gottfried Herder, *Werke*, ed. B. Suphan (Berlin 1877–1913), vol. 8 (1892), p. 340.

18 Ibid., vol. 4, p. 127.

19 Gotthold Ephraim Lessing, *Ausgewählte Werke*, ed. Wolfgang Stammler, 3 vols. (Munich, n.d.), vol. 3, p. 124 [trans. JL].

20 Ibid., p. 131.

21 Johann Joachim Winckelmann, *Werke in einem Bande*, ed. Helmut Holtzhauer (Berlin and Weimar, 1976), p. 167; Eng. trans., as *History of Ancient Art*, trans. Henry Lodge (London, 1881) [trans. JL].

22 Ibid., p. 196.

23 Ibid., p. 194.

24 Ibid., p. 144.

25 Ibid., p. 194.

26 Quoted in *Historisches Wörterbuch der Philosophie*, vol. 1, col. 561.

27 Jean Paul, *Vorschule der Ästhetik*, ed. Norbert Miller (Munich, 1963), p. 22.

28 Immanuel Kant, *Critique of Judgment*, trans. Werner S. Pluhar (Indianapolis and Cambridge, 1987).

29 Georg Wilhelm Friedrich Hegel, *The Philosophy of Fine Art*, trans. F. P. B. Osmaston, 4 vols. (New York, 1975), vol. 1, p. 83.

30 Ibid., p. 86.

31 See Lothar Pikulik, *Leistungsethik contra Gefühlskult: über das Verhältnis von Bürgerlichkeit und Empfindsamkeit in Deutschland* (Göttingen, 1984), p. 215ff.

32 Ernst Platner, *Anthropologie für Ärzte und Weltweise* (Leipzig, 1772 [repr. Hildesheim, 1998]), p. 80.

33 Jörg Krämer, 'Auge und Ohr: Rezeptionsweisen im deutschen Musiktheater des späten 18. Jahrhunderts', in Erika Fischer-Lichte and Jörg Schönert (eds), *Theater im Kulturwandel des 18. Jahrhunderts* (Göttingen, 1999), pp. 109–32 (p. 131).

34 See Barbara Maria Stafford, *Body Criticism: Imaging the Unseen in Enlightenment Art and Medicine* (Cambridge, MA, 1991), p. 392ff.
35 Jean-Jacques Rousseau, *Confessions* (1783–90), rev. A. S. B Glover (New York, 1955), p. 361.
36 Jean-Jacques Rousseau, *Essai sur l'origine des langues*, ed. C. Porset (Bordeaux, 1968), pp. 175–7.
37 Julius Bernhard von Rohr, *Einleitung zur Ceremoniel-Wissenschafft der Privat-Personen* (Berlin, 1728 [repr. Weinheim, 1990]), p. 102.
38 Jean-Louis Flandrin, 'Der gute Geschmack und die soziale Hierarchie', in Philippe Ariès and Roger Chartier (eds), *Geschichte des privaten Lebens* (Frankfurt am Main, 1991), vol. 3 (*Von der Renaissance zur Aufklärung*), pp. 269–312 (p. 291).
39 Voltaire, *Dictionnaire philosophique* (Paris, 1826), vol. 5, p. 398 [trans. JL].
40 Hans Robert Jauss, 'Ästhetische Normen und geschichtliche Reflexion der "Querelle des Anciens et des Modernes"', in *Charles Perrault, Parallèle des Anciens et des Modernes*, ed. Hans Robert Jauss (Munich, 1964), pp. 8–64 (p. 25).
41 Quoted in Ute Frackowiak, *Der gute Geschmack: Studien zur Entwicklung des Geschmacksbegriffs* (Munich, 1991), p. 191.
42 Quoted ibid., p. 193.
43 Quoted ibid., p. 203.
44 Quoted ibid., p. 212.
45 Eva Barlösius, 'Soziale und historische Aspekte der deutschen Küche', postscript to the German edn of Stephen Mennell, *Die Kultivierung des Appetits: die Geschichte des Essens vom Mittelalter bis heute*, trans. Rainer von Savigny (Frankfurt am Main, 1988) [orig. pubd as *All Manners of Food*, Oxford, 1985].
46 Jean-Anthelme Brillat-Savarin, *The Physiology of Taste*, trans. M. F. K. Fisher (New York, 1949), p. 163.
47 See Michel Onfray, 'Der Uterus, die Trüffel und der Philosoph', in Kunst- und Ausstellungshalle der Bundesrepublik Deutschland (ed.), *Geschmacksache* (Göttingen, 1996), pp. 112–39.

CHAPTER 8   THE EDUCATION OF THE SENSES

1 Thomas Adams, *The Workes: Being the Summe of his Sermones, Meditations, and Other Divine, and Morall Discourses* (London, 1629), p. 149.
2 Ignatius von Loyola, *Briefe und Unterweisung*, ed. Peter Knauer (Würzburg, 1993), p. 923 [trans. JL].

3 Ignatius of Loyola, *The Spiritual Exercises*, trans. Louis J. Puhl, SJ (New York, 2000). See also Hugo Rahner, *Ignatius von Loyola als Mensch und Theologe* (Freiburg/Breisgau, 1964), p. 344ff.

4 Joseph Maskell, *The Five Senses: God's Gift and Man's Responsibility: Addresses to Children* (London, 1888), p. 15.

5 Ibid., pp. 16–17.

6 Jean-Jacques Rousseau, *Emile, or Education*, trans. Barbara Foxley (London and New York, 1911), p. 193.

7 Ibid., p. 97.

8 Quoted by Peter Utz, *Das Auge und das Ohr im Text: literarische Sinneswahrnehmung in der Goethezeit* (Munich, 1990), p. 34.

9 Quoted by Katharina Rutschky (ed.), *Schwarze Pädagogik: Quellen zur Naturgeschichte der bürgerlichen Erziehung* (Frankfurt am Main, Berlin and Vienna, 1977), p. 337.

10 Carl Friedrich von Rumohr, *Schule der Höflichkeit für Alt und Jung* (Stuttgart and Tübingen, 1834), p. 25.

11 Quoted by Rutschky, *Schwarze Pädagogik*, p. 465.

12 Ibid., p. 241.

13 Carl Ernst Bock, *Kleine Gesundheitslehre*, 7th edn (Leipzig, 1890), p. 73.

14 S. A. Tissot, *Onanism*, ed. Randolph Trumbach (New York and London, 1985), p. 21. See also Ludger Lütkehaus, 'O Wollust, o Hölle': die Onanie: Stationen einer Inquisition (Frankfurt am Main, 1992), p. 175.

15 Ludwig Friedrich Froriep, *Über die Isolierung der Sinne als Basis eines neuen Systems der Isolierung der Strafgefangenen* (Weimar, 1846), p. 12.

16 Ibid., p. 23.

17 See Michael Ignatieff, *A Just Measure of Pain: The Penitentiary in the Industrial Revolution 1750–1850* (Harmondsworth, 1989), p. 5, and the illustration opposite p. 82.

18 Michel Foucault, *Discipline and Punish: The Birth of the Prison*, trans. Alan Sheridan (Harmondsworth, 1979), p. 171.

19 Marie-Anne Berr, *Technik und Körper* (Berlin, 1990), p. 49.

20 Martin Illi, *Von der Schîssgruob zur modernen Stadtentwässerung* (Zurich, 1987), p. 64.

21 Peter Reinhart Gleichmann, 'Die Verhäuslichung körperlicher Verrichtungen', in Peter Reinhart Gleichmann, Johan Goudsblom and Hermann Korte (eds), *Materialien zu Norbert Elias' Zivilisationstheorie* (Frankfurt am Main, 1979), pp. 254–78.

22 Quoted by Michael Hagner, 'Sinnlichkeit und Sittlichkeit: Spinozas "grenzenlose Uneigennützigkeit" und Johannes Müllers Entwurf einer Sinnespsychologie', in Michael Hagner and Bettina Wahrig-Schmidt (eds), *Johannnes Müller und die Philosophie* (Berlin, 1992), pp. 29–44 (p. 38).

23 Rumohr, *Schule der Höflichkeit*, p. 36.
24 August Schulze, *Die Regeln des äußern Anstandes oder die Kunst, sich im geselligen Leben mit Anstand und Anmuth zu bewegen* (Naumburg, 1857), p. 20.
25 See Joan Burbick, *Healing the Republic: The Language of Health and the Culture of Nationalism in Nineteenth-Century America* (Cambridge, 1994), p. 267.
26 Christian August Struve, *Der Gesundheitsfreund der Jugend, oder Praktische Anweisung, wie man in der Jugend den Grund zu einer dauerhaften Gesundheit erhalten könne* (Hannover, 1804), p. 183.
27 Tissot, *Onanism*, p. 29.
28 See Lütkehaus, 'O Wollust, o Hölle', pp. 203, 207.
29 John Baptist de la Salle, *The Rules of Christian Decorum and Civility*, trans. Richard Arnandez (Romeoville, IL, 1990), p. 45.
30 Abraham a Santa Clara, *In der Arche waren nicht nur Tauben*, ed. and introd. Franz Georg Brugsti (Stuttgart, 1988), p. 48.
31 *The Christian Physiologist: Tales Illustrative of the Five Senses: Their Mechanism, Uses, and Government . . .* (London, 1830).
32 Maskell, *The Five Senses*, p. 15.
33 Ibid., p. 26.
34 Johann Amos Comenius, *Informatorium Maternum: der Mutter Schul . . .* (Nuremberg, 1636 [repr. Leipzig, 1987]), p. 119.
35 Rousseau, *Emile*, pp. 112–13.
36 Quoted in Günter Henner, *Quellen zur Geschichte der Gesundheitspädagogik* (Würzburg, 1998), p. 159.
37 Quoted in Karl-Heinz Göttert, *Geschichte der Stimme* (Munich, 1998), p. 379.
38 Quoted in Hubert Gottfried Heilemann, 'Goethe: eine Krankengeschichte und kritische Darstellung der pathographischen Literatur' (MD dissertation, Freie Universität Berlin, 1989), p. 68.
39 Arthur Schopenhauer, *Die Welt als Wille und Vorstellung* (Zurich, 1977), vol. 2, p. 41 [trans. JL].
40 Quoted by Rutschky, *Schwarze Pädagogik*, p. 215.
41 Quoted by Lothar Machtan, 'Zum Innenleben deutscher Fabriken im 19. Jahrhundert', *Archiv für Sozialgeschichte* 21 (1981), pp. 179–236 (p. 200).
42 Dietmar Kamper and Christoph Wulf (eds), *Das Schwinden der Sinne* (Frankfurt am Main, 1984), p. 13. See also Eva Barlösius, 'Riechen und Schmecken – Riechendes und Schmeckendes', *Kölner Zeitschrift für Soziologie und Sozialpsychologie* 39 (1987), pp. 367–75 (p. 368).
43 Rousseau, *Emile*, p. 122.
44 Quoted by Rutschky, *Schwarze Pädagogik*, p. 467.
45 Bock, *Kleine Gesundheitslehre*, p. 76.

46 Illi, *Von der Schîssgruob zur modernen Stadtentwässerung*, p. 103. For the measures adopted against smells by other municipalities, see Gleichmann, 'Die Verhäuslichung körperlicher Verrichtungen'.

47 Quoted in Corinna Wernz, *Sexualität als Krankheit: der medizinische Diskurs zur Sexualität um 1800* (Stuttgart, 1993), p. 119.

48 Quoted by Stephen Mennell, *All Manners of Food: Eating and Taste in England and France from the Middle Ages to the Present* (Oxford, 1985), p. 126.

49 Friedrich Engels, *The Condition of the Working Class in England*, trans. Institute of Marxism-Leninism, Moscow, ed. E. J. Hobsbawm (London, 1969), p. 103.

50 Mennell, *All Manners of Food*, p. 214.

51 Rousseau, *Emile*, p. 118.

52 Quoted by Rutschky, *Schwarze Pädagogik*, p. 357.

53 Quoted by Jean-Louis Flandrin, 'Der gute Geschmack und die soziale Hierarchie', in Philippe Ariès and Roger Chartier (eds), *Geschichte des privaten Lebens* (Frankfurt am Main, 1991), vol. 3, p. 294.

54 Quoted by Peter Albrecht, 'Kaffeetrinken: dem Bürger zur Ehr' – dem Armen zur Schand', in Rudolf Vierhaus (ed.), *Das Volk als Objekt obrigkeitlichen Handelns* (Tübingen, 1992), pp. 57–100 (p. 89).

55 Sidney W. Mintz, *Sweetness and Power: The Place of Sugar in Modern History* (Harmondsworth, 1986), p. 214. See also Roman Sandgruber, *Bittersüße Genüsse: Kulturgeschichte der Genußmittel* (Vienna, Cologne and Graz, 1986); Hans Jürgen Teuteberg, 'Prolegomena zu einer Kulturpsychologie des Geschmacks', in Alois Wierlacher, Gerhard Neumann and Hans Jürgen Teuteberg (eds), *Kulturthema Essen: Ansichten und Problemfelder* (Berlin, 1993), pp. 103–36.

56 See Rutschky, *Schwarze Pädagogik*, p. 462.

57 See Roy Porter, 'The rise of physical examination', in William F. Bynum and Roy Porter (eds), *Medicine and the Five Senses* (Cambridge, 1993), pp. 179–97 (p. 187).

58 Quoted by Martin Beutelspacher, *Kultivierung bei lebendigem Leib: alltägliche Körpererfahrungen in der Aufklärung* (Weingarten, 1986), p. 98 [trans. JL].

59 Quoted by Susan C. Lawrence, 'Educating the senses: students, teachers and medical rhetoric in eighteenth-century London', in William F. Bynum and Roy Porter (eds), *Medicine and the Five Senses* (Cambridge, 1993), pp. 154–78 (p. 172).

60 Leopold von Auenbrugger, *Neue Erfindung, mittelst Anschlagens an den Brustkorb, als eines Zeichens, verborgene Brustkrankheiten zu entdecken* (1761), trans. and introd. V. Fossel (Leipzig, 1912), p. 1 [trans. JL].

61 Beutelspacher, *Kultivierung bei lebendigem Leib*, p. 28.
62 Louis-Sébastien Mercier, *The Waiting City: Paris 1782–88*, trans. Helen Simpson (London, 1933).
63 Julius Bernhard von Rohr, *Einleitung zur Ceremoniel-Wissenschafft der Privat-Personen* (Berlin, 1728 [repr. Weinheim, 1990]), p. 360.
64 J. Lehmann, *Die Regeln des Anstands, der Höflichkeit und der guten Sitte: für die deutschen Knaben- und Mädchenschulen in den Vereinigten Staaten von Amerika* (St Louis, 1867), p. 9.
65 Hasso Spode, *Die Macht der Trunkenheit: Kultur- und Sozialgeschichte des Alkohols in Deutschland* (Opladen, 1993), p. 28.
66 Ibid., p. 36.
67 Norbert Elias, *The Civilizing Process*, trans. Edmund Jephcott, 2 vols. (Oxford, 1978), vol. 1, p. 128.
68 Richard Sennett, *Flesh and Stone: The City in Western Civilization* (London, 1994), p. 23.
69 Quoted by Leo Schidrowitz, *Sittengeschichte der Liebkosung und Strafe: die Zärtlichkeitsworte, Gesten und Handlungen der Kulturmenschheit und ihr Gegenpol, die Strenge* (Vienna and Leipzig, 1928), p. 128.
70 Quoted by Hans Peter Duerr, *Der erotische Leib: der Mythos vom Zivilisationsprozeß* (Frankfurt am Main, 1997), p. 432, n. 13.
71 Rumohr, *Schule der Höflichkeit*, p. 25.

CHAPTER 9   THE TRANSFORMATION OF THE SENSES BY
INDUSTRIALIZATION AND TECHNOLOGY

1 Philipp Richter, *Ein Bauernleben*, 2nd edn, rev. and ed. Helmut Müller (Rheda-Wiedenbrück, 1991), pp. 41–2.
2 Walter Asmus, 'Nähe, Ferne, Geschwindigkeit: Wandlungen des Zeit-Raum-Empfindens im 19. Jahrhundert an Beispielen aus Schleswig-Holstein', in Martin Rheinsheimer (ed.), *Subjektive Welten: Wahrnehmung und Identität in der Neuzeit* (Neumünster, 1998), pp. 321–54 (p. 346).
3 Quoted by Martin Illi, *Von der Schîssgruob zur modernen Stadtent-wässerung* (Zurich, 1987), p. 72.
4 Quoted in Beatrix Mesmer (ed.), *Die Verwissenschaftlichung des Alltags: Anweisungen zum richtigen Umgang mit dem Körper in der schweizerischen Populärpresse 1850–1900* (Zurich, 1997), p. 233.
5 Théodore Vannod, *La fatigue intellectuelle et son influence sur la sensibilité cutanée* (Geneva, 1896), p. 15ff.
6 These statistics are taken from Theodor Weyl (ed.), *Handbuch der Arbeiterkrankheiten* (Jena, 1908), pp. i–lxix (pp. xxxii, xxxix).

7 Quoted in Christoph Hohmann, *Arbeitsmedizin und Umwelthygiene in der Gewerbeordnung des Norddeutschen Bundes vom 21. 06. 1869* (Düsseldorf, 1996), p. 122.

8 Sigmund Freud, *Standard Edition* (London, 1953–), vol. 9, pp. 183–4.

9 Willy Hellpach, *Mensch und Volk der Großstadt*, 2nd rev. edn (Stuttgart, 1952), p. 71.

10 Ibid., p. 69f.

11 Theodor Ziehen, 'Neurasthenie', in *Real-Encyclopädie der gesammten Heilkunde*, vol. 17 (Vienna and Leipzig, 1898), pp. 25–101 (p. 34). See also Joachim Radkau, *Das Zeitalter der Nervosität: Deutschland zwischen Bismarck und Hitler* (Munich, 1998), p. 174ff.

12 Karl Marx, *Capital*, Karl Marx–Friedrich Engels Gesamtausgabe (MEGA) (Berlin, 1990), pt II, vol. 9 [1], p. 369.

13 Ibid., p. 326.

14 See Thomas L. Hankins, *Instruments and the Imagination* (Princeton, 1995), p. 225.

15 Martin Jay, 'Scopic regimes of modernity', in Nicholas Mirzoeff (ed.), *Visual Culture Reader* (London and New York, 1998), pp. 66–9. See also David Michael Levin (ed.), *Modernity and the Hegemony of Vision* (Berkeley, 1993); Barabara Duden and Ivan Illich, 'Die skopische Vergangenheit Europas und die Ethik der Opsis: Plädoyer für eine Geschichte des Blickes und Blickens', *Historische Anthropologie* 3 (1995), pp. 203–21.

16 See David Howes and Marc Lalonde, 'The history of sensibilities: of the standards of taste in mid-eighteenth century England and the circulation of smells in post-revolutionary France', *Dialectical Anthropology* 16 (1992), pp. 125–35 (p. 132).

17 Quoted in Gudrun M. König, *Eine Kulturgeschichte des Spazierganges: Spuren einer bürgerlichen Praktik 1780–1850* (Vienna, 1996), p. 315.

18 See Clemens Alexander Wimmer, *Geschichte der Gartentheorie* (Darmstadt, 1989), p. 463.

19 *The Works of John Ruskin* (Cambridge, 1996), vol. 37, p. 153 [CD-ROM].

20 Carl Friedrich von Rumohr, *Schule der Höflichkeit für Alt und Jung* (Stuttgart and Tübingen, 1834), p. 39.

21 Georg Simmel, *Soziologie: Untersuchungen über die Formen der Vergesellschaftung*, ed. Otthein Rammstedt (Frankfurt am Main, 1992), p. 727.

22 *Zedlers Universal-Lexicon*, vol. 9 (1735), col. 591.

23 Quoted in Barbara Maria Stafford, *Body Criticism: Imaging the Unseen in Enlightenment Art and Medicine* (Cambridge, MA, 1991), p. 345.

24 *Zedlers Universal-Lexicon*, vol. 47 (1746), col. 766.

25 Quoted in H. Meyer and R. Suntrup, *Lexikon der mittelalterlichen Zahlenbedeutungen* (Munich, 1987), p. 45.

26 *Zedlers Universal-Lexicon*, vol. 47 (1746), col. 764.

27 Jonathan Crary, *Techniques of the Observer: On Vision and Modernity in the Nineteenth Century* (Cambridge, MA, and London, 1990), p. 39.

28 *Zedlers Universal-Lexicon*, vol. 16 (1737), col. 890.

29 Quoted in Friedrich von Zglinicki, *Der Weg des Films: die Geschichte der Kinematographie und ihrer Vorläufer* (Berlin, 1956), p. 86.

30 H. K. Browne, *Illustrations of the Five Senses* (London, 1852), illustration 1.

31 Crary, *Techniques of the Observer*, p. 98.

32 Hermann von Helmholtz, *Handbook of Physiological Optics*, 3 vols., trans. George T. Ladd (New York, 1962), vol. 3, p. 303.

33 Crary, *Techniques of the Observer*, p. 128.

34 See Heinz Buddemeier, *Panorama, Diorama, Photographie: Entstehung und Wirkung neuer Medien im 19. Jahrhundert* (Munich, 1970), p. 15ff.

35 Stephan Oettermann, 'Das Panorama – ein Massenmedium', in KABD, *Sehsucht: über die Veränderung der visuellen Wahrnehmung* (Göttingen, 1995), p. 79.

36 Quoted by Zglinicki, *Der Weg des Films*, p. 105 [trans. JL].

37 Quoted ibid., p. 144.

38 Quoted by Robert Castel, 'Bilder und Phantasiebilder', in Pierre Bourdieu et al., *Eine illegitime Kunst: die sozialen Gebrauchsweisen der Photographie*, trans. Udo Rennert (Frankfurt am Main, 1981), pp. 235–66 (p. 235).

39 Pierre Bourdieu, Luc Boltanski, Robert Castel et al., *Photography: A Middle-brow Art*, trans. Shaun Whiteside (Cambridge, 1990), p. 76.

40 Oliver Wendell Holmes, 'Stereoscope and the stereograph', in *Atlantic Monthly* (1859), pp. 738–48.

41 Daniel Breazeale, trans. and ed., *Philosophy and Truth: Selections from Nietzsche's Notebooks of the Early 1870s* (Atlantic Highlands, NJ, 1979), p. 80.

42 Wolfgang Schivelbusch, *Geschichte der Eisenbahnreise: zur Industrialisierung von Raum und Zeit* (Frankfurt am Main, 1979), p. 58ff.

43 Quoted in Klaus Beyer, *Die Postkutschenreise* (Tübingen, 1985), p. 248.

44 Quoted in Asmus, 'Nähe, Ferne, Geschwindigkeit', p. 335.

45 Anne Friedberg, *Window Shopping: Cinema and the Postmodern* (Berkeley, 1993), p. 57.

46 See Griselda Pollock, 'Modernity and the spaces of femininity', in Nicholas Mirzoeff (ed.), *The Visual Culture Reader* (London and New York, 1998), pp. 74–84 (p. 74ff.).

47 Walter Benjamin, *Illuminationen* (Frankfurt am Main, 1977), p. 248 [trans. JL]. The Berlin of this period is described by Peter Fritzsche in *Reading Berlin 1900* (Cambridge, MA, and London, 1996).

48 Michel Foucault, *The Birth of the Clinic*, trans. A. M. Sheridan Smith (New York, 1975), p. 115.

49 Ibid., p. 120.

50 Jörn Henning Wolf, 'Der Arzt und sein Spiegel', in Christa Habrich et al. (eds), *Medizinische Diagnostik in Geschichte und Gegenwart: Festschrift für Heinz Goerke zum 60. Geburtstag* (Munich, 1978), pp. 477–516 (p. 498).

51 Quoted by Jan Brügelmann, 'Der Blick des Arztes auf die Krankheit im Alltag 1779–1850' (PhD dissertation, Berlin, 1982), p. 29.

52 Quoted in Thomas Kleinspehn, *Der flüchtige Blick: Sehen und Identität in der Kultur der Neuzeit* (Reinbek, 1989), p. 255f.

53 Figures cited by [F.] Walther, 'Gewerbliche Augenerkrankungen', in *Handbuch der Arbeiterkrankheiten*, ed. Theodor Weyl (Jena, 1908), pp. 657–740 (p. 701ff.).

54 Figures cited by [?] Baumeister, in 'Über die zum Dienste in der Armee erforderliche Sehschärfe', *Klinisches Monatsblatt für Augenheilkunde* 13 (1875), pp. 504–12 (p. 506ff.).

55 Andreas Fischer, 'Okkulte Fotografie', in *Im Reich der Phantome: Fotografie des Unsichtbaren*, exhibition catalogue (Ostfildern, 1997), pp. 27–103 (p. 99).

56 Quoted by Richard Birkefeld and Martina Jung, in *Die Stadt, der Lärm und das Licht: die Veränderung des öffentlichen Raumes durch Motorisierung und Elektrifizierung* (Seelze, 1994), p. 9.

57 Quoted in Matthias Lentz, ' "Ruhe ist die erste Bürgerpflicht": Lärm, Großstadt und Nervosität im Spiegel von Theodor Lessings "Antilärmverein" ', *Medizin, Gesellschaft und Geschichte* 13 (1995), pp. 81–106 (p. 91).

58 Adolf Levenstein, *Die Arbeiterfrage: mit besonderer Berücksichtigung der sozialpsychologischen Seite des modernen Großbetriebes und der psychologischen Einwirkungen auf die Arbeiter* (Munich, 1912), p. 77.

59 Quoted by Siegfried Krömer, 'Lärm als medizinisches Problem im 19. Jahrhundert' (MD dissertation, Mainz, 1981), p. 28.

60 Edward Shorter, *Moderne Leiden: zur Geschichte der psychosomatischen Krankheiten* (Reinbek, 1994), p. 467f.

61 Quoted by Klaus Saul, 'Wider die "Lärmpest": Lärmkritik und Lärmbekämpfung im Deutschen Kaiserreich', in Ditmar Machule, Olaf Mischer and Arnold Sywottek (eds), *Macht Stadt krank? Vom Umgang mit Gesundheit und Krankheit* (Hamburg, 1996), pp. 151–92 (p. 154).

Notes to pp. 205–14

62 Arthur Schopenhauer, 'Über Lerm und Geräusch', in *Werke*, ed. Arthur Hübscher (Zurich, 1977), vol. 10, pp. 697–701 (p. 698).
63 *The Diaries of Franz Kafka*, ed. Max Brod, trans. Joseph Kresh and Martin Greenberg (London, 1992), p. 104.
64 Quoted by Saul, in 'Wider die "Lärmpest"', p. 168.
65 Alain Corbin, *Village Bells: Sound and Meaning in the Nineteenth-Century French Countryside*, trans. Martin Thom (London, 1999), p. 292.
66 Quoted by Michael Stolberg, *Ein Recht auf saubere Luft? Umweltkonflikte am Beginn des Industriezeitalters* (Erlangen, 1994), p. 23.
67 Quoted in Marianne Rodenstein, *'Mehr Licht, mehr Luft': Gesundheitskonzepte im Städtebau seit 1750* (Frankfurt am Main and New York, 1988), p. 103.
68 Paul Niemeyer, *Aerztliche Sprechstunden: Gesundheitslehre für jedermann* (Jena, 1878), vol. 1, p. 189.
69 Gerd Spelsberg, *Rauchplage: hundert Jahre Saurer Regen* (Aachen, 1984), p. 38.
70 Quoted in Ulrike Gilhaus, *'Schmerzenskinder der Industrie': Umweltverschmutzung, Umweltpolitik und sozialer Protest im Industriezeitalter in Westfalen 1845–1914* (Paderborn, 1995), p. 485.
71 Quoted by Illi, *Von der Schîssgruob zur modernen Stadtentwässerung*, p. 76.
72 Quoted by Gerd Göckenjan, *Kurien und Staat machen: Gesundheit und Medizin in der bürgerlichen Welt* (Frankfurt am Main, 1985), p. 114.
73 See Artur Kutzelnigg, 'Die Verarmung des Geruchswortschatzes seit dem Mittelalter', *Muttersprache* 94 (1983–4), pp. 328–46 (p. 340).
74 Eva Barlösius, 'Riechen und Schmecken – Riechendes und Schmeckendes', *Kölner Zeitschrift für Soziologie und Sozialpsychologie* 39 (1987), pp. 367–75 (p. 374f.).
75 P. Rullier, 'Geschmacksinn', in *Encyclopädie der medicinischen Wissenschaften nach dem Dictionnaire de médecine*, ed. Friedrich Ludwig Meissner, vol. 5 (Leipzig, 1831), pp. 305–9 (p. 308).
76 Quoted by Hasso Spode, *Die Macht der Trunkenheit* (Opladen, 1993), p. 155.
77 Quoted by Michael Grüttner, 'Alkoholkonsum in der Arbeiterschaft 1871–1939', in Toni Pierenkemper (ed.), *Haushalt und Verbrauch in historischer Perspektive: zum Wandel des privaten Verbrauchs in Deutschland im 19. und 20. Jahrhundert* (St Katharinen, 1987), pp. 229–73 (p. 240).
78 Hans Jürgen Teuteberg and Günter Wiegelmann, *Unsere tägliche Kost: Geschichte und regionale Prägung*, 2nd edn (Münster, 1988), p. 194.
79 Ibid., p. 213.

80 Johann Beckmann, *Beyträge zu einer Geschichte der Erfindungen*, pt 5 (Leipzig, 1805), p. 109.
81 Teuteberg and Wiegelmann, *Unsere tägliche Kost*, p. 149. See also Hans Medick, 'Süße und bittere Seiten der Weltgeschichte des Zuckers', *Geschichtswerkstatt* 12 (1987), pp. 8–19.
82 See Kirsten Schlegel-Matthies, 'Anfänge der modernen Lebens- und Genußmittelwerbung: Produkte und Konsumgruppen im Spiegel von Zeitschriftenannoncen', in Hans Jürgen Teuteberg (ed.), *Durchbruch zum modernen Massenkonsum: Lebensmittelmärkte und Lebensmittelqualität im Städtewachstum des Industriezeitalters* (Münster, 1987), pp. 277–308 (p. 279).
83 See Karl-Peter Ellerbrock, *Geschichte der deutschen Nahrungs- und Genußmittelindustrie 1750–1914* (Stuttgart, 1993).
84 Quoted in Hans Jürgen Teuteberg, *Die Rolle des Fleischextrakts für die Ernährungswissenschaften und den Aufstieg der Suppenindustrie* (Stuttgart, 1990), p. 44.
85 P. Rullier, 'Tastsinn', in *Encyclopädie der medicinischen Wissenschaften nach dem Dictionnaire de médecine*, ed. Friedrich Ludwig Meissner, vol. 12 (Leipzig, 1833), pp. 13–16 (p. 15).
86 Michael Giesecke, *Sinnenwandel, Sprachwandel, Kulturwandel: Studien zur Vorgeschichte der Informationsgesellschaft* (Frankfurt am Main, 1992), p. 224.
87 Rudolf Spitzer, 'Geographische Verteilung der Hautkrankheiten', in *Verschlemmte Welt: Essen und Trinken historisch-anthropologisch*, ed. Alexander Schuller and Jutta Anna Kleber (Göttingen, 1994), pp. 253–328 (p. 317f.).

CHAPTER 10   EXPERIMENTAL PHYSIOLOGY AND THE
SEPARATION OF THE SENSES

1 Rudolf Virchow, *Johannes Müller: eine Gedächtnisrede* (Berlin, 1858), p. 24.
2 Quoted by Martin Müller, 'Über philosophische Anschauungen des Naturforschers Johannes Müller', *Archiv für Geschichte der Medizin* 28 (1926), pp. 130–50, 209–34, 328–50 (p. 222).
3 Hermann von Helmholtz, *On the Sensations of Tone*, trans. Alexander Ellis (New York, 1954).
4 Karl Marx and Friedrich Engels, *Collected Works* (London, 1974–), vol. 3, p. 301.
5 See Edwin G. Boring, *Sensation and Perception in the History of Experimental Psychology* (New York, 1977), p. 10.

6 Quoted by Ernst Florey, 'Sinnesenergie, spezifische', in *Historisches Wörterbuch der Philosophie*, vol. 9 (Darmstadt, 1995), cols. 882–6.

7 Dieter Hoffmann-Axthelm, *Sinnesarbeit: Nachdenken über Wahrnehmung* (Frankfurt am Main and New York, 1984), p. 49.

8 A. Rollet, 'Muskel (physiologisch)', in *Real-Encyclopädie der gesammten Heilkunde*, vol. 16 (Vienna and Leipzig, 1898), pp. 175–244 (p. 234).

9 Quoted in Karl E. Rothschuh, *Physiologie: der Wandel ihrer Konzepte, Probleme, Methoden vom 16. bis 19. Jahrhundert* (Freiburg and Munich, 1968), p. 229. Some of these instruments are illustrated in Nicola Lepp, Martin Roth and Klaus Vogel (eds), *Der Neue Mensch: Obsessionen des 20. Jahrhunderts: Katalog zur Ausstellung im Deutschen Hygienemuseum Dresden 22. 4.–8. 8. 1999* (Ostfildern-Ruit, 1999), p. 210ff.

10 Jutta Schikore, ' "Worauf die Strahlen der sichtbaren Gegenstände wirken": mikroskopische Anatomie der Retina 1834–1841', *Medizinhistorisches Journal* 34 (1999), pp. 139–57 (p. 139f.).

11 Georg Elias Müller, *Zur Grundlegung der Psychophysik* (Berlin, 1878), p. 10.

12 Quoted in Timothy Lenoir, 'Das Auge des Physiologen: zur Entstehungsgeschichte von Helmholtz' Theorie des Sehens', in Philipp Sarasin and Jakob Tanner (eds), *Physiologie und industrielle Gesellschaft: Studien zur Verwissenschaftlichung des Körpers im 19. und 20. Jahrhundert* (Frankfurt am Main, 1998), pp. 99–128 (p. 104).

13 Ibid., p. 105.

14 Hermann von Helmholtz, *Treatise on Physiological Optics*, ed. J. P. C. Southall (Bristol 2000), vol. 2, p. 103.

15 See Steven R. Turner, *In the Eye's Mind: Vision and the Helmholtz–Hering Controversy* (Princeton, 1994).

16 Otto-Joachim Grüsser, 'Hermann von Helmholtz und die Physiologie des Sehvorganges', in Wolfgang U. Eckart and Klaus Volkert (eds), *Hermann Helmholtz* (Pfaffenweiler, 1996), pp. 119–76 (p. 147).

17 Quoted by Otto-Joachim Grüsser, *Justinus Kerner 1786–1862: Arzt – Poet – Geisterseher* (Berlin, 1987), p. 69.

18 Adam Politzer, *Geschichte der Ohrenheilkunde*, 2 vols., with an introduction by K. E. Rothschuh (Hildesheim, 1967), vol. 1, p. 425.

19 Ibid., vol. 2, p. 45.

20 Hippolyte Cloquet, *Ophrésiologie: ou, Traité des odeurs, du sens et des organs de l'olfaction: avec l'histoire détailée des maladies du nez et des fosses nasals, et des opérations qui leur conviennent* (Paris, 1820) [trans. JL].

21 Ibid., p. 173.

22 See Klaus Seifert, 'Geschichte und Bibliographie der Erforschung des peripheren Geruchsorgans', *Clio Medica* 4 (1969), pp. 303–37 (p. 309f.).

23 Quoted by Elisabeth Kaufmann, in *Gustav Jäger 1832–1917: Arzt, Zoologe und Hygieniker* (Zurich, 1984), p. 31.

24 Ibid.

25 Quoted by Heinrich Weinreich, in *Duftstofftheorie: Gustav Jaeger (1832–1917): vom Biologen zum 'Seelenriecher'* (Stuttgart, 1993), p. 196.

26 Wilhelm Horn, *Über den Geschmackssinn des Menschen: ein Beitrag zur Physiologie desselben* (Heidelberg, 1825), p. 83f.

27 Ernst Heinrich Weber, *Tastsinn und Gemeingefühl*, ed. Ewald Hering (Leipzig, 1905), p. 1.

28 Ibid., p. 10f.

29 See Ursula Bueck-Rich, *Ernst Heinrich Weber (1795–1878) und der Anfang einer Physiologie der Hautsinne* (Zurich, 1970); Edwin G. Boring, *Sensation and Perception in the History of Experimental Psychology* (New York, 1977).

30 Quoted by Peter Becker, 'Die Rezeption der Physiologie in der Kriminalistik und Kriminologie: Variationen über Norm und Ausgrenzung', in Jakob Tanner and Philipp Sarasin (eds), *Physiologie und industrielle Gesellschaft: Studien zur Verwissenschaftlichung des Körpers im 19. und 20. Jahrhundert* (Frankfurt am Main, 1998), pp. 453–90 (p. 473).

CHAPTER 11   TOUCHING – OR THE NEW PLEASURE
IN THE BODY

1 Hermann Friedmann, *Die Welt der Formen: System eines morphologischen Idealismus*, 2nd rev. and expanded edn (Munich, 1930), p. 33.

2 Geza Révész, *Die Formenwelt des Tastsinnes* (The Hague, 1938), and *Die menschliche Hand: eine psychologische Studie* (Basel and New York, 1944).

3 Jean Baudrillard, *The System of Objects*, trans. James Benedict (London and New York, 1996), p. 53.

4 See Helmut Milz, *Der wiederentdeckte Körper: vom schöpferischen Umgang mit sich selbst* (Munich, 1994), p. 28.

5 Derrick de Kerckhove, 'Touch versus Vision: Ästhetik neuer Technologien', in Wolfgang Welsch (ed.), *Die Aktualität des Ästhetischen* (Munich, 1993), pp. 135–68 (p. 148).

6 Quoted by Hans-Dieter Hentschel, 'Über die Massage in ihren Anfängen', *Physikalische Therapie in Theorie und Praxis* 7 (1986), pp. 506–9 (p. 505) [trans. JL].

7 Alan Switzer et al., 'Die Rolle des Körpers in der Feeling Therapy', in Hilarion G. Petzold (ed.), *Die neuen Körpertherapien* (Paderborn, 1977), pp. 376–87 (p. 378).

8 Ibid., p. 379.
9 Quoted in Georg Hünerfauth, *Handbuch der Massage* (Leipzig, 1877), p. 22.
10 Friedrich Eduard Bilz, *Das neue Naturheilverfahren* [jubilee edn], 2 vols. (Leipzig, 1902), vol. 2, p. 1728.
11 Sabine Ruth Welti, *Massage und Heilgymnastik in der ersten Hälfte des 20. Jahrhunderts* (Bern, 1997), p. 58.
12 H. Ernst, *Die Ehre des Weibes und die Thure-Brandt'sche Massage: ein Mahnwort an alle Männer zum Schutze unserer Frauen und Töchter* (Leipzig, n.d.), p. 57.
13 Ibid., p. 58.
14 Quoted in Rachel P. Maines, *The Technology of Orgasm: 'Hysteria', the Vibrator and Women's Sexual Satisfaction* (Baltimore and London, 1999), p. 103.
15 M. Platen, *Die neue Heilmethode: Lehrbuch der naturgemäßen Lebensweise, der Gesundheitspflege und der naturgemäßen Heilweise* (Berlin, 1907), vol. 1, p. 807.
16 Novalis, *Schriften*, ed. Richard Samuel, vol. 3 (Darmstadt, 1968), p. 264.
17 See Liz Stanley, *Sex Surveyed, 1949–1994: From Mass Observation's 'Little Kinsey' to the National Survey and the Hite Reports* (London, 1995).
18 This and the following quotations are taken from *The Standard Edition of the Complete Works of Sigmund Freud*, trans. under the general editorship of James Strachey (London, 1953–66): vol. 7, pp. 233, 210, 150; vol. 18, p. 137; vol. 20, p. 132.
19 Leo Schidrowitz, *Sittengeschichte der Liebkosung und Strafe: die Zärtlichkeitsworte, Gesten und Handlungen der Kulturmenschheit und ihr Gegenpol, die Strenge* (Vienna and Leipzig, 1928), p. 58.
20 Iwan Bloch, *Das Sexualleben unserer Zeit in seinen Beziehungen zur modernen Kultur*, 12th rev. edn (Berlin, 1919), p. 32 [trans. JL].
21 Havelock Ellis, *Studies in the Psychology of Sex* (New York, 1936), vol. 2, p. 41.
22 See Stephen Thayer, 'Social touching', in William Schiff and Emerson Foulke (eds), *Tactual Perception: A Sourcebook* (Cambridge, 1982), pp. 263–304 (p. 283). See also Anthony Synnott, *The Body Social: Symbolism, Self and Society* (London and New York, 1993), p. 165ff.
23 Wilhelm Reich, *Die frühen Schriften*, ed. Mary Boyd Higgins and Chester M. Raphael, 2 vols. (Frankfurt am Main, 1983–5), vol. 2, p. 142 [trans. JL].
24 Wilhelm Reich, 'The therapeutic significance of genital libido', in Reich, *Early Writings*, trans. Philip Schmitz (New York, 1975), vol. 1, p. 217.

25 Johann C. Becker, *Der Rathgeber vor, bei und nach dem Beischlafe*, 6th edn (Reutlingen, 1816 [repr. Wiesbaden, 1993]), p. 76.

26 Promotional blurb on the back cover of Christine Unseld-Baumanns's *Partner-Massage: Streicheleinheiten für Körper und Seele* (Niederhausen/ Taunus, 1994).

27 Ulrich Stock, 'Bitte berühren!', *Die Zeit*, 8 November 1996, p. 76.

28 Willi Aeppli, *Sinnesorganismus, Sinnesverlust, Sinnespflege: die Sinnes-lehre Rudolf Steiners in ihrer Bedeutung für die Erziehung* (Stuttgart, 1996), p. 109.

CHAPTER 12   TASTING – OR WHAT DO FAST FOOD AND
NOUVELLE CUISINE HAVE IN COMMON?

1 Quoted in Eva Barlösius, *Soziologie des Essens: eine sozial- und kulturwis-senschaftliche Einführung in die Ernährungsforschung* (Weinheim and Munich, 1999), p. 86.

2 Nicolaus Hein, 'Hungern und sattes Leben: zur sozialen Modellierung von Ernährungsbedürfnissen', in Alexander Schuller and Jutta Anna Kleber (eds), *Verschlemmte Welt: Essen und Trinken historisch-anthropologisch* (Göttingen, 1994), pp. 89–102 (p. 90).

3 Ernst Günter Schenck, *Grundlagen und Vorschriften für die Regelung der Krankenernährung im Kriege* (Berlin and Vienna, 1940), p. 10.

4 Gustavo Corni and Horst Gies, *Brot, Butter, Kanonen: die Ernährungs-wirtschaft unter der Diktatur Hitlers* (Berlin, 1997), p. 572.

5 Quoted in Arne Andersen, *Der Traum vom guten Leben: Alltags- und Konsumgeschichte vom Wirtschaftswunder bis heute* (Frankfurt am Main, 1999), p. 36.

6 Michael Wildt, 'Die Zeichen des Geschmacks', *Geschichtswerkstatt* 12 (1987), pp. 43–8 (p. 47).

7 Quoted in Michael Wildt, 'Der Abschied von der "Freßwelle" oder: die Pluralisierung des Geschmacks: Essen in der Bundesrepublik Deutschland der fünfziger Jahre', in Alois Wierlacher, Gerhard Neumann and Hans Jürgen Teuteberg (eds), *Kulturthema Essen: Ansichten und Problemfelder* (Berlin, 1993), pp. 211–26 (p. 222).

8 See Gerda Bos et al., '85 jaar voedingsmiddelen advertenties in Neder-landse tijdschriften', in Annemarie de Knecht van Eekelen and Marian Stasse-Wolthuis (eds), *Voeding in onze semenleving, een cultuurhistorisch perspectief* (Alphen aan den Rijn and Brussels, 1987), pp. 135–9.

9 Pierre Bourdieu, *Distinction: A Social Critique of the Judgement of Taste* (London, 1984), p. 372.

10 Quoted in Stephen Mennell, *All Manners of Food* (Oxford, 1985), p. 326.

11 Jörg Maier and Gabi Troeger-Weiss, 'Kulinarische Fremdenverkehrs-
   und Freizeitkultur: Freizeittrends und Lebensstile in der Bundesrepublik
   Deutschland', in Alois Wierlacher et al. (eds), *Kulturthema Essen*,
   pp. 227–41 (p. 235).
12 Eva Barlösius, 'Riechen und Schmecken', *Kölner Zeitschrift für Soziologie
   und Sozialpsychologie* 39 (1987), p. 371.
13 Quoted in Karl Möckl, 'Die große deutsche Küche: Formen des
   Eßverhaltens seit den 1970er Jahren', in Wolfgang Protzner (ed.), *Vom
   Hungerwinter zum kulinarischen Schlaraffenland* (Wiesbaden, 1987),
   pp. 49–64 (p. 59).
14 Barlösius, *Soziologie des Essens*, p. 157.
15 Ibid., p. 160.
16 Quoted in Christoph Wagner, *Fast schon Food: die Geschichte des
   schnellen Essens* (Frankfurt am Main and New York, 1995), p. 170.
17 Quoted ibid., p. 198.
18 Barlösius, 'Riechen und Schmecken', p. 373.
19 See H[einz] Vetter et al., *Qualität pflanzlicher Nahrungsmittel* (Darmstadt,
   1983).

CHAPTER 13   SCENTING – OR FROM DEODORIZATION
             TO REODORIZATION

1 Annick Le Guérer, *Scent*, trans. R. Miller (London, 1993), p. 205.
2 Gerd Spelsberg, *Rauchplage: hundert Jahre saurer Regen* (Aachen, 1984),
  p. 75.
3 Quoted ibid., p. 152.
4 Quoted ibid., p. 211.
5 Quoted in Klaus-Georg Wey, *Umweltpolitik in Deutschland: kurze
  Geschichte des Umweltschutzes in Deutschland seit 1900* (Opladen,
  1982), p. 115.
6 Quoted ibid., p. 50.
7 Quoted ibid., p. 99.
8 Dietmar Klenke, 'Bundesdeutsche Verkehrspolitik und Umwelt: von
  der Motorisierungseuphorie zur ökologischen Katerstimmung', in
  Werner Abelshauser (ed.), *Umweltgeschichte: Umweltverträgliches
  Wirtschaften in historischer Perspektive* (Göttingen, 1994), pp. 163–89
  (p. 184).
9 Peter Payer, *Der Gestank von Wien* (Vienna, 1997), p. 13.
10 Georg Simmel, *Soziologie* (Frankfurt am Main, 1992), p. 736.
11 John M. Efron, 'Der reine und der schmutzige Jude', in Sander L. Gilman,
   Robert Jütte and Gabriele Kohlbauer-Fritz (eds), *'Der schejne Jid'*:

das Bild des *'jüdischen Körpers'* in *Mythos und Ritual* (Vienna, 1998), pp. 75–85 (p. 76).

12 Quoted in Robert Jay Lifton, *The Nazi Doctors: Medical Killing and the Psychology of Genocide* (New York, 1986), p. 319.

13 Ibid., p. 164.

14 Ibid., p. 197.

15 Mynona [Salomo Friedländer], *Rosa die schöne Schutzmannsfrau und andere Grotesken*, ed. Ellen Otten (Zurich, 1965), p. 20.

16 Martin Roth, Manfred Scheske and Hans-Christian Täubrich (eds), *In aller Munde: einhundert Jahre Odol* (Ostfildern-Ruit, 1993), p. 110.

17 Ibid., p. 155.

18 Ibid., p. 99.

19 Robert Walser, *Prosa-Stücke* (Berlin, 1978), p. 360.

20 Kurt Tucholsky, *Gesammelte Werke*, ed. Mary Gerold-Tucholsky and Fritz J. Raddatz, 10 vols. (Reinbek, 1975), vol. 9, p. 206.

21 Stephan J. Jellinek, 'Der Planet der Parfums im Sternbild der Düfte', in Kunst- und Ausstellungshalle der Bundesrepublik Deutschland (ed.), *Das Riechen: von Nasen, Düften und Gestank* (Göttingen, 1995), p. 128.

22 Anne Paech, 'Das Aroma des Kinos: Filme mit der Nase gesehen: vom Geruchsfilm und Düften und Lüften im Kino', <www.uni-konstanz.de/FuF/Philo/LitWiss/MedienWiss/Texte/duft.htm>.

23 Ibid., p. 2.

24 Quoted ibid., p. 5.

25 Werner Kühni-Ramisch, *Sanftes Heilen mit edlen Düften: ein praktisches Handbuch der Aromatherapie* (Heidelberg, 1993), p. 9.

26 Constance Classen, *Worlds of Sense: Exploring the Senses in History and Across Cultures* (London and New York, 1993), p. 35.

CHAPTER 14   LISTENING EFFECTS – OR THE ART AND
POWER OF NOISES

1 Luigi Russolo, *The Art of Noises*, trans. with an introduction by Barclay Brown (New York, 1986), p. 28.

2 Wolfgang Kaschuba, 'Arbeitskörper und Freizeitmensch: der industrielle Habitus und seine postindustriellen Metamorphosen', in Michael Dauskardt and Helge Gerndt (eds), *Der industrialisierte Mensch* (Hagen, 1993), p. 55.

3 Christoph Wulf, 'Das mimetische Ohr', *Paragrana* 2, nos. 1/2 (1993), pp. 9–14 (p. 9).

4 Stephan Marks, *Es ist zu laut! Ein Sachbuch über Lärm und Stille: mit einem Text von Robert Gernhardt* (Frankfurt am Main, 1999), p. 122.

5 Quoted ibid., p. 14.
6 All quotations from Kurt Tucholsky, *Gesammelte Werke* (Reinbek, 1975), vol. 9, p. 248.
7 *Deutsches Ärzteblatt* 96 (1999), A-1081.
8 See Hans-Peter Zenner et al., 'Gehörschäden durch Freizeitlärm', in *HNO* 47 (1999), pp. 236–48.
9 Quoted in Marks, *Es ist zu laut!*, p. 14.
10 Doris Schuhmacher-Chilla, 'Wenn das Auge das Ohr übermannt: Erleben im künstlerischen Prozeß', *Paragrana* 2, nos. 1/2 (1993), pp. 44–55 (p. 51).
11 Quoted in Brian Duguid, 'The pre-history of industrial music' (1995), at <www.synesthesie.com/heterophonics/historique/Duguid-Prehistorytxt.html>.
12 Quoted ibid.
13 Manfred Mixner, 'Der Aufstand des Ohrs', *Paragrana* 2, nos. 1/2 (1993), pp. 29–39 (p. 37).
14 Quoted in Duguid, 'Pre-history of industrial music'.
15 Jacques Attali, *Noise: The Political Economy of Music* (Manchester, 1985), p. 6.
16 See Jon Savage, 'Industrial principles' (1983) <www.hyperreal.org/music/epsilon/info/industrial_principles.html>, p. 1.
17 Duguid, 'Pre-history of industrial music'.
18 Frank Fölsch, Florian Hayler and Shelly Kupferberg, 'Jugend-Kultur-Ur-Suppe Techno: Entwicklung und Erscheinungsformen einer Jugendkultur', in-house publication of the Department of Journalism and Communication Studies, Freie Universität Berlin (1995–6), <www.virtualc.prz.tu-berlin.de./essay/techno5.htm>, p. 7. See also Martin M. Coers, *Friede, Freude, Eierkuchen: die Technoszene* (Munich, 2000).
19 Quoted in Regina Bendix, 'Symbols and Sounds, Senses and Sentiments: Notizen zu einer Ethnographie des (Zu-)Hörens', in Rolf Wilhelm Brednich and Heinz Schmitt (eds), *Symbole: zur Bedeutung der Zeichen in der Kultur* (Münster, 1997), pp. 42–57 (p. 53).
20 Quoted in Mixner, 'Der Aufstand des Ohrs', p. 36.
21 Quoted in Martin Geck, *Musiktherapie als Problem der Gesellschaft* (Stuttgart, 1973), p. 54.
22 Siegfried Zielinski, *Audiovisionen: Kino und Fernsehen als Zwischenspiele in der Geschichte* (Reinbek, 1989), p. 114.
23 Richard Murray Schafer, *The Tuning of the World* (New York, 1977), pp. 4–5.
24 Karl-Josef Pazzini, ' "Wer nicht hören will, muß fühlen": einige Diskussionsbeiträge zum Hören in der Psychoanalyse in der Pädagogik', *Paragrana* 2, nos. 1/2 (1993), pp. 15–28.

CHAPTER 15   WAYS OF SEEING – OR THE HUMAN RIGHTS
OF THE EYE

1 Martin Heidegger, *Holzwege* (Frankurt am Main, 1950), p. 246f.
2 Guy Debord, *The Society of the Spectacle*, trans. Donald Nicholson-Smith (New York, 1994), pp. 12–13.
3 Ibid., p. 23.
4 Ibid., p. 18.
5 Jean-Claude Kaufmann, *Corps de femmes regards d'hommes: sociologie des seins nus* (Paris, 1995), p. 107 [trans. JL].
6 Ibid., p. 113.
7 *Real-Encyclopädie der gesammten Heilkunde*, vol. 20 (1899), p. 461.
8 Debord, *Society of the Spectacle*, p. 20.
9 Quoted in Julius Kayer-Petersen, 'Über Reihenuntersuchungen mit Röntgenstrahlen', in *Ergebnisse der gesamten Tuberkuloseforschung* (Leipzig, 1937), pp. 71–158 (p. 73).
10 Quoted ibid., p. 143.
11 Jean-Claude Kaufmann, *Corps de femmes*, p. 108.
12 Vilém Flusser, *Ins Universum der technischen Bilder* (Göttingen, 1989), p. 14.
13 Hans-Georg Soeffner and Jürgen Raab, 'Sehtechniken: die Medialisierung des Sehens: Schnitt und Montage als Ästhetisierungsmittel medialer Kommunikation', in Werner Rammert (ed.), *Technik und Sozialtheorie* (Frankfurt am Main, 1998), pp. 121–48 (p. 129).
14 Quoted in Carl Aigner, 'Das Gespenst der Sichtbarkeit: Notizen zum Verhältnis von Fotografie und Epiphanie', in *Im Reich der Phantome: Fotografie des Unsichtbaren*, exhibition catalogue (Ostfildern, 1997), pp. 104–8 (p. 104).
15 Laszlo Moholy-Nagy, *Vision in Motion* (Chicago, 1947), p. 12.
16 Quoted in Wibke von Bonin, 'Vom Künstlerfilm zum Videoclip', in Wolfgang Welsch (ed.), *Die Aktualität des Ästhetischen* (Munich, 1993), pp. 169–91 (p. 172).
17 *The Diaries of Franz Kafka*, ed. M. Brod (Harmondsworth, 1972), p. 238.
18 Quoted in Bruno Fischli, 'Das goldene Zeitalter der Kölner Kinematographie (1896–1918)', in Fischli (ed.), *Vom Sehen im Dunkeln: Kinogeschichten einer Stadt* (Cologne, 1990), pp. 7–38 (p. 22f.).
19 Quoted in Jürgen Kinter, ' "Durch Nacht zum Licht" – vom Guckkasten zum Filmpalast: die Anfänge des Kinos und das Verhältnis der Arbeiterbewegung', in Dagmar Krift (ed.), *Kirmes – Kneipe – Kino: Arbeiterkultur im Ruhrgebiet zwischen Kommerz und Kontrolle (1850–1914)* (Paderborn, 1992), pp. 119–46 (p. 138).

20 Quoted in Siegfried Zielinski, *Audiovisionen* (Reinbek, 1989), p. 144.
21 Quoted ibid., p. 150.
22 Quoted ibid., p. 152.
23 Quoted in Knut Hickethier, 'Der Fernseher: zwischen Teilhabe und Medienkonsum', in Wolfgang Rupert (ed.), *Fahrrad, Auto, Fernsehschrank: zur Kulturgeschichte der Alltagsdinge* (Frankfurt am Main, 1993), pp. 162–87 (p. 168f.).
24 Quoted ibid., p. 175.
25 Paul Virilio, *Guerre et Cinéma 1, logistique de la perception* (Paris, 1984), p. 26.
26 Dorothea McEwan, *Ausreiten der Ecken: die Aby Warburg–Fritz Saxl Korrespondenz 1910–1919* (Hamburg, 1998), p. 110.
27 Bernd Hüppauf, 'Schlachtenmythen und die Konstruktion des "Neuen Menschen"', in Gerhard Hirschfeld and Gerd Krumeich (eds), *'Keiner fühlt sich mehr als Mensch...'* (Essen, 1993), pp. 43–84 (p. 65).
28 Marie-Anne Berr, *Technik und Körper* (Berlin, 1990), p. 91f.
29 Ibid., p. 95.
30 Freud, *Standard Edition* (London, 1953–), vol. 20, p. 156.
31 *Das große Wörterbuch der deutschen Sprache* (1980), vol. 5, p. 1964.
32 <www.jura.uni-sb.de/FB/LS/Grupp/Faelle/peepshow-fall.htm>.

CHAPTER 16   PSI PHENOMENA – OR THE EXPLORATION OF
EXTRA-SENSORY PERCEPTION

1 Eberhard Bauer and Walter von Lucadou, 'Parapsychologie in Freiburg – Versuch einer Bestandsaufnahme', *Zeitschrift für Parapsychologie und Grenzgebiete der Psychologie* 29 (1987), pp. 241–82 (p. 242). The following descriptions are based for the most part on: Robert Amadou, *Das Zwischenreich: vom Okkultismus zur Parapsychologie* (Baden-Baden, 1957); Lawrence L. Moore, *In Search of White Crows: Spiritualism, Parapsychology and American Culture* (New York, 1977); H. Seymour Mauskopf and Michael R. McVaugh, *The Elusive Science: Origins of Experimental Psychical Research* (Baltimore and London, 1980); Eberhard Bauer, '100 Jahre parapsychologische Forschung – die Society for Psychical Research', in Eberhard Bauer and Walter von Lucadou (eds), *Psi – was verbirgt sich dahinter?* (Freiburg/Breisgau, 1984), pp. 51–75; Janet Oppenheim, *The Other World: Spiritualism and Psychical Research in England 1850–1914* (Cambridge, 1985); Martin Stute, *Hauptzüge wissenschaftlicher Erforschung des Aberglaubens und seiner populärwissenschaftlichen Darstellungen der Zeit von 1800 bis in die Gegenwart* (Frankfurt am Main, 1997); Barbara Wolf-Braun, 'Zur

Rezeptionsgeschichte der Parapsychologie im Rahmen der akademischen Psychologie: die Stellungnahmen von Wilhelm Wundt (1832–1920) und Hugo Münsterberg (1863–1916)', in J. Jahnke et al. (eds), *Psychologiegeschichte – Beziehungen zu Philosophie und Grenzgebieten* (Munich and Vienna, 1998), pp. 405–19. I should like to record my indebtedness to Eberhard Bauer (Freiburg/Breisgau) and Barbara Wolf-Braun (Bonn) for many valuable suggestions.

2 D. Scott Rogo, *Parapsychology: A Century of Inquiry* (New York, 1975), p. 56.

3 Albert Moll, *Ein Leben als Arzt der Seele: Erinnerungen* (Dresden, 1936), p. 91.

4 Quoted in Clément Chéroux, 'Ein Alphabet unsichtbarer Strahlen: Fluidalfotografie am Ausgang des 19. Jahrhunderts', in *Im Reich der Phantome: Fotografie des Unsichtbaren*, exhibition catalogue (Ostfildern, 1997), pp. 11–22 (p. 20).

5 Moll, *Leben als Arzt der Seele*, p. 116.

6 Rudolf Tischner, *Ergebnisse okkulter Forschung: eine Einführung in die Parapsychologie* (Stuttgart, 1950), p. 152.

7 Eberhard Bauer, 'Parapsychologie', in *Illustrierte Geschichte der Psychologie*, ed. Helmut E. Lück and Rudolf Miller (Munich, 1993), pp. 295–300 (p. 296).

8 Rogo, *Parapsychology*, p. 72.

9 Ibid., p. 81.

10 Ibid., p. 100.

11 Quoted in Eberhard Bauer, 'Hans Bender und die Gründung des "Instituts für Grenzgebiete der Psychologie und Psychohygiene" ', in J. Jahnke et al., (eds), *Psychologiegeschichte – Beziehungen zu Philosophie und Grenzgebieten* (Munich and Vienna, 1998), pp. 461–6 (p. 466).

12 Bauer and Lucadou, 'Parapsychologie in Freiburg', p. 251.

13 Hans Bender, *Unser sechster Sinn: Telepathie, Hellsehen und Psychokinese in der parapsychologischen Forschung* (Stuttgart, 1971), p. 83.

14 Bauer and Lucadou, 'Parapsychologie in Freiburg', p. 255.

CHAPTER 17   CYBERSPACE AND THE FUTURE OF
THE SENSES

1 Mynona [Salomo Friedländer], *Der verliebte Leichnam*, ed. Klaus Konz (Hamburg, 1985), p. 34.

2 Ibid.

3 Mark Dery, *Escape Velocity: Cyberculture at the End of the Century* (London, 1996), p. 75.

4 Hans Moravec, 'Körper, Roboter, Geist', in *Die Zukunft des Körpers II*, ed. Florian Rötzer (special number of the journal *Kunstforum*, vol. 133, 1996), pp. 98–112 (p. 110).

5 Achim Bühl, 'Cyberspace und Virtual Reality: Sozialwissenschaftlicher Forschungsbedarf' (1995), <http://staff-www.uni-marburg.de/~buehlach/forum195.htm>, p. 2.

6 Derrick de Kerckhove, 'Touch versus Vision', in Wolfgang Welsch (ed.), *Die Aktualität des Ästhetischen* (Munich, 1993), pp. 135–68 (p. 153).

7 Paul Virilio, *Art of the Motor*, trans. Julie Rose (Minneapolis, 1995), p. 110.

8 Kerckhove, 'Touch versus Vision', p. 164.

9 Quoted in Constance Classen, *Worlds of Sense: Exploring the Senses in History and Across Cultures* (London and New York, 1993), p. 6.

10 Quoted in Nathalie Waehlisch, 'Elektronische Supernasen', *Frankfurter Rundschau*, 25 August 1998, p. 32.

11 Elke Heitmüller, 'Kybernetische Sinnlichkeit: SM-Körper – Authentizität – Digitalisierung', *Ästhetik und Kommunikation* 23 (1994), pp. 14–21 (p. 17).

12 <http://www.time.com/time/reports/v21/tech/mag_sex.html>.

13 Florian Rötzer, 'Von der Lust vernetzt zu sein', <www.heise.de/tp/deutsch/inhalt/co/2018/1.html> (undated), p. 2.

14 Donna J. Haraway, *Simians, Cyborgs and Women: The Reinvention of Nature* (London, 1991), p. 152.

15 Hans Magnus Enzensberger, 'Das digitale Evangelium', *Der Spiegel*, 10 January 2000, pp. 92–101 (p. 101).

Index

Page numbers in italics refer to illustrations.

Abaelardus, Peter 121
Die Abderiten (Christoph Martin
   Wieland) 57–8
Ackermann, Diane 12
Adams, Thomas 157
Addison, Joseph 172
Adorno, Theodor W. 293
aesthetics
   birth of 145–51
   and concept of taste 152–6
   practice of 151–2
Agathodämon (Christoph Martin
   Wieland) 56–7
Agricola, Johann 87, 91–2
Albertus Magnus 42, 45, 47, 48,
   49–50, 55, 56, 60, 67, 95
Albilda, Moses 59, 75
Albo, Joseph 60, 64
Albucasis 120
Alcmaeon of Croton 32
alcohol consumption 212–13
Alcuin 65
Alexander, Frederick Matthias
   242

Algarotti, Francesco 188
Alhazen (Ibn Al-Haytham) 39,
   50, 111–12
Almosnino, Moses 61
Altar of the Passion, Marienthal
   zu Netze 92
Ambrose, St 87
American Society for Psychical
   Research 310
Anders, Günter 303
Annales school 11
Anti-Claudianus (Alanus ab
   Insulis) 63
anti-Semitism 269–71
Aquinas, St Thomas 42, 45, 47,
   48, 50–1, 59, 69–70
Arama, Isaac 75
Arcades Project (Walter
   Benjamin) 198–9
Arcadious, Stelios (Stelarc)
   328–30, *329*, 332
Aristotle 34, 36–43, 55, 56,
   58–9, 59–60, 61, 64, 67, 68,
   69, 70–1, 110

aromatherapy 278–80
Aronsohn, Emil 230
The Art of Noises (Luigi Russolo) 281–2, 286, 288
Ashley Cooper, Anthony 142–3
Atharvaveda (Veda of the Spells) 21, 24
Attali, Jacques 288–9
'Audio-Visuality Before and After Gutenberg' (conference) 5–6
Auenbrugger, Leopold von 176–7
Augustine of Hippo 45–6, 64–5, 77, 86, 87, 117–18
Auschwitz 270
Autenrieth, Johann Heinrich Ferdinand von 226
automata 129–33
Averroes (Ibn Rušd) 47–9, 56
Avicenna (Ibn Sînâ) 47, 50, 51, 58, 59, 67, 68, 69
Ayurveda (The Wisdom of Long Life) 21, 23–5

Bachja ben Ascher 67
Bacon, Francis 146
Bacon, Roger 51, 112
bad breath 271–4
Balde, Jakob 63, 85
Baraduc, Hippolyte 311–12
Barker, Robert 194
Barlösius, Eva 212, 259, 263
Barre, Poullain de la 137
Barrett, Sir William 310
Bartisch, Georg 112
Basel Museum of Design 2
Bataille, Georges 295
Batteux, Charles 143
Baudelaire, Charles 198, 199
Baudrillard, Jean 239

Baumeister, Friedrich Christian 145
Baumgarten, Alexander Gottlieb 145–6, 150, 151
Beauvoir, Simone de 252
Beckmann, Johann 214
Bede, the Venerable 118
Bell, Charles 223, 233
Bender, Hans 317–18, 319, 320
Benjamin, Walter 10, 146, 196, 198–9
Bentham, Jeremy 165, 307
Berkeley, George 127–8
Bermúdez, Juan Antonio Ceán 144
Bernard of Clairvaux 65, 77
Berr, Marie-Anne 165, 305
bestiaires d'amour 80
Bethke, Bruce 325
Bibago, Abraham ben Schemtov 71, 75
Bichat, Marie-François-Xavier 212
'Big Brother' (TV programme) 308
Billroth, Theodor 242
Bilz, Friedrich Eduard 243
Blix, Magnus Gustaf 234
Bloch, Iwan 246–7
Boccioni, Umberto 286
Bock, Carl Ernst 171
Bocuse, Paul 259
Bodmer, Johann Jakob 130–1, 145, 182
body odour 274–5
body therapy 240–5
Boetius 87
Bonnaterre, Pierre-Joseph 134
Bonnet, Charles 130
Borel, Pierre 189

Bosch, Hieronymus 92
Bosch, Robert 232
Boucher, François 130
Boulez, Pierre 287
Bourdieu, Pierre 196, 254, 257
Boureau-Deslandes, André
  François 131
Bouvelles, Charles 58–61
Boyle, Robert 146
Bräker, Ulrich 176
Brandt, Thure 243
Brandt, Willy 267
Brave New World (Aldous
  Huxley) 277
Brecht, Bertolt 292
Breinholt, Niels Buch 198
Breitinger, Johann Jacob 145
Brentano, Clemens von 136
Breuer, Joseph 172
Breughel, Jan 94
Breysig, Johann Adam 194
Brillat-Savarin, Jean-Anthelme
  57, 140, 155–6
Brin, David 307–8
Brockes, Barthold Heinrich 85,
  91, 96
Brouwer, Adriaen 101
Browne, Hablot Knight 191
Brugmans, Henri Johan 313
Büchlein der Weisheit (Heinrich
  von Seuse) 76
Buffon, Georges-Louis Leclerc
  130
Bühl, Achim 327
Bulwer, John 106, 118
Buñuel, Luis 300
Bygraves, Max 289

Cabanis, Pierre-Jean Georges
  136–7, 139

Caelius Aurelianus 119
Cage, John 287–8
Calderón, Pedro 81
camera obscura 190
Campanella, Tommaso 52
Campe, Johann Heinrich 160
Canon of Medicine (Avicenna) 47
Capital (Karl Marx) 185
Capivacco, Hieronymus 116
Caraka 21
Caravaggio 101
Cardano, Girolamo 52
Carràs, Carlo 286
Carríon, Ramirez de 118
Carus, Carl Gustav 139
Cassirer, Ernst 72
Cazazza, Monte 289
Celsus 108, 116
Certeau, Michel de 295
Cesti, Marc-Antonio 62
Chanel, Coco 275
Charles, Daniel 287–8
Chartier, Roger 15, 72
Chauliac, Guy de 112
Cheselden, William 133
'The Chess-Playing Turk'
  (Wolfgang von Kempelen)
  131
Un Chien Andalou (film) 300
Chinese natural philosophy
  25–31
Chrysippus 43
Chun Chiu Fan Lu 28
Cicero 77, 106–7
cinemas, scents 277–8
Civilization and its Discontents
  (Sigmund Freud) 12
clairvoyance 309, 314
Classen, Constance 279–80
Cleveland Public Library 3

'clinical gaze' (Foucault)
199–200
Clinton, Bill 249
Cloquet, Hippolyte 229–30
'clouded gaze' 200–2
Clynes, Manfred 335
Coca-Cola 261–2
Coleridge, Samuel Taylor 186
Collaert, Adriaen 83, 97
collective hyperaesthesia 15–16
Colloquia (Erasmus of
Rotterdam) 106
Comenius, Johannes Amos 168
Condillac, Etienne Bonnot de
127, 129–30, 131, 133, 134
*The Condition of the Working
Class in England* (Friedrich
Engels) 172–3
Confessions (Augustine of Hippo)
65
Confessions (Jean-Jacques
Rousseau) 152
Confucianism 30
Cook, James 241
Corbin, Alain 12, 15, 207–8,
210, 279
Corneille, Thomas 144
Crary, Jonathan 11, 190, 191–2
Critique of Judgement (Immanuel
Kant) 146, 150, 155
Croiset, Gerard 319–20
Croon, Bree 2
Crousaz, Jean-Pierre de 153–4
'La Cucina Futuristica' 253
culinary pluralism 258–9
cyber art 327–30
cyberpunk 325
cyberspace 326, 327
cyborgs 335
Czermak, Joseph 230–1

Daguerre, Louis Jacques Mandé
195
d'Alembert, Jean Le Rond 128–9
Dali, Salvador 300
Dalton, John 111
Damian, Peter 77
Darget, Louis 312
d'Auvergne, Guillaume 69
David of Augsburg 89
Davies, Sir John 54
De anima (Albertus Magnus) 42
De anima (Thomas Aquinas) 42
De anima (Aristotle) 36–7, 39,
40, 42, 55, 69
De audibilibus (Aristotle) 40
De civilitate morum puerilium
(Erasmus of Rotterdam) 166
De remediis utriusque fortunae
(Petrarch) 114
De sensibus (Theophrastus) 32
De sensu (Aristotle) 40
De sensu (Theophrastus) 34, 55
De trinitate (Augustine of Hippo)
46
*De unitate intellectus contra
Averroem* (Albertus Magnus)
48
*De unitate intellectus contra
Averroistas* (Thomas
Aquinas) 48
De universo (Hrabanus Maurus)
55
Debord, Guy 295–6, 297
Democritus 33–4, 39
Descartes, René 41, 44, 52–3,
68, 127
Dessoir, Max 310, 311
d'Estrées, Gabrielle 100, *101*
Le devin du village (Jean-Jacques
Rousseau) 152

—— 381 ——

Dictionnaire philosophique (Voltaire) 152
Diderot, Denis 129, 130, 133, 142, 143–4, 167
Diepenbrock, Melchior von 72
Dincklage, Emmy von 205
Dioptrics (René Descartes) 44
Discipline and Punish (Michel Foucault) 295
'disembodied gaze' 190
Dobelle, William A. 331
Dohm, Christian Wilhelm 174
domestic noise 206–7
Domman, Monika 297
Dubos, Jean-Baptiste 154
Duden, Barbara 8
Duguid, Brian 289
Dumas, Alexandre 156
Duns Scotus, Johannes 51
Duran, Simon 56
Dürer, Albrecht 100

ear-trumpets *117*
early modern natural philosophy 52–3
Ebberfeld, Ingelore 274
Ebers Papyrus 115–16
Eckermann, Johann Peter 136
Eckhart, Meister 67, 77
École Militaire, Paris 165
Efron, John 269
electrotherapy 244–5
Elements of Physiology (Johannes Müller) 219
Elias, Norbert 12, 97, 165, 178
Ellis, Henry Havelock 247–8
Emblemata (Johannes Sambucus) 90–1
Emerson, Ralph Waldo 166, 330

Emile, or Education (Jean-Jacques Rousseau) 157, 159–60
Emmerick, Katharina 136
Empedocles 32–3, 36, 39, 86
Ems, Rudolf von 88, 94
Encyclopédie 128–9, 167
Engels, Friedrich 172–3
Ense, Karl August Varnhagen von 226
environmental protection 265–9
Enzensberger, Hans Magnus 253, 335
Epicharmos 31
Erasmus of Rotterdam 106, 166
Erasmus Quellinus 82
Erb, Wilhelm 184
Erlangen manuscript, Heilbronn 78, 79
erogenous zones 245–8
Erxleben, Dorothea von 137
Escalante, Juan Antonio 81–2
Eschenbach, Wolfram von 114
Esra, Abraham ben Meir Ibn 56, 68
An Essay Concerning Human Understanding (John Locke) 127, 133
An Essay Towards a New Theory of Vision (George Berkeley) 127–8
Estabrooks, George 314
Euclid 44
extra-sensory perception 17, 309–21

Faber, Zachäus 105–6
Fabre, Pierre 144
Fabricius de Aquapendente, Hieronymus 40

factory noise 203–5
Faraday, Michael 192
fast food 261–2
Febvre, Lucien 11–12
Fechner, Gustav 224, 230
Federal Exhibition Hall, Bonn 2,
    5
females, sensitivity of 137–41
Ferrari, Luc 287
Feuerbach, Anselm von 134
Feuerbach, Ludwig 9
Fichte, Johann Gottlieb 72
Finsonius, Ludovicus 83
Fisher, Scott 334
Fließ, Wilhelm 95, 172
Flusser, Vilém 299
'Flute Player' (Jacques
    Vaucanson) 131
Forster, Georg 57
Foucault, Michel 10, 162, 165,
    199–200, 295
Fouquet, Henri 129, 138
Francis of Sales 94
Franck, Bernhard Matthias
    41
Frank, Johann Peter 168
Frauenlob, Heinrich 90
Freud, Sigmund 12, 172, 184,
    246–8, 305
Frey, Max von 234, 235
Friedländer, Salomo (Mynona)
    270–1, 324–5
Friedman, Hermann 239
Fritz, Kurt von 34
Fröbel, Friedrich Wilhelm August
    161
Froriep, Ludwig Friedrich 162–5,
    170
Frugardi, Roger 120
Fuller Brooch 80

Galen 33–4, 39, 40, 41, 43–4,
    47, 60, 103, 116, 121
Galileo 188
Galle, Philipp 82
Garden of Delights (Hieronymus
    Bosch) 92
Gattefossé, René-Maurice 279
Gault, Henri 259
Gay, Peter 246
*Genitality in the Theory and
    Therapy of Neurosis*
    (Wilhelm Reich) 248
German Museum of Hygiene
    250, 272
Gernhardt, Robert 283, 285
Gessner, Conrad 40
Gibson, William 326
Giesecke, Michael 216
Gilman, Sander 99
Ginzburg, Carlo 14
Goethe, Johann Wolfgang von
    15, 86, 98, 114, 136, 169,
    176, 188
Goldscheider, Alfred 234
Göpel, Wolfgang 333
Gorgias (Plato) 34
Gottsched, Johann Christoph
    145
gourmet tourism 258
Goya, Francisco 144
Graaf, Reinier de 189
Graeco-Roman natural
    philosophy 31–46
Le Grand Bleu (film) 278
Grant, Horace 161
Grau, David 104
Great Book of Painting (Gerard
    de Lairesse) 85
Gregory the Great 87, 88
Grenzen von Utopia (film) 324

Grewel der Verwüstung Menschlichen Geschlechts (Hippolytus Guarinonius) 66
Grimmelshausen, Hans Jacob Christoffel von 92
Grosseteste, Robert 51
Gruber, Max 213
Grunewald, Fritz 312
Grüsser, Otto-Joachim 226
Guarinonius, Hippolytus 66
Gubisch, Wilhelm 320
Guérard, Michel 259
Guide for the Perplexed (Maimonides) 70
Gurney, Edmund 310
Gutsmuths, Johann Christoph 160–1, 175
gynaecology, massage in 243
Gyphantie, oder Die Erdbeschreibung (Tiphaigne de la Roche) 195

Häberlin, Paul 259
Hadrian, Emperor 116
Halberstadt, Albrecht von 89
Halevi, Salomo 68, 75
Haller, Albrecht von 232, 233
Hamann, Johann Georg 15, 147
Hamburg Speicherstadtmuseum 3
Handbook of Physiological Optics (Hermann von Helmholtz) 225
Handke, Peter 291
Haraway, Donna 335
Harig, Georg 44
Harsdörffer, Georg Philipp 85–6, 88
Hartmann, Eduard von 310
Hauffe, Frederike 135–6
Hauptmann, Gerhard 238

Hauser, Kaspar 134–5, 156
'head mounted display' (HMD) 330–1
hearing
ailments 114–18
Aristotle on 40
imagery of 90–3
and listening 293–4
and noise 202–7
physiology of 226–9
status of 66–7
training of 167–70
Hegel, Georg Wilhelm Friedrich 150–1
Heidegger, Martin 295, 296
Heiderich, Friedrich 233
Heim, Nicolaus 253
Heister, Lorenz 111
Hellpach, Willy 184
Helmholtz, Hermann von 176, 193, 220, 223, 224–5, 228–9
Henry I, Bishop of Breslau 104
Heraclitus 31
Herder, Johann Gottfried 57, 147, 149, 150
Hering, Ewald 221, 223, 225–6
Hermann, Ludimar 230
Hermes Trismegistos 99
Herodotus 109
Herophilus 43
Herrenberg altar 17
Hesiod 31
Hildegard of Bingen 65, 76, 87
Hillmann, Howard 263
Hippocrates 43, 103
Hippolytus of Rome 77–8
Hirschfeld, Magnus 247
Historia animalum (Aristotle) 59

The History of the Eye (Georges Bataille) 295
history of the gaze 10–11
Hitler, Adolf 270
Hobbes, Thomas 90
Hoffmann, E. T. A. 185–6
Hoffmann, Johann Moritz 41
Hoffmann-Axthelm, Dieter 221–2
Holmes, Oliver Wendell 196
Homer 31, 88, 93
Honegger, Arthur 286, 287
Horn, Wilhelm 232–3
Horner, William G. 192
Howard, Jane 241
Hsü Ch'un-fu 30
Hsun Tzu 30
Hugo of Saint-Victor 77
Hume, David 128, 143
Hunterian Museum, Glasgow 2
Hüppauf, Bernd 304
Hutcheson, Francis 142, 143
Huxley, Aldous 277
Huygens, Christian 190
Hyett, Barbara 265

I Ching (Book of Changes) 25
Iconologia (Cesare Ripa) 101
Ignatius Loyola 82, 157–8
Indian natural philosophy 20–5
industrialization 180–2
Institute of Fringe Areas of Psychology, Freiburg 312, 317–21
Insulis, Alanus ab 63
Interim Age 15
Internet, sensory experiences on 4, 251–2, 307
Isidor of Seville 65, 68–9, 88
Isserles, Moses 71, 75

Jacob of Voragine 76
Jäger, Gustav 231–2
Jandl, Ernst 281
Jansen, Zacharias 188
Jaquet-Droz, Pierre 131
Jaucourt, Louis Chevalier de 129
Jauss, Hans Robert 153
Jay, Martin 186
Jean Paul (Johann Friedrich Richter) 131–2, 140–1, 149
Jellinek, J. Stephen 276
Jerome, St 65, 90
Jerusalem, Karl Wilhelm 148
John of Genoa 65
Juan II of Aragon 71

Kafka, Franz 206, 300
Kagel, Mauricio 292
Kamper, Dietmar 5, 291
Kant, Immanuel 57, 106, 114, 127, 136, 146, 150, 155
Karle, Werner 242
Kaschuba, Wolfgang 282
Kaufmann, David 76, 95
Kaufmann, Hans 83, 84
Kaufmann, Jean-Claude 296, 299
Kaysersberg, Geiler von 105
Kempelen, Wolfgang von 131
Kepler, Johannes 44, 53, 188, 190
Kerckhove, Derrick de 240, 327, 330
Kerner, Justinus 135–6, 226–7
Kieser, Dietrich Georg 135
Kitab al-amanat wa al-i 'tiqadat (Saadia ben Josef) 56, 64
Klee, Paul 299
Klein, Calvin 276
Klenke, Dietmar 267
Klinger, Friedrich Maximilian 56

Kluge, Alexander 304
Koch, Robert 105
König, Johann Ulrich 154–5
Kortum, Carl Georg Theodor
 208
Kraftwerk 289–90
Krall, Karl 312
Krämer, Jörg 151
Kranken-Examen (Samuel
 Gottlieb Vogel) 103
Ku-chin i-t'ung ta-ch'üan
 (Comprehensive System of
 Medicine of All Times)
 29–30
Kuhn, Paul 241
Kükelhaus, Hugo 251
Kulm, Tilo von 77
Külpe, Oswald 221
Kung-sun Lung 30
Kutschmann, Werner 82–3

La Bruyère, Jean de 153
La Mettrie, Julien Offray de 126,
 131
Laarmann, Jürgen 291
Lady with the Unicorn 80, 94
Lagerfeld, Karl 276
Lairesse, Gerard de 85
Lamprecht, Karl 203
Landgrave Henry I, tomb of
 92–3
Lanfranc of Milan 116
Langhans, Carl Ferdinand 195
Lasker-Schüler, Else 266
last rites 104–5
laterna magica 190–1
Laube, Hans E. 277
Lavater, Johann Caspar 189
Lavater, Johannes 118
Le Guérer, Annick 265

Le Pansif, Jacques 62, 71
Ledermüller, Martin Frobenius
 189
Leewenhoek, Antoni van 188–9
Legenda aurea (Jacob of
 Voragine) 76
LeGoff, Jacques 14
Leibniz, Gottfried Wilhelm 145
Leonardo da Vinci 40, 66, 107
Lessing, Gotthold Ephraim
 147–8, 149
Lessing, Theodor 206
Lettre sur les aveugles (Denis
 Diderot) 133, 143–4
Leviathan (Thomas Hobbes) 90
Lewinsky, Monica 249
*L'Homme machine: A Study in
 the Origins of an Idea*
 (Julien Offray de La Mettrie)
 126, 131
Liber ad Almansorem (Rhazes)
 91
Libido sexualis (Albert Moll) 246
Liesegang, Paul Eduard 191
Lifton, Robert Jay 270
Liguori, Alphons Maria di 179
Lindner, Rolf 303–4
Linger, Karl August Ferdinand
 271–2
*Lingua, or The Combat of the
 Tongue and the Five Senses
 for Superiority* (Thomas
 Tomkis) 62
Linnard, Jacques 85
Linné, Karl von 229, 232
Lipperhey, Hans 188
Locke, John 127, 128, 129,
 132–3
Lodge, David 6
Loenhoff, Jens 245

Lohenstein, Daniel Casper von 57
Lombroso, Cesare 235
Loo, Charles André van 130
Louis IX of France 110
Lovén, Otto Christian 233
Löw, Rabbi 91
Lucadou, Walter von 321
Lucy, St 109
Ludwig, Carl 234
LumiTest 332
Luther, Martin 91, 105, 114

McDonald's 261
McDougall, William 314
Mach, Ernst 228
Macho, Thomas 5
Machover, Tod 325
Mackenzie, John Noland 172
McLuhan, Marshall 10, 240, 304
Magdeburg, Mechthild von 89
Magen avot (Simon Duran) 56
Magendie, François 42, 226
Maimonides 61, 65, 70
Malpighi, Marcello 42
Marat, Jean Paul 126, 127
Marcus Aurelius 116
Marinetti, Filippo Tommaso 253
Marjan, Marie-Luise 241
Marks, Stephan 283
Marx, Karl 8, 9–10, 17, 180, 185, 216, 220, 296
Maskell, Joseph 159, 168, 171, 175
massage 240–5
masturbation 162, 167
Maurus, Hrabanus 55, 78, 88, 94
Maury, Marguerite 279
Mayer, Helmut 186

Mayer, Johannes 134
medieval natural philosophy 46–52
The Medium is the Message (Marshall McLuhan) 240
Megenberg, Konrad von 67–8, 89, 91
Melanchthon, Philipp 52
Mellenkamp, Patricia 278
Mendelssohn, Moses 131, 146–7, 148
Mennell, Stephen 258
Mercier, Louis-Sébastien 177
Messiaen, Olivier 287
Metamorphoses (Ovid) 64, 88
Le Miasme et la jonquille (Alain Corbin) 208
microphysiology 223
microscopes 188–90
Millau, Christian 259
Miller, Willoughby Dayton 272
Mintz, Sidney W. 10, 174–5
Miracula Sancte Elyzabet 109, 122
Mischo, Johannes 320
Mixner, Manfred 287
Mo Ti 30
Mo Tzu (Book of the Master) 30
Möckl, Karl 257, 260
Mohist school (of Chinese philosophy) 30
Moholy-Nagy, Laszlo 299
Mohrmann, Ruth E. 178
Molenaer, Jan 101
Moll, Albert 246, 310, 311, 312
Molyneux, William 132
Montaigne, Michel de 52, 97
Moravec, Hans 5, 326
Moscherosch, Johann Michael 85, 178

Motte, Dr 291
Müller, Johannes 16, 166,
 218–20, 224–5, 227, 233
Munich Psychological Society
 310
muscular sensation 222–3
Museum of Medical History,
 Ingolstadt 2–3
museums, sensual exhibitions
 1–3, 249–51
music
 industrial 289–90
 listening to 293–4
 and noise 286–8
 techno 290–1
musique concrète 287
Myers, Frederic 310
Mynona (Salomo Friedländer)
 270–1, 324–5

Naisbitt, John 239
Nam June Paik 303
A Natural History of the Senses
 (Diane Ackerman) 12
Needham, Joseph 26, 28, 30
Negt, Oskar 5, 304
Nemesius 45, 60
Neues Arzneibuch (Christoph
 Wirsung) 119
neurasthenia 184–5
New Romancer (William Gibson)
 326
Nicomachean Ethics (Aristotle)
 70–1, 110
Niepce, Josephe-Nicéphore 195
Nietzsche, Friedrich 126, 167,
 197
noise 202–7
 aircraft 282–4
 in music 286–8

post-industrial 281–2
 recreational 284–5
*Noise: The Political Economy
 of Music* (Jacques Attali)
 288–9
Noort, Adam van 83
Nordau, Max 185
nouvelle cuisine 259–60
Novalis 140, 245
El nuevo palacio del Retiro
 (Pedro Calderón) 81

Odol (mouthwash) 271–2, 273,
 274
Ohm, Georg Simon 228
Olat Tamid (Moses Albilda) 59
Olivier, Raymond 259
On Nature (Alcmaeon of Croton)
 32
On the Sensations of Tone
 (Hermann von Helmholtz)
 220, 228
L'Onanisme (Samuel Auguste
 André David Tissot) 162
Oosterwijck, Maria van 85
Origen 76
*The Origin, Nature and
 Immortality of the Soul*
 (Sir John Davies) 54
Ortmann, Günther 307
Orwell, George 308
Oshima, Nagisa 6
Osiander, Friedrich Benjamin
 175–6
Ottilie, St 109
Ovid 64, 82, 88

Pacific 231 (Arthur Honegger)
 286
Paech, Anne 277–8

Palais de la Découverte, Paris 2
panopticon 165
panoramas 194–5
Paracelsus 91, 93, 96
paralysis 120–3
parapsychology 17, 309–21
Paré, Ambrose 110
Paris, John 192
Parmenides 31
Parzival (Wolfram von
    Eschenbach) 114
Pasteur, Louis 105
Paulinus of Nola 76, 77
Payer, Peter 268
Pazzini, Karl-Josef 294
peep-shows 191, 305–6
Pelo, H. 252
Pemberton, John S. 261–2
perception
  of the beautiful 142–5
  sensualistic theories of 126–41
perfume 275–6
Perfume (Patrick Süßkind) 119
Pergolesi, Giovanni Battista
    151–2
Perrault, Charles 153
Pestalozzi, Johann Heinrich 160
Petrarch 114, 118, 120
Pettenkofer, Max von 211
Pfalz, Elisabeth Charlotte von der
    113
Phaedrus (Plato) 63
Phenakistoscope 192
Pheron 109
Philo of Alexandria 66, 73, 75
Philocopus, or The Deafe and
    Dumbe Mans Friend (John
    Bulwer) 106, 118
Philosophy of Fine Art (G. W. F.
    Hegel) 150

The Philosophy of Symbolic
    Forms (Ernst Cassirer) 72
Photodram Opus I (Walther
    Ruttmann) 300
photography 195–6
physiotherapy 242–3
Pinel, Philippe 134
Plateau, Joseph 192
Platner, Ernst 151
Plato 34–6, 39, 55, 63, 64, 86
Platter, Felix 106, 122
Pleorama 195
Pleßner, M. 206
Plotinus 44–5
Pneumatics 43
Poetischer Trichter (Georg Philipp
    Harsdörffer) 88
Polansky, Fanciscus 227
Polemon 95
Politzer, Adam 227, 228–9
Polyester (film) 278
Il pomo d'oro (Marc-Antonio
    Cesti) 62
Porta, Giovanni Battista della 95,
    190
Porter, Roy 128
Pratella, Ballila 286
precognition 309
Preißler, Daniel 85
Prel, Carl du 310
Preu, Paul Sigmund Karl 134, 135
Priestley, Joseph 111, 127
Process of Civilization (Norbert
    Elias) 12
psi phenomena 309–21
psychokinesis 17, 309
Ptahhotep 102
Punarvasu Atreya 24
Purkyně, Johannes Evangelista
    218, 221

Pygmalion and Elise (Johann Jakob Bodmer) 130–1
Pythagoras 31–2

Raab, Jürgen 299
Racine, Jean 144
radio 291–2
Rahn, Johann Heinrich 136
Railway Concerto (John Cage) 287
railway travel 197–8
Rapports du physique et du morale de l'homme (Pierre-Jean Georges Cabanis) 136–7
Ratgeb, Jerg 17
Rayleigh, Lord 310
Recco, Giuseppe 85
Redeker, Franz 298
Regensburg, Berthold von 90
Reich, Wilhelm 242, 244, 248–9
Reischer, Jacob 118
Rembrandt 98
Der Renner (Hugo von Trimberg) 86
Republic (Plato) 36, 64
The Return of the Prodigal Son (Ludovicus Finsonius) 83–4, *84*
Révész, Geza 239
Reynière, Alexandre Balthazar-Laurent Grimond de la 156
Ṛgveda (Veda of Verses) 21, 24
Rhazes (Ar-razi) 91
Rheingold, Howard 334
Rhine, Joseph B. 314, 317
Rhine, Louisa 314
Richet, Charles 312–13
Richter, Johann Friedrich (Jean Paul) 131–2, 140–1, 149

Richter, Philipp 180
Ripa, Cesare 101
Risala fi n-nafs (Avicenna) 47
Roberts, Lissa 103
robotics 326
Roche, Tiphaigne de la 195
Roemer, Paul 308
Rogo, D. Scott 310, 313
Rohr, Julius Bernhard von 166, 177
Rollet, Alexander 222
Röntgen, Wilhelm Conrad 297, 311
Röse, Carl 272, 274
Rosenstock-Huessy, Eugen 294
Rothschuh, Karl E. 9
Rötzer, Florian 334
Rousseau, Jean-Jacques 129, 152, 157, 159–60, 162, 167, 168, 170, 172, 173, 175
Roussel, Pierre 138
Rubens, Peter Paul 98
Rules of Christian Decorum and Civility (Jean-Baptiste de la Salle) 167
Rumohr, Friedrich von 161, 166
Ruskin, John 187
Russolo, Luigi 202, 281–2, 286, 288
Ruttmann, Walther 299, 300

Saadia ben Josef 56, 64
Sachs, Hans 98
Saint-Evremond, Charles de 153
Saint Laurent, Yves 276
Salle, Jean-Baptiste de la 167
salt consumption 213–14
Sambucus, Johannes 90–1
Saṃhitās 21

The Sandman (E. T. A. Hoffman) 185–6
Sansovino, Francesco 41
Santa Clara, Abraham a 92, 94, 167
Sartre, Jean-Paul 252
Savage, Jon 289
Saxl, Fritz 304
Sbarra, Francesco 62
Scarpa, Antonio 41
Scent of Mystery (film) 277
'scented TV' 277
Sceptics 43
Schaeffer, Pierre 287
Schafer, Richard Murray 294
Scheerer, Eckart 53
Scheiner, Christoph 188
Schelhammer, Günther Christoph 116
Schelling, Friedrich Wilhelm Joseph 135, 149
Schemtov, Joseph Schemtov ibn 71
Schenk, Ernst Günter 254
Schiller, Friedrich 91, 98, 150–1, 169
Schivelbusch, Wolfgang 197
Schlegel, Friedrich 17, 140
Schneider, Conrad Victor 41
Schöne, Johann Heinrich 161
Schopenhauer, Arthur 169, 205
Schrader, Ludwig 73, 157
Schreber, Daniel J. 161, 170–1, 175
Schrenck-Notzing, Albert von 310, 312
Schuhmacher-Chilla, Doris 286
Schultze, Max 230, 233
Schwalbe, Gustav 233
Scivias (Hildegard of Bingen) 76

scopic regime 10–11, 186–7
Sedan-Panorama 194
Die Seherin von Prevorst (Justinus Kerner) 135–6
Sennett, Richard 178
'The Sense of the Senses' (exhibition) 2, 5
Senseless (film) 5
senses
  ailments 102–23
  in Chinese natural philosophy 25–31
  classification of 58–61
  computer simulation of 330–5
  in early modern natural philosophy 52–3
  in Graeco-Roman natural philosophy 31–46
  hierarchy of 61–71
  iconographic symbols 74
  imagery of 72–101
  in Indian natural philosophy 20–5
  industrialization, effects of 182–217
  in medieval natural philosophy 46–52
  modern interest in 1–6, 16
  number of 54–8
  physiology of 9, 12, 16, 218–36
  training of 157–79
sensory energy 218–21
sensory isolation 162–5
sensualism 15, 126–41
Sentencia libri de sensu et sensato (Thomas Aquinas) 51
Sermon, Paul 327
La serva padrona (Giovanni Battista Pergolesi) 151–2

Seuse, Heinrich von 76, 87
Sexual Selection in Man (Henry
  Havelock Ellis) 247
Das Sexualleben unserer Zeit
  (Iwan Block) 247
'Sexy Egg' 250–1
Sèze, Paul-Victor de 139
Shakespeare, William 106
Shore, Lewis E. 233
Sidgwick, Henry 310
Siegwarth, Günter 293
sight
  ailments 107–14
  Aristotle on 39–40
  and art 299
  Augustine of Hippo on 46
  and the cinema 300–1
  critique of primacy of 295–6
  enhancement of 187–90
  imagery of 86–90
  industrialization, effects of
    200–2
  physiology of 224–6
  pre-eminence of 64–6
  scopic regime 10–11, 186–7
  and television 301–4
  training of 165–7
  and X-rays 296–8
Simmel, Georg 187, 269
Simplicissimus (Grimmelshausen)
  92
Six Senses Spa 4
sixth sense 56–7, 309–10
The Sixth Sense (film) 321
skin diseases 216–17
Slade, Henry 311
Small World (David Lodge) 6
smell
  and anti-Semitism 269–71
  Aristotle on 40

Corbin on 207–8, 210
Galen on 41
imagery of 93–5
loss of 118–19
physiology of 229–32
pollution 207–11, 265–9
status of 67–8
training of 170–2
Smell (Jan Breughel) 94
Society for Psychical Research
  310
Society of Experimental
  Psychology 310
The Society of the Spectacle (Guy
  Debord) 295–6
Socrates 34, 35
Soeffner, Hans-Georg 299
Soemmering, Thomas 45
Spiritual Exercises (Ignatius
  Loyola) 158
Stampfer, Simon 192
The State of the Sun (Tommaso
  Campanella) 52
Steen, Jan 84
Steiner, Rudolf 250
Stelarc (Stelios Arcadious)
  328–30, *329*, 332
stereoscopy 192–3
Sternberg, Wilhelm 120
Stoics 43
Stoskopff, Sebastian 85
stroboscope 192
Struve, Christian August 166
Stubbes, George 142
Stuttgart University 17
subjective seeing 191–2
sugar consumption 214–15
surveillance cameras 307–8
Suśruta 21
Süßkind, Patrick 119

Sutherland, Ivan 331
Swift, Jonathan 115
Switzer, Alan 242

Taktschreibmethode 161
Tangerine Dream 289–90
taste
 Aristotle on 41–2
 artificial 262–4
 changes in 212–16
 imagery of 96–8
 internationalization of 260–2
 loss of 120
 physiology of 232–3
 status of 68–9
 training of 172–5
'taste of necessity' 253–5
*Der Tastsinn und das
 Gemeingefühl* (Ernst
 Heinrich Weber) 234
Telematic Dreaming (Paul
 Sermon) 327
telepathy 309
telescopes 187–8
Tellkamp, Jörg 51
tellurism 135
Teniers, David 101
Teuteburg, Hans Jürgen 213
Thaumatrope 192
Theaetetus (Plato) 34–5
Theophrastus 32, 33, 34, 55, 86
Theory of Colour (Goethe) 86
Thierry, Guillaume de 78
Thomas, Antoine Léonard 138
Thompson, Henry 176
Thoreau, Henry David 166
Three Essays on Sexual Theory
 (Sigmund Freud) 246, 305
Throbbing Gristle 289
Tiedemann, Friedrich 223

Timaeus (Plato) 35–6
The Time Machine (H. G. Wells)
 325
Tischner, Rudolf 312
Tissot, Samuel Auguste André
 David 162, 167
Titchener, Edward 221
Todd, Mike 277
Tomkis, Thomas 62
touch
 Aristotle on 42
 and the 'haptic age' 238–40
 imagery of 98–101
 industrialization, effects of
  216–17
 loss of 120–3
 physiology of 233–6
 status of 69–71
 training of 175–9
Touch Me! (Jane Howard) 241
Toulouse-Lautrec, Henri Marie de
 199
traffic noise 205–6
Traité des sensations (Etienne
 Bonnot de Condillac)
 129–30
Tralles, Alexander von 116
Transatlantic Wrestling 327–8
The Transparent Society (David
 Brin) 307–8
*Treatise Concerning the Principles
 of Human Knowledge*
 (George Berkeley) 128
A Treatise of Human Nature
 (David Hume) 128
Treatise on Painting (Leonardo
 da Vinci) 107
Treviranus, Gottfried Reinhold
 223
Trimberg, Hugo von 86

Index

'The Triumph of Faith over the Senses' (Juan Antonio Escalante) 81–2, *81*
Troisgros, Jean and Pierre 259
Troland, Leonard Thompson 313–14
Tsou Yen 26, 28
Tucholsky, Kurt 1, 274, 283–4
Tung Chung 28
Tusculan Disputations (Cicero) 106–7

Über das Organ der Seele (Thomas Soemmering) 45
Upaniṣads 21

Vaerst, Friedrich Christian Eugen von 156
Vāgbhaṭa 21
Valloires 3
Vannod, Théodore 183, 217
Varèse, Edgar 288
Vaucanson, Jacques 131
Vedas 20–5
Velde, Esais van den 84
Vergé, Roger 259
Vertov, Dziga 292
video surveillance 307–8
Villanova, Arnaldus de 116
Vintschgau, Maximilian von 232
Virchow, Rudolf 218
Virilio, Paul 304
virtual reality 327
VIVED (virtual visual environment display) 331
Vogel, Samuel Gottlieb 103
Vogelweide, Walther von der 89
Voltaire 152
Vos, Marten de 93, 97, 99, 109
Vostell, Wolf 303

Wagner, Richard 167
Wagner, Rudolf 230
Walser, Robert 274
Wang Chung 28
Warburg, Aby 304
Waters, John 278
'wave of gluttony' 255–7
Weber, Ernst Heinrich 222, 223, 227, 233–5
Weber, Max 82
Weinsberg, Hermann 13–14, 112–13, 115, 119, 120, 121
Weiss, Charles 277
Weissenburg, Otfrid von 77
Wells, H. G. 325
Welsch, Wolfgang 293
Der welsche Gast (Thomasin von Zerclaere) 65
Weltharmonik (Johannes Kepler) 53
Welti, Sabine Ruth 243
Wheatstone, Charles 193
Wiegelmann, Günter 214, 215
Wieland, Christoph Martin 56, 57–8
Wildt, Michael 256
Wilmenrod, Clemens 256
Winckelmann, Johann Joachim 148–9
Wirsung, Christoph 119
Witzigmann, Eckart 259–60
'wolf-children' 133–4
Wolff, Christian 145
The Work of Art in the Age of Mechanical Reproduction (Walter Benjamin) 146
'The Writer' (Pierre Jaquet-Droz) 131
Wulf, Christoph 282

Wundt, Wilhelm 217, 223, 231, 311

X-rays 296–8
Xenophanes 31

The Yellow Emperor's Classic of the Interior 25–6, 29
Yellowstone National Park 4
yin–yang principle 25, 29
Young, Thomas 225

Zedler's Universal Lexicon 20, 102, 104, 107, 119, 120, 121, 122, 188, 189
Zenner, Hans-Peter 332
Zerclaere, Thomasin von 65
Ziehen, Theodor 184–5
Zielinski, Siegfried 301, 304
Zierold, Maria Reyes de 309
Zöllner, Karl Friedrich 311
Zootrope 192
Zwaardemaker, Hendrik 223–4, 230